Facial Reconstructive Controversies

Editor

MARK K. WAX

FACIAL PLASTIC SURGERY CLINICS OF NORTH AMERICA

www.facialplastic.theclinics.com

Consulting Editor
J. REGAN THOMAS

August 2016 • Volume 24 • Number 3

ELSEVIER

1600 John F. Kennedy Boulevard • Suite 1800 • Philadelphia, Pennsylvania, 19103-2899

http://www.theclinics.com

FACIAL PLASTIC SURGERY CLINICS OF NORTH AMERICA Volume 24, Number 3
August 2016 ISSN 1064-7406, ISBN-13: 978-0-323-45963-1

Editor: Jessica McCool
Developmental Editor: Alison Swety

Facial Plastic Surgery Clinics of North America (ISSN 1064-7406) is published quarterly by Elsevier Inc., 360 Park Avenue South, New York, NY 10010-1710. Months of issue are February, May, August, and November. Business and Editorial Offices: 1600 John F. Kennedy Blvd., Suite 1800, Philadelphia, PA 19103-2899. Periodicals postage paid at New York, NY, and additional mailing offices. Subscription prices are $390.00 per year (US individuals), $575.00 per year (US institutions), $445.00 per year (Canadian individuals), $716.00 per year (Canadian institutions), $535.00 per year (foreign individuals), $716.00 per year (foreign institutions), $100.00 per year (US students), and $255.00 per year (foreign students). Foreign air speed delivery is included in all *Clinics* subscription prices. All prices are subject to change without notice. POSTMASTER: Send address changes to *Facial Plastic Surgery Clinics*, Elsevier Health Sciences Division, Subscription Customer Service, 3251 Riverport Lane, Maryland Heights, MO 63043. **Customer service: 1-800-654-2452 (US and Canada); 1-314-447-8871 (outside US and Canada); Fax: 314-447-8029; E-mail: journalscustomerservice-usa@elsevier.com (for print support); journalsonline support-usa@elsevier.com (for online support).**

Reprints. For copies of 100 or more of articles in this publication, please contact the Commercial Reprints Department, Elsevier Inc., 360 Park Avenue South, New York, NY 10010-1710. Tel.: 212-633-3874; Fax: 212-633-3820; E-mail: reprints@elsevier.com.

Facial Plastic Surgery Clinics of North America is covered in *MEDLINE/PubMed* (*Index Medicus*).

Contributors

CONSULTING EDITOR

J. REGAN THOMAS, MD, FACS
Professor and Chairman, Department of
Otolaryngology, University of Illinois at
Chicago, Chicago, Illinois

EDITOR

MARK K. WAX, MD, FACS, FRCS(C)
Professor Otolaryngology, Professor Oral
Maxillofacial Surgery, Program Director,
Director Microvascular Reconstruction, Past
President American Head and Neck Society,
Past President Otolaryngology Program
Directors Organization, Oregon Health and
Sciences University, Portland, Oregon

AUTHORS

DANE M. BARRETT, MD
Fellow/Clinical Instructor, Department of
Otolaryngology–Head and Neck Surgery,
Oregon Health and Science University,
Portland, Oregon

ADITI BHUSKUTE, MD
Department of Otolaryngology, University of
California, Davis, Davis, California

LOU BUCKY, MD
Division of Plastic Surgery, Hospital of the
University of Pennsylvania, Philadelphia,
Pennsylvania

PATRICK J. BYRNE, MD, MBA
Professor and Division Director of Facial
Plastic and Reconstructive Surgery, Johns
Hopkins Medicine, Baltimore, Maryland

STEVEN B. CANNADY, MD
Assistant Professor, Otorhinolaryngology
Head and Neck Surgery, University of
Pennsylvania, Philadelphia, Pennsylvania

FERNANDO J. CASANUEVA, MD
Observational Fellow, Department of
Otolaryngology–Head and Neck Surgery,
Oregon Health and Science University,
Portland, Oregon

TED A. COOK, MD, FACS
Division of Facial Plastic and Reconstructive
Surgery, Professor, Department of
Otolaryngology–Head and Neck Surgery,
Oregon Health and Science University,
Portland, Oregon

RAJ DEDHIA, MD
Department of Otolaryngology–Head and Neck
Surgery, UC Davis Medical Center,
Sacramento, California

FRED G. FEDOK, MD, FACS
Adjunct Professor, Department of Surgery, The
University of South Alabama, Mobile, Alabama;
Professor, Facial Plastic and Reconstructive
Surgery, Otolaryngology/Head and Neck
Surgery, The Hershey Medical Center, The
Pennsylvania State University, Hershey,
Pennsylvania

OREN FRIEDMAN, MD
Department of Otorhinolaryngology–Head and
Neck Surgery, University of Pennsylvania,
Philadelphia, Pennsylvania

MICHAEL A. FRITZ, MD
Head and Neck Institute, Cleveland Clinic;
Associate Professor, Cleveland Clinic Lerner
College of Medicine, Cleveland, Ohio

ERIC M. GENDEN, MD, MHCA, FACS
Department of Otolaryngology–Head and Neck
Surgery, Icahn School of Medicine at Mount
Sinai, New York, New York

DENIZ GERECCI, MD
Resident, Department of Otolaryngology–Head
and Neck Surgery, Oregon Health and Science
University, Portland, Oregon

JAVIER GONZÁLEZ-CASTRO, MD
Assistant Professor, Otolaryngology–Head
and Neck Surgery, University of Puerto Rico,
San Juan, Puerto Rico

KYLE HATTEN, MD
Fellow, Head and Neck Surgery, Department of
Otorhinolaryngology–Head and Neck Surgery,
University of Pennsylvania, Philadelphia,
Pennsylvania

TSUNG-YEN HSIEH, MD
Department of Otolaryngology–Head and Neck
Surgery, UC Davis Medical Center,
Sacramento, California

LISA E. ISHII, MD, MHS
Associate Professor, Department of
Otolaryngology–Head and Neck Surgery,
Johns Hopkins School of Medicine, Baltimore,
Maryland

JARROD KEELER, MD
Division of Facial Plastic and Reconstructive
Surgery, Stanford University School of
Medicine, Stanford, California

ROBERT M. KELLMAN, MD, FACS
Chair, Department of Otolaryngology, SUNY
Upstate, Syracuse, New York

LESLIE KIM, MD, MPH
Instructor in Facial Plastic and Reconstructive
Surgery, Johns Hopkins Medicine, Baltimore,
Maryland

P. DANIEL KNOTT, MD
Associate Professor, Department of
Otolaryngology–Head and Neck Surgery,
University of California San Francisco,
San Francisco, California

JESSYKA G. LIGHTHALL, MD
Assistant Professor, Division of
Otolaryngology–Head and Neck Surgery,
Director of Facial Plastic and Reconstructive
Surgery, Penn State Hershey Medical Center,
Hershey, Pennsylvania

SAM P. MOST, MD
Division of Facial Plastic and Reconstructive
Surgery, Stanford University School of
Medicine, Stanford, California

REGINA E. RODMAN, MD
Facial Plastics and Craniofacial Surgery, SUNY
Upstate, Syracuse, New York

ERIC S. ROSENBERGER, MD
Fellow, Facial Plastic and Reconstructive
Surgery, Department of Otolaryngology,
University of Illinois Chicago, Chicago, Illinois

JACK E. RUSSO, MD, MS
Department of Otolaryngology–Head and
Neck Surgery, Icahn School of Medicine at
Mount Sinai, New York, New York

CRAIG SENDERS, MD
Department of Otolaryngology, University of
California, Davis, Davis, California

RAHUL SETH, MD
Assistant Professor, Department of
Otolaryngology–Head and Neck Surgery,
University of California San Francisco, San
Francisco, California

MIKA SUMIYOSHI, MD
Department of Otolaryngology, University of
California, Davis, Davis, California

MATTHEW TAMPLEN, MD
Resident Physician, Department of
Otolaryngology–Head and Neck Surgery,
University of California San Francisco,
San Francisco, California

SHERARD TATUM, MD
Professor of Otolaryngology and Pediatrics,
Division of Facial Plastic Surgery, Cleft and
Craniofacial Center, Upstate Medical
University, Syracuse, New York

WILLIAM WALSH THOMAS, MD
Department of Otorhinolaryngology–Head
and Neck Surgery, University of Pennsylvania,
Philadelphia, Pennsylvania

TRAVIS T. TOLLEFSON, MD, MPH, FACS
Professor, Facial Plastic and Reconstructive
Surgery, Department of Otolaryngology–Head
and Neck Surgery, UC Davis Medical Center,
Sacramento, California

DEAN M. TORIUMI, MD
Professor, Facial Plastic and Reconstructive
Surgery, Department of Otolaryngology,
University of Illinois Chicago, Chicago, Illinois

TOM D. WANG, MD, FACS
Division of Facial Plastic and Reconstructive
Surgery, Professor, Department of
Otolaryngology–Head and Neck Surgery,
Oregon Health and Science University,
Portland, Oregon

MARK K. WAX, MD, FACS, FRCS(C)
Professor Otolaryngology, Professor Oral
Maxillofacial Surgery, Program Director,
Director Microvascular Reconstruction, Past
President American Head and Neck Society,
Past President Otolaryngology Program
Directors Organization, Oregon Health and
Sciences University, Portland, Oregon

Contents

presurgical period. Proponents of nasoalveolar molding claim several benefits, including improved aesthetic outcome, reduced overall costs, and a psychosocial benefit to the family. Research on these outcomes is not conclusive.

Evidence-based medicine (EBM) encompasses the evaluation and application of best available evidence, incorporation of clinical experience, and emphasis on patient preference and values. Different scales are used to rate levels of evidence. Translating available data for interventions to clinical practice guidelines requires an assessment of both the quality of evidence and the strength of recommendation. Essential to the practice of EBM is evaluating the effectiveness of an intervention through outcome measures. This article discusses principles essential to EBM, resources commonly used in EBM practice, and the strengths and limitations of EBM in facial plastic and reconstructive surgery.

 Video content accompanies this article at http://www.facialplastic.theclinics.com

Facial palsy is a devastating condition with profound functional, aesthetic, and psychosocial implications. Although the complexity of facial expression and intricate synergy of facial mimetic muscles are difficult to restore, the goal of management is to reestablish facial symmetry and movement. Facial reanimation surgery requires an individualized treatment approach based on the cause, pattern, and duration of facial palsy while considering patient age, comorbidities, motivation, and goals. Contemporary reconstructive options include a spectrum of static and dynamic procedures. Controversies in the evaluation of patients with facial palsy, timing of intervention, and management decisions for dynamic smile reanimation are discussed.

Facial trauma is a significant cause of morbidity in the United States. Despite the large volume of trauma surgeries at most academic institutions, there is still controversy regarding management of many traumatic injuries. The literature lacks clear-cut best practices for most fractures. In orbital trauma, there is debate about the optimal timing of repair, preferred biomaterial to be used, and the utility of evaluation afterward with intraoperative computed tomographic scan. In repair of mandible fractures, there is debate regarding open versus closed reduction of subcondylar fractures, or alternatively, endoscopic repair.

Free tissue transfer is the gold standard for reconstructing head and neck defects. Free flap success approaches 95% in centers with experience, affording unparalleled ability to restore form and function in cancer, trauma, or other major composite tissue loss. It is critical to manage the perioperative variables that predict success; several areas of controversy have not yet reached consensus. This review focuses on postoperative anticoagulation, fluid management, and flap monitoring methods. These areas of controversy potentially influence flap survival. We review published practices considered within the standard of care, why controversy remains, and future directions to reach standardization.

The nose and the nasal airway is highly complex with intricate 3-dimensional anatomy, with multiple functions in respiration and filtration of the respired air. Nasal airway obstruction (NAO) is a complex problem with no clearly defined "gold-standard" in measurement. There are 3 tools for the measurement of NAO: patient-derived measurements, physician-observed measurements, and objective measurements. We continue to work towards finding a link between subjective and objective nasal obstruction. The field of evaluation and surgical treatment for NAO has grown tremendously in the past 4-5 decades and will continue to grow as we learn more about the pathophysiology and treatment of nasal obstruction.

Rhinoplasty is inherently a difficult procedure given the complexity of its structure and the functional and aesthetic impact of this anatomy. This report explores some of the remaining questions regarding the use of spreader grafts and autospreader flaps in the management of the middle vault in rhinoplasty, the performance of the open approach versus the endonasal rhinoplasty approach, corrective rhinoplasty in the younger patient, the use of the rib and other cartilage donor sites for grafting in rhinoplasty, and the use of filler materials in rhinoplasty.

Revision rhinoplasty is a complex operation with many variables that may influence the final esthetic and functional outcome of the procedure. Cartilage forms the structural framework of the lower two-thirds of nose and is essential for long-term support and maintenance of a patent nasal airway. The use of autologous cartilage grafting is the primary source of this material, limited by donor site quantity, quality, and harvest morbidity. Alloplastic materials, solid and injectable, are often used for augmentation purposes and may have devastating consequences. This article discusses past and current treatment concepts for various nasal deformities using available autologous grafting techniques.

Prophylactic antibiotic use in facial plastic surgery is a highly controversial topic primarily due to the lack of evidence in support of or against antibiotic use. In this section the authors present the available literature on the most commonly performed procedures within facial plastic surgery in an attempt to see if the data support or contradict the need for antibiotic prophylaxis in facial plastic surgery.

FACIAL PLASTIC SURGERY CLINICS OF NORTH AMERICA

RELATED INTEREST

Otolaryngologic Clinics, October 2015 (Vol. 48, No. 5)
Medical and Surgical Complications in the Treatment of Chronic Rhinosinusitis
James A. Stankiewicz, *Editor*
http://www.oto.theclinics.com/

THE CLINICS ARE AVAILABLE ONLINE!
Access your subscription at:
www.theclinics.com

FACIAL PLASTIC SURGERY CLINICS
OF NORTH AMERICA

Preface
Facial Reconstructive Controversies

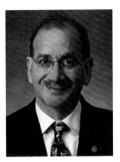

Mark K. Wax, MD, FACS, FRCS(C)
Editor

The field of Facial Plastic and Reconstructive Surgery continues to expand on many different fronts. Teaching in this area of surgical expertise has become a fundamental part of all residency programs. The knowledge base of Facial Plastics comprises up to 20% of the Otolaryngology requirements of the certifying exam. Not only do most Otolaryngologists utilize the knowledge that has been taught by the facial plastic surgeons but also they use the skills learned in their residency on a day-to-day basis. Whether it is for the pediatric patient who needs a cleft revised, or the otology patient who needs tissue rearrangement to cover a cochlear implant, facial plastic surgery is a fundamental part of patient care in the many subspecialties of Otolaryngology. With the integration of facial plastic and reconstructive surgery into the armamentarium of most Otolaryngologists has come a burgeoning in the knowledge of what once were rare fields in Facial Plastic Reconstructive Surgery. This in turn has led to the expansion of knowledge and technical approaches to many areas of facial plastic and reconstructive surgery that were only practiced by a few in academic centers.

The facial plastic reconstructive surgeon is now faced with an array of management tools that can be offered to patients. Along with this has come interest in evidence-based medicine. Not only is the number of publications concerning evidence-

based medicine in the field increasing but also textbooks, such as a recent *Facial Plastic Surgery Clinics of North America*, was dedicated to the subject of evidence-based medicine in facial plastic reconstructive surgery.

A review of the literature in this area reveals that more and more authors are not only reviewing their own results but also analyzing and comparing, on an evidence-based method, what are some of the benefits or drawbacks to current management paradigms of a broad variety of diseases. With this has come the natural development of controversy. In each of many different areas, some more common than others, there are topics in the management of the patient that are not well defined. The maturing of the specialty has seen a critical analysis of the pros and cons of many techniques and foundations of knowledge.

This issue of *Facial Plastic Surgery Clinics of North America* has asked a number of experts in various subspecialties to analyze the controversial areas in their area of expertise. By discussing the pros, cons, and future directions, we will continue to learn what is the best option for the treatment of our patients. We also should be able to discuss and discover when different options offer the same outcomes. It has been a pleasure to work with such esteemed experts on such a controversial project.

I can only end by acknowledging the leaders in the field of facial plastic and reconstructive surgery

Facial Plast Surg Clin N Am 24 (2016) xiii–xiv
http://dx.doi.org/10.1016/j.fsc.2016.03.015

who have always examine their outcomes and results and sought to improve patient care. Continuing evaluation of outcomes is essential to maintaining the best possible practices for our patients. The field is strong and will only continue to grow as younger surgeons are taught by such exemplary professionals.

Mark K. Wax, MD, FACS, FRCS(C)
Oregon Health and Sciences University
3181 SW Sam Jackson Park Road PV-01
Portland, OR 97239, USA

E-mail address:
waxm@ohsu.edu

Management of the Nasal Valve

Dane M. Barrett, MD[a],*, Fernando J. Casanueva, MD[b], Ted A. Cook, MD[c],*

KEYWORDS

- Nasal obstruction • Functional rhinoplasty • Nasal valve • External valve • Internal valve
- Spreader grafts • Butterfly graft • Batten grafts

KEY POINTS

- The nasal valve is frequently a contributor or sole cause of nasal obstruction and must be clinically evaluated in any patient presenting with nasal obstruction.
- Understanding of nasal valve anatomy with critical assessment of the site of obstruction is essential to effective nasal valve management.
- Validated outcome measures, such as the Nasal Obstruction Symptom Evaluation score, are helpful for preoperative evaluation of the severity of obstruction and postoperative assessment of success.
- Technique selection should be individualized to the locale and type of valve dysfunction. Spreader grafts are seldom adequate as a lone intervention for nasal valve dysfunction.
- High-quality research, ideally directly comparing techniques, is needed to both simplify and improve nasal valve management.

INTRODUCTION

The ability to breathe through the nasal passages is a noticeable feature of healthiness and well-being. The nasal airway plays a central role in air heating and humidification, olfaction, and, most importantly, airflow.[1] Obstruction of the nasal airway is a common complaint in the otolaryngologic practice and has a dramatic impact on patient quality of life.[2] Although several medical and surgical treatments exist to address this common patient complaint, developing the best therapeutic strategy targeting the sources of the problem can be challenging. Often, there are multiple contributing factors complicating treatment.

The causes of nasal airway obstruction are legion, though they can typically be broken down to mucosal or structural causes. Structural causes of obstruction may be posttraumatic, idiopathic, or iatrogenic at the hands of the nasal surgeon.[3,4] Underpinning all of this is an anatomic malformation or dysfunction. In fact, up to 75% to 85% of people have some type of anatomic deformity of the nose.[5] Only a subset of these individuals experience a severe enough impact on quality of life to prompt a clinical evaluation.

Most otolaryngologists are adept at diagnosing anatomical deformities of the septum and turbinates. However, nasal obstruction from nasal valve dysfunction (NVD) may be overlooked as a

Disclosures: None of the authors have any commercial or financial conflicts of interest.
[a] Department of Otolaryngology, Head and Neck Surgery, Oregon Health and Science University, 3181 Southwest Sam Jackson Park Road, SJH01, Portland, OR 97239, USA; [b] Department of Otolaryngology, Head and Neck Surgery, Oregon Health and Science University, 3181 Southwest Sam Jackson Park Road, Portland, OR 97239, USA; [c] Division of Facial Plastic & Reconstructive Surgery, Department of Otolaryngology, Head and Neck Surgery, Oregon Health and Science University, 3181 Southwest Sam Jackson Park Road, SJH01, Portland, OR 97239, USA
* Corresponding authors.
E-mail addresses: Barredan@ohsu.edu; Cookt@ohsu.edu

Facial Plast Surg Clin N Am 24 (2016) 219–234
http://dx.doi.org/10.1016/j.fsc.2016.03.001

facialplastic.theclinics.com

contributor or sole cause of nasal obstruction. NVD has been implicated in having a role in up to 13% of adults complaining of chronic nasal obstruction.[3] Moreover, the nasal valve has been implicated as the cause of persistent nasal obstruction after septoplasty in up to 95% of cases.[6]

NVD is a distinct cause of symptomatic nasal obstruction, yet there are several ambiguities surrounding the diagnosis and management of this process.[7] The literature has often been confusing and occasionally contradictory in almost every aspect of management of the nasal valve. Discrepancies exist over the nomenclature and terminology, anatomy of the nasal valve, the desired effects of a particular technique, and appropriate outcome measures, just to name a few. In most outcomes studies, adjunctive procedures are often performed in addition to directed nasal valve correction, which potentially confounds the results. There is significant heterogeneity in study designs and lack of randomized controlled trials. Most studies are uncontrolled case series, which only recently have used validated outcome measures.[7–9] This problem in the literature serves as an unfortunate imposition to quality clinical decision-making.

Although confusion may exist in the literature, there is in fact a good body of evidence supporting treatment of the nasal valve.[8,9] Most of the evidence has been overwhelmingly positive. This article reviews the management of the nasal valve, highlighting the controversial aspects of this topic and addressing the current best practices available. The goal is not only to help the reader understand the challenges in the literature but also to provide a framework for thoughtful and effective management of this problem (**Box 1**).

ANATOMY

The nasal valve is an anatomically complex concept and is nonspecific in its original description. First suggested by Mink,[10] the nasal valve was described as the region of maximal nasal resistance.[10] It was later described by Bridger[11]

Box 1
Controversies in nasal valve management

Anatomy

Terminology

Diagnosis

Objective outcome measures

Technique selection

---

as the flow-limiting segment of the nasal airway located at the triangular aperture between the upper lateral cartilage (ULC) and septum. From the author's perspective, the nasal valve is much more generic. In reality, the nasal valve encompasses the column of air housed by the mucosa, cartilage, and soft tissue of the nose external to the piriform aperture. This area is typically modified in some fashion during nasal valve surgery (**Fig. 1**).

The two major components that comprise the nasal valve, the internal and external valves, are classically described in more anatomically specific terms. In most texts, the internal valve is the triangular cross-sectional area between the caudal border of the ULCs, the septum, the head of the inferior turbinate, and nasal floor. The normal angle at the junction of the caudal ULC and septum is 10° to 15° in the caucasian nose and usually more obtuse in asians and african americans.[12,13] Of the entire nasal valve area, the internal valve is generally considered to be the narrowest portion and is the site of maximal airway resistance.[5,14]

The external valve has classically referred to the area in the nasal vestibule, under the alar lobule, formed by the caudal septum, medial crura of the alar cartilages, alar rim, and nasal sill.[15] It is important to note that, though the location and anatomy of the internal valve has been largely consistent in the literature, this has not been universally true regarding the external valve.

As an alternative to the classic definition of the external valve, Khosh and colleagues[4] referred to the external valve as bound superolaterally by the caudal edge of the upper lateral cartilages, laterally by the piriform aperture and fibrofatty tissues of the ala, and the nasal floor. Spielmann and colleagues[8] described the external nasal valve as being formed by the septum, the medial and lateral crura of the lower lateral cartilage (LLC), and the premaxilla. Ballert and Park[13] used a separate term to describe the area between the internal and external valves. The intervalve area was defined as the caudal-lateral aspect of the lateral crus, including the fibrofatty tissue, which extends to the piriform aperture and immediately deep to the supra-alar crease.

Yet another way to consider the anatomy of the nasal valve is to divide it into 2 zones, as described by Most.[16] In order to better characterize the points of lateral wall collapse, he described 2 zones where lateral wall collapse occurs. Zone 1 corresponds to the scroll region and inferior portion of the upper lateral cartilage, whereas zone 2 corresponds to the skin and soft tissues of the nasal ala, similar to the traditionally described external valve[16] (**Fig. 2**).

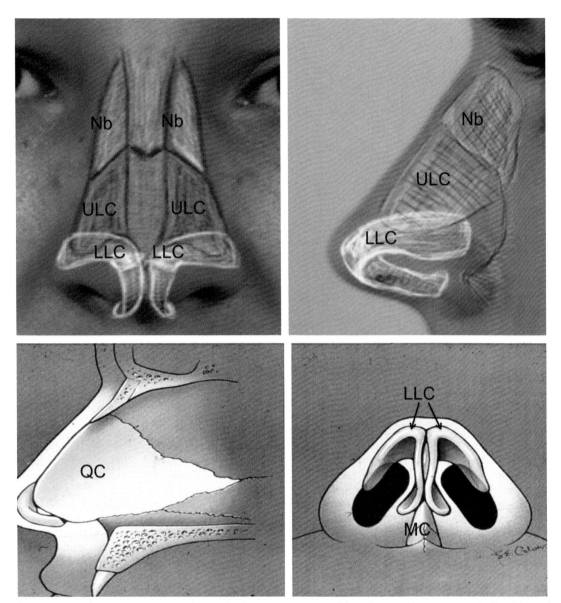

Fig. 1. Key nasal anatomic structures in nasal valve management. All but the nasal bones are typically addressed in nasal valve surgery. LLC, lower lateral cartilage; MC, maxillary crest; Nb, nasal bones; QC, quadrangular cartilage.

It is obvious that the anatomy of this region is complex, which has led to difficulties characterizing it in such a way that it can be treated in a standardized fashion. It is the authors' opinion that, though using the characterizations of the internal and external valves can be helpful for communication and surgical planning, it is important to be as specific as possible in regard to the anatomic structures affected by the pathologic process in order to select the best possible surgical technique.

PHYSIOLOGY

Normal airflow through the nasal valve depends on the Bernoulli principle and Poiseuille's law. The Bernoulli principle states that as the flow of air increases through a fixed space, the pressure in that space decreases. If the decrease in pressure overcomes the inherent rigidity of the flexible nasal sidewall, collapse can occur resulting in obstruction.[11,12] Clinically, the collapse of the nasal sidewall during inspiration is termed *dynamic obstruction*.

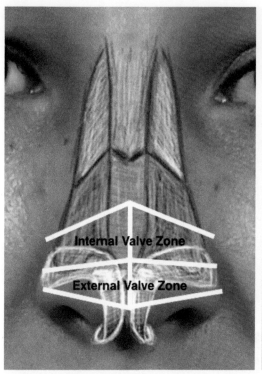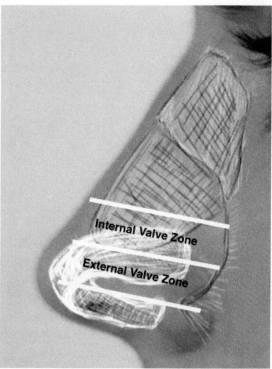

Fig. 2. Zones of lateral nasal sidewall collapse. The internal valve zone corresponds to the inferior portion of the ULC and scroll region. The external valve zone corresponds to the soft tissues of the nasal ala.

Pouseille's law states that flow is inversely proportional to the fourth power of the radius, which means that small decreases in the radius of a space have dramatic impacts on the flow of air through the nose. In the clinical setting, an anatomically narrowed portion of the nasal valve is defined as a static obstruction.

All surgical techniques in the management of the nasal valve are focused on optimizing the aforementioned physical principles. Surgical maneuvers either increase the cross-sectional area of the valve, strengthen the nasal sidewall to resist dynamic collapse, or both.

TERMINOLOGY

The terminology regarding nasal valve management is varied, confusing, and in need of standardization. There are several terms in the literature that reference pathology of the nasal valve as well as its component structures, the internal and external nasal valves. Some of the terms in the literature referencing the valve include NVD,[7] nasal valve collapse,[8] nasal valve compromise (NVC),[15] and nasal valve stenosis.[17] Similar terms have been applied to both the internal and external valves.

The use of some of these terms can be misleading. For example, nasal valve collapse

has been used to reference both insufficiency and weakness of the nasal sidewall and narrowing of the internal nasal valve. The former is a function of a dynamic problem whereby the sidewall collapses with inspiration, whereas the latter is a static and constant narrowing of the valve. Both clinical entities are managed differently. This point highlights the need for standardized nomenclature that accurately describes the clinical problem at hand.

The use of the terms NVC or NVD when referencing a general pathologic issue affecting the nasal valve is least confusing. The former is the term used in a recent clinical consensus statement,[15] whereas the latter has been proposed as an alternative that avoids confusion with the term nasal valve collapse if abbreviated.[7]

When referencing the pathology of the internal or external nasal valves, it is important to distinguish between narrowing, which is a static process, or collapse, which is dynamic. In regard to the internal nasal valve, in most cases, the process is static. The main components of the internal valve, the caudal ULC, septum, and inferior turbinate, typically do not vary dynamically during nasal inspiration. Therefore, internal valve narrowing is preferred[16] in such cases. This narrowing often results from trauma or previous rhinoplasty in which weakening of the ULC support structures resulted in a narrowed angle. If indeed there is dynamic collapse of the caudal ULC with inspiration at the internal valve, then internal nasal valve collapse should be used instead. Dynamic collapse of the internal nasal valve can be seen in patients with an overprojected septal cartilage seen commonly in tension nose deformities. These patients have thin skin and weak ULC prone to dynamic collapse with inspiration, which can be seen on frontal inspection as collapse of the middle third with inspiration.

Dysfunction of the external valve is more commonly the result of a dynamic process. As it is classically described, external valve collapse occurs at the alar rim and is visible externally, most notably on the base view (**Fig. 3**). However, collapse of the nasal sidewall can in fact occur at different points and is not simply confined to the classically described external valve. Ballert and Park[13] noted that the epicenter of nasal sidewall collapse is often at the intervalve area, which is cephalic to the classically defined external valve and immediately deep to the supra-alar crease. Most[16] and Lee and Most[18] described 2 zones of lateral sidewall collapse. In his description, Most[16] noted that collapse can occur either in zone 2 at the area of the classic external valve or in zone 1, which is more cephalad at the scroll region and corresponds to the Ballert and Park[13] intervalve area. If the term *external valve collapse* is used to describe dynamic collapse in this region, it would be helpful to also provide a more specific description of the location of collapse as suggested by Most.[16] In cases of a static problem involving the external valve, such as a severe caudal septal deviation or lateralization of the medial crura without a dynamic problem, external valve narrowing should be used.

HISTORICAL PERSPECTIVE

Traditionally, treatment of nasal obstruction centered on a septoplasty. The original submucous resection (SMR) consisted of removal of the deviated portion of the septum with preservation of a dorsal and caudal strut (L-strut). The SMR was made popular by Killian[19] and Freer[20] in early 1900s; however, this technique failed to address the dorsal or caudal portions of the septum. In 1948, Cottle and Loring[21] advocated an incision at the mucocutaneous junction instead of the Killian incision as well as addressing all deviated portions of the bony and cartilaginous septum.[21] Multiple techniques have since developed to address various types and locations of septal deviations while preserving structural support.[22] Unfortunately, both the literature and experience have shown that septoplasty alone is often an insufficient means of treating nasal obstruction in isolation. Success rates of septoplasty have ranged from 43% to 85% depending on the assessment tool used.[2,23–25]

The inferior turbinates were another surgical target identified causing nasal obstruction. Many techniques have been described to treat enlarged turbinates.[26] Initial procedures centered around inferior turbinate resection, though this resulted in significant morbidity, including empty nose syndrome, rhinitis sicca, and atrophic rhinitis.[27]

More recently, surgery for the inferior turbinate has shifted to reductive techniques with better outcomes and less morbidity. Inferior turbinate reduction has shown to be effective in improving nasal obstruction due to inferior turbinate hypertrophy, though many of the studies had a short follow-up period.[28] A study by Garzaro and colleagues[29] showed improvement in the Nasal Obstruction Symptom Evaluation (NOSE) scores

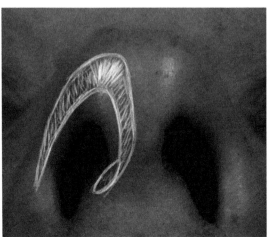
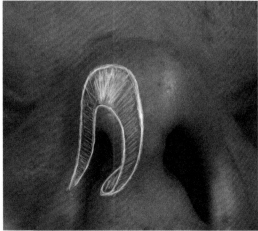

Fig. 3. Dynamic external nasal valve collapse occurring at the alar rim.

at the 2-year mark in patients who underwent inferior turbinate reduction by radiofrequency ablation. It is important to note that the preoperative symptom severity of this group preoperatively was relatively low (mean preoperative NOSE score: 23.14). A recent randomized controlled trial of patients undergoing septorhinoplasty with or without inferior turbinate reduction showed no improvement in quality-of-life outcome measures between the groups.[30] Although turbinate reduction is a useful adjunctive technique where indicated, it is unlikely to be effective when used in isolation, especially with other concomitant pathologies.

The need to address the nasal valve as a contributor to nasal obstruction was not recognized until 1984, when Sheen[31] first described the use of spreader grafts to open the internal nasal valve. Sheen recognized the need to correct the nasal dorsum following hump reduction and avoid a narrowed middle vault and inverted V deformity. The spreader graft was noted to increase the angle of the internal valve by laterally displacing the ULC subsequently recreating aesthetic lines.[31] Since Sheen's article, the spreader graft has become the gold standard for management of the internal nasal valve. However, this technique alone is often not sufficient in isolation to effectively manage the nasal valve. Today, there are several surgical techniques to target specific areas of NVC.[32,33]

DIAGNOSIS

Diagnosis of NVD is based on history and physical examination. Subjective assessment should include onset, laterality, duration, exacerbating and alleviating factors, trauma, history of nasal surgery, and impact on daily life. A history of use of nasal splints, such as BreatheRight Strips (CNS Inc, Minneapolis, MN), and their effectiveness is helpful as it may provide an indication of surgical success. Physical examination should include inspection of the outward appearance, palpation, and intranasal examination. External inspection should include evaluation of the nose on frontal, lateral, and base views in both the natural state and during inspiration. A pinched middle third, evident on frontal view, should provoke suspicion of internal valve dysfunction. Tip bossae, deep supra-alar creases, and medial sidewall movement on deep inspiration indicate a potential nasal sidewall issue.[4] Manual palpation should also be performed, as this provides information on the inherent strength of the nasal cartilages, alar rim strength, and nasal tip support.

Internal inspection should be performed to evaluate septal deviation, inferior turbinate hypertrophy, lateral crural recurvature, lateral wall collapse, and valve narrowing. Some advocate the use of nasal endoscopy to evaluate the internal nasal valve[34,35]; however, there is no consensus regarding routine usage.[15]

The Cottle maneuver has historically been a popular examination technique and involves stenting the nasal sidewall with lateral traction on the cheek. This maneuver is nonspecific in that it enhances nasal airflow even in patients without NVC.[4,13,36] The modified Cottle maneuver involves the use of an ear curette or Q-tip to stent the lateral nasal sidewall and has been proposed as an alternative diagnostic tool.[37] This maneuver is thought to be predictive of surgical outcomes.[38] Interestingly, only one study was found in the authors' review supporting the predictive ability of the modified Cottle on postoperative outcomes. Fung and colleagues[39] used the rhinoplasty outcomes evaluation, a validated quality-of-life survey, to show that the modified Cottle maneuver was predictive of positive surgical outcomes.

OBJECTIVE OUTCOME MEASURES

Objective measures in nasal valve surgery serve 2 purposes. They are useful in the assessment of clinical outcomes determining whether surgery accomplished the goal of improving patient outcomes. Secondly, and perhaps most importantly, these measures would theoretically have diagnostic utility in predicting surgical success. Such measures would ideally be inexpensive, readily accessible, and easy to administer. Unfortunately, no such tool currently exists. Most objective measures are cumbersome and difficult to administer, belying their clinical utility. Likewise, objective measures have been often incongruous with patient-reported severity of nasal valve obstruction.[40]

Although measures may show an effective surgical change, the correlation with improved patient symptoms has not been definitively shown with any objective measure. A recent systematic review correlating objective outcome measures with subjective sense of nasal patency found several studies with conflicting findings.[41] Likewise, in a consensus statement by Rhee and colleagues,[15] a panel of experts did not find imaging, acoustic rhinometry, or rhinomanometry useful in clinical diagnosis.

Nonetheless, the current perspective on objective measures in nasal valve surgery may change as new methods are designed and better clinical investigations are performed. The objective measures currently used in assessment of NVC include acoustic rhinometry, rhinomanometry, peak nasal inspiratory flow, and computed tomography (CT) imaging.

Acoustic rhinometry uses reflected acoustic pulses to calculate the nasal cross-sectional area. Nasal volumes can be calculated from a series of cross-sectional area measurements.[40] Acoustic rhinometry has been found to correlate well with other objective measures; consequently, hundreds of studies have used this objective measure in clinical research. Acoustic rhinometry has not been found to correlate well with subjective outcomes.[41,42]

Rhinomanometry is an objective physiologic measure that evaluates transnasal pressure and nasal airflow volume to calculate nasal airway resistance during inspiration. Nasal peak inspiratory flow is another noninvasive physiologic tool that measures maximum airflow during a forced nasal inspiration. Although this method has been validated against rhinomanometry, this tool depends on patient effort and pulmonary function and, therefore, may not be consistently reliable.[40,43]

CT imaging has shown promise as an objective measure as it is readily available to the clinician and can directly measure nasal dimensions and the angle of the internal nasal valve. It has been successfully validated against acoustic rhinometry.[44] However, as with the other objective measures, there has been limited evidence supporting the correlation of CT imaging to subjective outcomes. One study by Menger and colleagues[45] did find a correlation between improved postoperative NOSE scores and the change in minimal cross-sectional area on CT, though the validity of this correlation is questioned as the statistical analysis seems to have violated the principle of statistical independence in their analysis.[46,47]

Recently, clinician-derived measures have been developed to allow the clinician to standardize physical examination findings in assessing surgical outcomes. Tsao and colleagues[48] developed a methodology for description of lateral sidewall insufficiency. In this method, the clinician evaluates each nasal sidewall zone, as previously defined earlier, and rates collapse on a scale of 0 to 3. This measure has been validated in reporting surgical outcomes, though its use has remained limited.[48]

SUBJECTIVE OUTCOME MEASURES

Perhaps more important than objective measures of the nasal valve is the subjective experience of obstruction and self-reported assessment of efficacy. Although subjective assessments are not helpful in the specific diagnosis of a nasal valve problem, they can be helpful in indicating the degree of impact on a patient's quality of life. They also serve as an indicator of surgical success. The most commonly accepted patient-reported outcome measure in use is the NOSE scale. Initially developed to assess surgical outcomes for patients undergoing septoplasty, the NOSE scale is a validated disease-specific quality-of-life questionnaire that measures nasal obstruction.[49] The NOSE scale has been used in several nasal valve studies since its inception and has been useful in proving the effectiveness of nasal valve surgery in quality-of-life improvements as they relate to nasal obstruction.[2,7,9]

CONTROVERSY IN TECHNIQUE SELECTION

Long-term correction of NVD requires surgical intervention.[15]

Correction typically involves the use of various grafts or suture techniques to enlarge and/or support the nasal valve. Selection of the appropriate technique largely depends on the location and type of dysfunction (dynamic/static). Often, multiple techniques need to be used in the same surgical procedure.

Selection of the appropriate technique poses a significant challenge to the nasal valve surgeon. Most techniques have been shown to have positive effects on postoperative outcomes[2,4,6,37,45,50–52]; however, there have been few studies directly comparing techniques.[9] Additionally, adjunctive procedures, such as septoplasty and turbinoplasty, are almost universally performed in most of the studies. This use potentially confounds the accurate assessment of any nasal valve technique, as septoplasty and turbinoplasty inherently alters the nasal valve. Even studies looking at nasal valve correction after failed septoplasty often had to correct previously unaddressed deviations in the septum in addition to valve surgery.[6]

Another important consideration is that many of the maneuvers can impact both the internal and external valves. Some techniques are traditionally thought of as impacting the internal valve alone, with the primary effect of increasing the valve angle and altering static narrowing. Spreader grafts, autospreader flaps, and flaring sutures typically fall into this category. Most of the remaining techniques can impact both the internal and/or external valves depending on the location of placement along the lateral nasal sidewall. These grafts, such as alar batten grafts, alar struts, and alar rim grafts, primarily impact dynamic collapse (**Table 1**).

Table 1
Characteristics of Nasal Valve altering techniques

Technique	Valve Impacted		Type of Collapse Impacted		Advantages	Disadvantages	Placement Location
	Internal Nasal Valve	External Nasal Valve	Static	Dynamic			
Spreader graft	+	−	+	−	Cosmetic utility	Widens dorsum	Between dorsal septum and ULC
Autospreader	+	−	+	−	Cartilage sparing	Insufficient to expand the dorsum/stent the INV	Cranial ULC infolded medially toward dorsal septum
Flaring sutures	+	−	+	+	Simplicity	Lack of suture durability, widened middle third	Horizontal mattress suture from one ULC to the other over the nasal dorsum
Alar batten graft	+	+	−	+	Precise correction of area of collapse	Visibility	Pocket along lateral wall depending on the point of maximal collapse
Lateral nasal wall suspension	+	−	+	+	Cartilage sparing	Increased zone of dissection	Suture from the lateral alar and/or ULC to the bone of the infraorbital rim
Lateral crura strut graft	−	+	+	+	Corrects intrinsic concavities of the LLC	Visibility	Underlay or overlay graft between the lateral crura and vestibular mucosa extending past the cephalic edge of the lateral crus
Lateral crura turn-in	−	+	+	+	Cartilage sparing, improved tip contour	Weak, thin cartilage for valve support	Express cartilage along the cephalic lateral crura during a cephalic trim folded into a vestibular mucosal pocket
Alar rim graft	−	+	+	+	Improves contour and strength of rim	Visibility	Alar margin pocket
Butterfly graft	+	+	+	+	Single graft that can treat both internal and external valve dysfunction	Ear cartilage needed, visibility	Superficial to the anterior septal angle and caudal edge of the upper lateral cartilage; caudal aspect of the graft positioned deep to the cephalic margin of the lower lateral cartilage

Abbreviation: INV, internal nasal valve.

Although it may be cognitively helpful to classify pathology and treatments based on the distinction of the internal and external valves for sake of simplicity, it is likely more realistic to consider the nasal sidewall as a continuum, with placement of these grafts having different effects based on their specific location in relation to the patients' pathology. Nonetheless, the authors review the commonly used techniques for management of the nasal valve, categorizing each technique by whether it exerts its primary effect on the internal valve, external valve, or both. The review evaluates the advantages and disadvantages of each technique with mention of efficacy in relation to surgical outcome and in comparison with other techniques where possible.

SPREADER GRAFTS

Spreader grafts have been the workhorse technique for repairing the internal nasal valves and correcting abnormalities of the midvault. These grafts directly address static internal valve narrowing. Generally derived from septal cartilage, these grafts are secured to the dorsal septum increasing the angle and cross-sectional area of the internal nasal valve by lateral displacement of the ULC (**Fig. 4**). The grafts also have a cosmetic impact, often augmenting the concave side of the nasal dorsum to create asymmetry.[34] The main disadvantage is that spreader grafts typically widen the nasal dorsum. In a systematic review of nasal valve surgery, 24 of 44 studies evaluated spreader grafting as a component of the surgical techniques used with all studies finding functional surgery effective in improving outcomes.[9]

AUTOSPREADER GRAFTS

A recently discovered alternative technique to the classic spreader grafts is the use of spreader flaps, or autospreader grafts. Autospreader grafts use the same principles, primarily impacting internal nasal narrowing. Contrary to spreader grafts, autospreader grafts involve infolding of the ULC to act as a spacer (**Fig. 5**). First described by Lerma[53] in the late 1990s, the dorsal edge of the ULC is scored or left alone and infolded medially, occupying the space that a spreader graft would otherwise occupy.[53] The graft theoretically

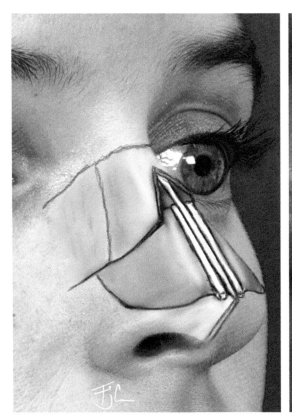
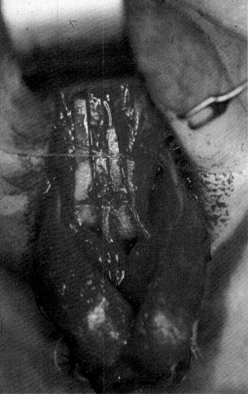

Fig. 4. Spreader grafts are placed just caudal to the nasal bones lateral to the dorsal septum and medial to the cranial portion of the upper lateral cartilage. Left: depiction of the location of spreader grafts. Right: spreader grafts secured to the dorsum during a functional rhinoplasty.

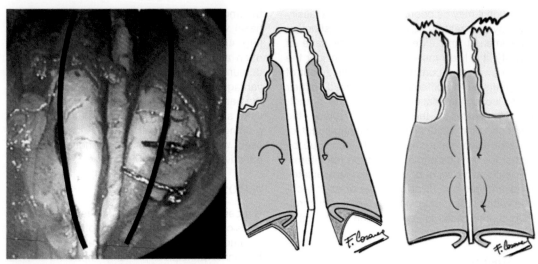

Fig. 5. Autospreader flaps. With autospreader flaps, the ULC are infolded, acting as spacers for the internal nasal valves. Left: intraoperative image of the autospreader flaps. Right: depiction of the autospreader flaps.

provides the same benefit as a spreader graft by increasing the angle and cross-sectional area of the internal valve. The benefit over the conventional technique is that it is cartilage sparing, allowing septal cartilage to be left alone or used for other purposes. Additionally, the ULC is typically thinner than the classic spreader graft, potentially avoiding the unwanted effect of a widened dorsum (0.5 mm compared with 2.0 mm).[54]

Interestingly, there have been conflicting reports regarding the efficacy of autospreader grafts. In a prospective observational outcomes study, Yoo and Most[55] found a significant improvement in mean postoperative NOSE scores in patients undergoing both functional and cosmetic rhinoplasty. Contradicting this finding, a recent randomized controlled trial evaluated postoperative improvement in nasal obstruction in patients undergoing rhinoplasty with or without autospreader flaps.[33] This study found no statistically significant difference in postoperative visual analog scale (VAS) scores regarding nasal obstruction between groups. However, they did not define whether patients in their cohorts had preoperative complaints of nasal obstruction.

FLARING SUTURES

The flaring suture is another method of primarily correcting internal NVC. The flaring suture is a horizontal mattress suture that extends from one ULC to the other over the nasal dorsum (**Fig. 6**). Once tightened, both ULCs are flared dorsally increasing the angle and cross-sectional area of the internal valve. This technique can impact both static narrowing and dynamic collapse. The suture widens

the internal valve, whereas the suture tension resists sidewall collapse. The main advantage of this technique is the ease of application and the fact it is cartilage sparing. The valve expansion gained by insertion of the flaring suture is significantly enhanced by the simultaneous insertion of spreader grafts. Critics of this technique argue that the result is temporary as the tension placed by the suture ultimately relaxes.

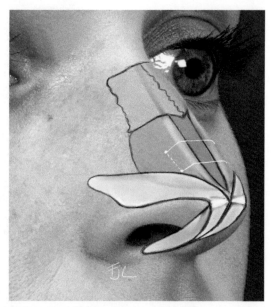

Fig. 6. The flaring suture. This suture is placed through the ULC spanning the dorsum to flare the cartilages and increase the cross-sectional area of the internal nasal valve.

A cadaver study by Schlosser and Park[32] demonstrated that the combination of spreader grafts and flaring sutures significantly increased the minimal cross-sectional area of the internal nasal valve as measured by acoustic rhinometry. Although each technique used in isolation created improvements in minimal cross-sectional area (MCA), these values were not statistically significant. Another cadaver study by Shadfar and colleagues[56] evaluated the changes in nasal airflow and nasal resistance through the internal nasal valve using a digital nasal model created from fine-cut CT scans. Similar to the study by Schlosser and Park,[32] this cadaver study found greater gains in nasal airflow using combinations of flaring suture and spreader graft techniques over the use of any individual technique in isolation. A recent prospective study comparing spreader grafts and flaring sutures in patients undergoing rhinoplasty for aesthetic concerns found similar improvements in nasal airway resistance between the groups. This study was not randomized or blinded.[57]

ALAR BATTEN GRAFTS

Alar batten grafts are cartilaginous grafts typically composed of conchal cartilage that are placed in precise pockets along the point of maximal nasal sidewall collapse. The lateral aspect of the graft overlaps the piriform aperture in order to support the nasal sidewall and prevent dynamic collapse (**Fig. 7**). The location of graft placement should depend on preoperative evaluation of the site of the nasal sidewall collapse as determined by the modified Cottle maneuver.[58] Typically this is deep to the supra-alar crease and just cephalad to the lateral crura. However, placement may need to be caudal to the lateral crura if the crura are cephalically malpositioned. The primary disadvantages of this technique include undesired fullness along the insertion site as well as technical difficulty in placement. If the graft is not placed precisely in the location of collapse, or if it does not overlap the piriform, the graft may exacerbate the nasal sidewall collapse. Several studies have validated alar batten grafting as an effective surgical technique.[4,6,7,9,51,59,60]

LATERAL CRURAL STRUT GRAFTS

Lateral crural strut grafts are useful in cases of inherent weakness, concavity, or cephalic malposition of the lateral crura resulting in dynamic nasal sidewall collapse. These grafts are ideally fashioned from septal cartilage as thin and straight grafts. They may be placed as an overlay or

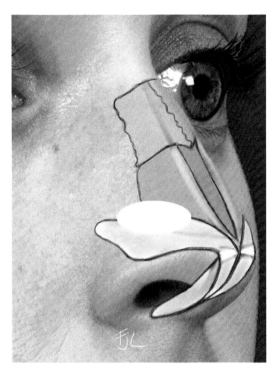

Fig. 7. Alar batten grafts. These grafts are placed in precise pockets along the point of maximal collapse in the nasal sidewall overlapping the piriform aperture.

underlay graft between the lateral crura and vestibular mucosa extending past the cephalic edge of the lateral crus (**Fig. 8**). It is important to place these grafts in a precisely dissected pocket, and the graft should be affixed to the lateral crus with suture. The main effects are to stiffen the lateral crura preventing collapse of the nasal sidewall and straightening intrinsic concavities in the shape of the lateral crus.[58]

This graft also provides tip support by strengthening the lateral components of the tripod. The main disadvantage of this technique is a noticeable contour edge along the vestibule if placed as an underlay or a noticeable fullness of the skin envelope if placed as an overlay.[34] The latter is more problematic in a thin-skinned individual. Lateral crural strut grafting has been used in the armamentarium of nasal valve techniques in prior studies and has proven effective in managing the external valve.[6]

LATERAL CRURAL TURN-IN GRAFTS

Lateral crural turn-in grafts are a novel technique first described by Tellioglu and Cimen[61] in 2007 and later Murakami and colleagues[62] in 2009. This technique takes advantage of the excess cartilage along the cephalic lateral crura during a cephalic trim. Instead of discarding the cartilage,

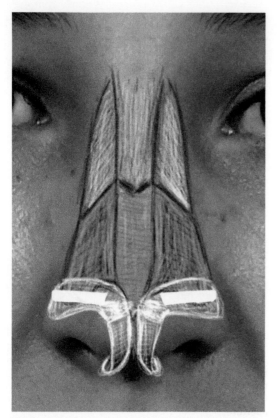

Fig. 8. Lateral crural strut grafts. These grafts may be placed as an underlay or overlay and provide support to the lower lateral cartilages resisting collapse. The grafts are also useful in correcting concavities of the lateral crura.

the cephalic cartilage is scored, infolded into a vestibular mucosal pocket, and secured with horizontal mattress sutures. The advantages of this technique are that it can improve nasal tip contour without compromising the scroll area. The infolded cartilage reinforces the lateral crus improving the nasal sidewall support and resisting dynamic collapse. Additionally, the infolded cartilage can improve intrinsic concavities of the lateral crura theoretically increasing the cross-sectional area of the external valve.

A recent prospective cohort study compared the efficacy of lateral crural strut grafts with cephalic turn-in for correction of external valve dysfunction.[63] They found that at a mean follow-up of 10 months, all patients in both groups had significantly improved VAS, sino-nasal outcome test (SNOT-22), NOSE, patient-reported function, and cosmesis scores. Nasal peak inspiratory flow also significantly improved in both groups when compared with preoperative measurements. All patients did undergo concomitant septoplasty and turbinoplasty.

ALAR RIM GRAFTS

Alar rim grafts are useful when contour deformities and collapse of the alar rim exist. Alar rim collapse may result from congenital weakness or malposition or as a result of overzealous cephalic trimming of the LLC in prior surgery. In these cases, the alar rim lacks rigid support and is subject to static or dynamic collapse. The alar rim graft is a thin cartilage graft, 1 to 3 mm in thickness placed in a non-anatomic fashion spanning the alar rim margin (**Fig. 9**). The medial aspect of the cartilage may be bruised to help camouflage the graft. In similar fashion to a collar stay, the graft sits in the alar margin improving the contour and strength of the rim. Boahene and Hilger[64] noted improvements in external valve dysfunction in a series of patients undergoing alar rim grafting.

LATERAL NASAL SIDEWALL SUSPENSION

Lateral nasal sidewall suspension involves placement of a permanent suture from the lateral alar cartilage to the bone of the infraorbital rim. As it was first described in the mid 1990s, the suture was placed using a combination of a small intranasal incision and an external incision on the medial lower eyelid or via transconjunctival incision.[65] Disadvantages of this technique included risk of ectropion, external incisions, and unclear efficacy. A similar technique has been described through a standard open rhinoplasty approach with dissection carried laterally onto the maxillary buttress and infraorbital rim. The suture is anchored to the infraorbital rim and secured to the lower and upper lateral cartilages.[16] Improved results compared with the original technique were attributed to the fact that the tissue planes were dissected allowing scar formation to hold the sidewall in the suspended position. Most[66] noted significant improvement in postoperative NOSE scores in patients who had lateral nasal sidewall suspension.

BUTTERFLY GRAFT

The butterfly graft is a structurally supportive onlay graft harvested from the conchal cartilage of the ear (**Fig. 10**). The graft is carved into the shape of a wedge and positioned superficial to the anterior septal angle and caudal edge of the upper lateral cartilage. The caudal aspect of the graft is positioned deep to the cephalic margin of the lower lateral cartilage. Acting as an internal BreatheRight Strip (CNS Inc, Minneapolis MN), the graft provides an outward spring effect both widening and supporting the upper lateral cartilages while also supporting the lower lateral cartilage.

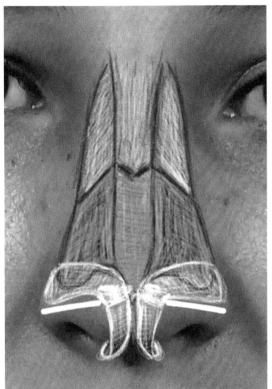
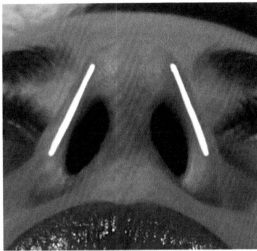

Fig. 9. Alar rim grafts. Alar rim grafts are placed along the alar rim in a nonanatomic fashion to provide external valve support and resist dynamic valve collapse.

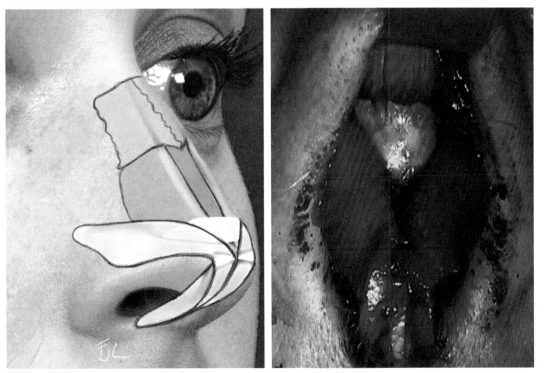

Fig. 10. Butterfly graft. This graft spans the nasal dorsum providing rigid support to the ULC and stenting the lower lateral cartilages.

This technique has been evaluated in both revision and primary functional rhinoplasty. Clark and Cook[67] found that 97% of their patients who underwent revision rhinoplasty with butterfly graft reported complete resolution of their nasal obstruction (N = 72). Eighty-six percent had notable improvement in cosmesis. Those who did not have a satisfactory cosmetic result valued the improved functional result over any apparent detriment to cosmesis. A similar study by Friedman and Cook[68] also evaluated this technique in primary functional rhinoplasty finding improved nasal breathing in 90% of patients and satisfactory cosmesis in 88% of their cohort.

This graft has many functional advantages making it a preferred technique in the authors' surgical armamentarium for nasal valve management. Placing the graft so the cephalic edge of the graft overlies the caudal aspect of the ULCs allows the inherent springlike effect of the cartilage to stent and lateralizes the ULC. This technique results in widening of the internal valve angle and an increase in internal valve cross-sectional area. Positioning the caudal aspect of the graft deep to the cephalic edge of the LLC allows the graft to support and stent the external valve. This dual effect underscores both the versatility and impact this graft has on the nasal valve.

The main criticism of this graft is poor cosmesis. There is fear that placement of a bulky graft over the dorsum will result in middle-third widening and graft visibility. Refinements in technique circumvent this problem. Beveling the edges of the graft helps prevent a palpable step-off over the dorsum. Although many patients have supratip saddling, which the butterfly graft corrects, fullness over the dorsum can be ameliorated by shaving down the dorsum of the caudal septum about 1.5 mm, which creates a depression for the graft to fill. Finally, placing crushed cartilage over the dorsum to ensure a smooth contour can help camouflage the graft.

SUMMARY

The nasal valve plays an important role in nasal airflow. It is important for the otolaryngologist to not only consider but also fully evaluate the nasal valve when seeing a patient with nasal obstruction. If not the primary cause of obstruction, it is often a contributing factor. If NVD is discovered, it should be addressed during surgical intervention to avoid a suboptimal outcome.

There is some controversy regarding the anatomy, terminology, evaluation, and management of the nasal valve. Both anatomy and terminology are in need of standardization so that future research may be consistent in describing how techniques impact the nasal valve. Many objective tools have been developed to evaluate nasal airflow, though the correlation with subjective patient outcomes has been inconsistent in the literature. Most nasal valve surgeons rely on history and physical examination to determine candidacy for surgery.

Regarding the management of the nasal valve, there are innumerable options available to the surgeon. Most of the techniques described have been shown to have positive effects, though there is a lack of randomized controlled trials directly comparing techniques. A large part of the problem is that the selection of the surgical method has to be tailored to the patients and their specific pathology. There is no one-size-fits-all approach. Nonetheless, the authors have found that the butterfly graft is a versatile option that has been useful for many patients.

Future research using standardized definitions and validated outcome measures can help increase the quality of evidence currently in the literature. Direct comparison of techniques would be optimal, though difficult to accomplish. Nonetheless, improvements in the quality of evidence will undoubtedly impact surgical decision-making.

REFERENCES

1. Franciscus RG, Trinkaus E. Nasal morphology and the emergence of homo erectus. Am J Phys Anthropol 1988;75(4):517–27.
2. Rhee JS, Poetker DM, Smith TL, et al. Nasal valve surgery improves disease-specific quality of life. Laryngoscope 2005;115(3):437–40.
3. Elwany S, Thabet H. Obstruction of the nasal valve. J Laryngol Otol 1996;110(3):221–4.
4. Khosh MM, Jen A, Honrado C, et al. Nasal valve reconstruction: experience in 53 consecutive patients. Arch Facial Plast Surg 2004;6(3):167–71.
5. Haight JS, Cole P. The site and function of the nasal valve. Laryngoscope 1983;93(1):49–55.
6. Chambers KJ, Horstkotte KA, Shanley K, et al. Evaluation of improvement in nasal obstruction following nasal valve correction in patients with a history of failed septoplasty. JAMA Facial Plast Surg 2015; 17(5):347–50.
7. Lindsay RW. Disease-specific quality of life outcomes in functional rhinoplasty. Laryngoscope 2012;122(7): 1480–8.
8. Spielmann PM, White PS, Hussain SS. Surgical techniques for the treatment of nasal valve collapse: a systematic review. Laryngoscope 2009;119(7):1281–90.
9. Rhee JS, Arganbright JM, McMullin BT, et al. Evidence supporting functional rhinoplasty or nasal

valve repair: a 25-year systematic review. Otolaryngol Head Neck Surg 2008;139(1):10–20.

10. Mink PJ. Physiologie der oberen Luftwege. Leipzig: F. Vol 4. CLeipzig: FCW Vogel; 1920. p. 150.

11. Bridger GP. Physiology of the nasal valve. Arch Otolaryngol 1970;92(6):543–53.

12. Kasperbauer JL, Kern EB. Nasal valve physiology. Implications in nasal surgery. Otolaryngol Clin North Am 1987;20(4):699–719.

13. Ballert JA, Park SS. Functional rhinoplasty: treatment of the dysfunctional nasal sidewall. Facial Plast Surg 2006;22(1):49–54.

14. Bridger GP, Proctor DF. Maximum nasal inspiratory flow and nasal resistance. Ann Otol Rhinol Laryngol 1970;79(3):481–8.

15. Rhee JS, Weaver EM, Park SS, et al. Clinical consensus statement: diagnosis and management of nasal valve compromise. Otolaryngol Head Neck Surg 2010;143(1):48–59.

16. Most SP. Trends in functional rhinoplasty. Arch Facial Plast Surg 2008;10(6):410–3.

17. Bae JH, Most SP. Cadaveric analysis of nasal valve suspension. Allergy Rhinol (Providence) 2012;3(2): e91–3.

18. Lee MK, Most SP. Evidence-based medicine: rhinoplasty. Facial Plast Surg Clin North Am 2015;23(3): 303–12.

19. Killian G. Die submucosa Fensterresektion der Nasencheidewand. Arch Laryngologic Rhinologic 1904;16:362–87.

20. Freer OT. The correction of defections of the nasal septum with a minimum of traumatization. JAMA 1902;38:636.

21. Cottle MH, Loring RM. Surgery of the nasal septum; new operative procedures and indications. Ann Otol Rhinol Laryngol 1948;57(3):705–13.

22. Dobratz EJ, Park SS. Septoplasty pearls. Otolaryngol Clin North Am 2009;42(3):527–37.

23. Stewart MG, Smith TL, Weaver EM, et al. Outcomes after nasal septoplasty: results from the Nasal Obstruction Septoplasty Effectiveness (NOSE) study. Otolaryngol Head Neck Surg 2004;130(3):283–90.

24. Bohlin L, Dahlqvist A. Nasal airway resistance and complications following functional septoplasty: a ten-year follow-up study. Rhinology 1994;32(4): 195–7.

25. Siegel NS, Gliklich RE, Taghizadeh F, et al. Outcomes of septoplasty. Otolaryngol Head Neck Surg 2000;122(2):228–32.

26. Hol MK, Huizing EH. Treatment of inferior turbinate pathology: a review and critical evaluation of the different techniques. Rhinology 2000; 38(4):157–66.

27. Moore GF, Freeman TJ, Ogren FP, et al. Extended follow-up of total inferior turbinate resection for relief of chronic nasal obstruction. Laryngoscope 1985; 95(9 Pt 1):1095–9.

28. Bhandarkar ND, Smith TL. Outcomes of surgery for inferior turbinate hypertrophy. Curr Opin Otolaryngol Head Neck Surg 2010;18(1):49–53.

29. Garzaro M, Pezzoli M, Landolfo V, et al. Radiofrequency inferior turbinate reduction: long-term olfactory and functional outcomes. Otolaryngol Head Neck Surg 2012;146(1):146–50.

30. Lavinsky-Wolff M, Camargo HL Jr, Barone CR, et al. Effect of turbinate surgery in rhinoseptoplasty on quality-of-life and acoustic rhinometry outcomes: a randomized clinical trial. Laryngoscope 2013; 123(1):82–9.

31. Sheen JH. Spreader graft: a method of reconstructing the roof of the middle nasal vault following rhinoplasty. Plast Reconstr Surg 1984;73(2):230–9.

32. Schlosser RJ, Park SS. Surgery for the dysfunctional nasal valve. Cadaveric analysis and clinical outcomes. Arch Facial Plast Surg 1999;1(2):105–10.

33. Saedi B, Amali A, Gharavis V, et al. Spreader flaps do not change early functional outcomes in reduction rhinoplasty: a randomized control trial. Am J Rhinol Allergy 2014;28(1):70–4.

34. Antunes MB, Goldstein SA. Surgical approach to nasal valves and the midvault in patients with a crooked nose. Facial Plast Surg 2011;27(5):422–36.

35. Miman MC, Deliktas H, Ozturan O, et al. Internal nasal valve: revisited with objective facts. Otolaryngol Head Neck Surg 2006;134(1):41–7.

36. Teymoortash A, Fasunla JA, Sazgar AA. The value of spreader grafts in rhinoplasty: a critical review. Eur Arch Otorhinolaryngol 2012;269(5):1411–6.

37. Constantinides M, Galli SK, Miller PJ. A simple and reliable method of patient evaluation in the surgical treatment of nasal obstruction. Ear Nose Throat J 2002;81(10):734–7.

38. Constantinides MS, Adamson PA, Cole P. The long-term effects of open cosmetic septorhinoplasty on nasal air flow. Arch Otolaryngol Head Neck Surg 1996;122(1):41–5.

39. Fung E, Hong P, Moore C, et al. The effectiveness of modified Cottle maneuver in predicting outcomes in functional rhinoplasty. Plast Surg Int 2014;2014: 618313.

40. Lam K, Tan BK, Lavin JM, et al. Comparison of nasal sprays and irrigations in the delivery of topical agents to the olfactory mucosa. Laryngoscope 2013;123(12):2950–7.

41. Andre RF, Vuyk HD, Ahmed A, et al. Correlation between subjective and objective evaluation of the nasal airway. A systematic review of the highest level of evidence. Clin Otolaryngol 2009;34(6):518–25.

42. Lal D, Corey JP. Acoustic rhinometry and its uses in rhinology and diagnosis of nasal obstruction. Facial Plast Surg Clin North Am 2004;12(4):397–405, v.

43. Angelos PC, Been MJ, Toriumi DM. Contemporary review of rhinoplasty. Arch Facial Plast Surg 2012; 14(4):238–47.

44. Dastidar P, Numminen J, Heinonen T, et al. Nasal airway volumetric measurement using segmented HRCT images and acoustic rhinometry. Am J Rhinol 1999;13(2):97–103.

45. Menger DJ, Swart KM, Nolst Trenite GJ,. et al. Surgery of the external nasal valve: the correlation between subjective and objective measurements. Clin Otolaryngol 2014;39(3):150–5.

46. Ranstam J. Repeated measurements, bilateral observations and pseudoreplicates, why does it matter? Osteoarthritis Cartilage 2012;20(6):473–5.

47. Park MS, Kim SJ, Chung CY, et al. Statistical consideration for bilateral cases in orthopaedic research. J Bone Joint Surg Am 2010;92(8):1732–7.

48. Tsao GJ, Fijalkowski N, Most SP. Validation of a grading system for lateral nasal wall insufficiency. Allergy Rhinol (Providence) 2013;4(2):e66–8.

49. Stewart MG, Witsell DL, Smith TL, et al. Development and validation of the Nasal Obstruction Symptom Evaluation (NOSE) scale. Otolaryngol Head Neck Surg 2004;130(2):157–63.

50. Kalan A, Kenyon GS, Seemungal TA. Treatment of external nasal valve (alar rim) collapse with an alar strut. J Laryngol Otol 2001;115(10):788–91.

51. Toriumi DM, Josen J, Weinberger M, et al. Use of alar batten grafts for correction of nasal valve collapse. Arch Otolaryngol Head Neck Surg 1997; 123(8):802–8.

52. Hussein WK, Elwany S, Montaser M. Modified autospreader flap for nasal valve support: utilizing the spring effect of the upper lateral cartilage. Eur Arch Otorhinolaryngol 2015;272(2):497–504.

53. Lerma J. The "lapel" technique. Plast Reconstr Surg 1998;102(6):2274–5.

54. Gruber RP, Park E, Newman J, et al. The spreader flap in primary rhinoplasty. Plast Reconstr Surg 2007;119(6):1903–10.

55. Yoo S, Most SP. Nasal airway preservation using the autospreader technique: analysis of outcomes using a disease-specific quality-of-life instrument. Arch Facial Plast Surg 2011;13(4):231–3.

56. Shadfar S, Shockley WW, Fleischman GM, et al. Characterization of postoperative changes in nasal airflow using a cadaveric computational fluid dynamics model: supporting the internal nasal valve. JAMA Facial Plast Surg 2014;16(5):319–27.

57. Jalali MM. Comparison of effects of spreader grafts and flaring sutures on nasal airway resistance in rhinoplasty. Eur Arch Otorhinolaryngol 2015;272(9): 2299–303.

58. Kim DW, Rodriguez-Bruno K. Functional rhinoplasty. Facial Plast Surg Clin North Am 2009; 17(1):115–31, vii.

59. Cervelli V, Spallone D, Bottini JD, et al. Alar batten cartilage graft: treatment of internal and external nasal valve collapse. Aesthetic Plast Surg 2009; 33(4):625–34.

60. Millman B. Alar batten grafting for management of the collapsed nasal valve. Laryngoscope 2002; 112(3):574–9.

61. Tellioglu AT, Cimen K. Turn-in folding of the cephalic portion of the lateral crus to support the alar rim in rhinoplasty. Aesthetic Plast Surg 2007;31(3):306–10.

62. Murakami CS, Barrera JE, Most SP. Preserving structural integrity of the alar cartilage in aesthetic rhinoplasty using a cephalic turn-in flap. Arch Facial Plast Surg 2009;11(2):126–8.

63. Barham HP, Knisely A, Christensen J, et al. Costal cartilage lateral crural strut graft vs cephalic crural turn-in for correction of external valve dysfunction. JAMA Facial Plast Surg 2015;17(5):340–5.

64. Boahene KD, Hilger PA. Alar rim grafting in rhinoplasty: indications, technique, and outcomes. Arch Facial Plast Surg 2009;11(5):285–9.

65. Paniello RC. Nasal valve suspension. An effective treatment for nasal valve collapse. Arch Otolaryngol Head Neck Surg 1996;122(12):1342–6.

66. Most SP. Analysis of outcomes after functional rhinoplasty using a disease-specific quality-of-life instrument. Arch Facial Plast Surg 2006;8(5):306–9.

67. Clark JM, Cook TA. The 'butterfly' graft in functional secondary rhinoplasty. Laryngoscope 2002;112(11): 1917–25.

68. Friedman O, Cook TA. Conchal cartilage butterfly graft in primary functional rhinoplasty. Laryngoscope 2009;119(2):255–62.

Controversies in Parotid Defect Reconstruction

Matthew Tamplen, MD[a], P. Daniel Knott, MD[a], Michael A. Fritz, MD[b], Rahul Seth, MD[a],*

KEYWORDS

- Parotid defects • Parotidectomy • Reconstruction • Facial nerve • Microvascular surgery

KEY POINTS

- Multiple reconstructive options are available for parotidectomy defect reconstruction. These vary depending on the extent of parotidectomy—superficial, total, or radical.
- Reconstructive considerations include facial contour, avoidance of Frey syndrome, skin coverage, tumor surveillance, potential adjuvant therapy, and facial reanimation.
- Parotidectomy reconstruction should be tailored to the patient, specific to the defect, and within the comfort level of the reconstructive surgeon.
- Facial reanimation should be performed in radical parotidectomy reconstruction while giving consideration to patient age, comorbidities, prognosis, goals of treatment, and future adjuvant radiation therapy.

INTRODUCTION

Effective and aesthetically pleasing reconstruction of the parotidectomy defect requires full understanding of both facial form and function. To appropriately discuss the varying reconstructive methods available, defects created by superficial parotidectomy, total parotidectomy, and radical parotidectomy are addressed separately. Overall, reconstructive emphasis is placed on recreating facial contour, avoiding Frey syndrome, providing skin coverage, minimizing deleterious effects of adjuvant therapy, and restoring facial function. Areas of controversy are highlighted and discussed.

SUPERFICIAL PAROTIDECTOMY

Reconstruction of the superficial parotidectomy defect is usually easiest when performed primarily, because the defect and facial nerve are exposed. The greatest risk of secondary reconstruction is inadvertent facial nerve injury. Options for addressing facial asymmetry after superficial parotidectomy include abdominal fat grafting, use of injectable fillers, placement of acellular dermal matrix (ADM), sternocleidomastoid rotational flap, temporoparietal fascia (TPF) rotational flap, and superficial muscular aponeurotic system (SMAS) advancement flaps.

Although usually of minor significance, the contour defect after superficial parotidectomy can be disfiguring. In addition to facial asymmetry, Frey syndrome, also known as gustatory sweating, commonly affects patients undergoing superficial parotidectomy and is caused by aberrant reinervation of severed parasympathetic fibers to sweat glands of elevated cheek skin.[1,2] The incidence of Frey syndrome ranges from 38% to 86% depending on if subjective or objective measures are used.[3]

Frey syndrome can be treated secondarily with botulinum toxin type A; however, the therapeutic effect after injection with botulinum toxin type A is temporary and patients most affected by Frey syndrome may require lifelong recurrent injections. Secondary surgical procedures offering potential permanent solutions for Frey syndrome may place the exposed

Disclosures: M.A. Fritz: Consultant to Stryker; All the other authors in this article have nothing to disclose.
[a] Department of Otolaryngology–Head and Neck Surgery, University of California San Francisco, 2233 Post Street, 3rd Floor, San Francisco, CA 94115, USA; [b] Head and Neck Institute, Cleveland Clinic, CCLCM, 9500 Euclid Avenue, Desk A71, Cleveland, OH 44195, USA
* Corresponding author.
E-mail address: Rahul.Seth@ucsf.edu

Facial Plast Surg Clin N Am 24 (2016) 235–243
http://dx.doi.org/10.1016/j.fsc.2016.03.002
1064-7406/16/$ – see front matter © 2016 Elsevier Inc. All rights reserved.

facial nerve at risk. Measures taken at the time of primary surgical treatment of the parotid to prevent the development of Frey syndrome provide optimal results. Several surgical techniques may be used, all of which involve placement of a barrier between remaining parotid tissue and the elevated skin flap. As an added benefit, this barrier can provide varying degrees of volume to the defect site to improve facial contour. Barrier options include abdominal fat, ADM, and autogenous vascularized tissue, such as sternocleidomastoid rotational flap, TPF rotational flap, and SMAS advancement flaps. There is some debate regarding the success rates of each technique (discussed later).

Abdominal Fat Grafting

Autologous fat transfer is a widely used technique for moderate contour defect restoration that has the benefits of simplicity, minimal donor site morbidity, and little additional operative time. Abdominal fat is typically harvested via a lower abdominal incision, and placed into the defect site en bloc (**Fig. 1**). High patient satisfaction, correction of contour defect, and avoidance of Frey syndrome have been demonstrated in patients undergoing superficial or total parotidectomy with single-stage en bloc abdominal fat grafting.[4,5]

A composite of de-epithelialized dermis with an en bloc fat graft, known as a dermofat graft, may likewise be applied to the parotid defect site.[6,7] It is thought that inclusion of the dermis prevents fat necrosis and minimizes graft resorption. Dermofat grafts require larger harvest incisions, typically positioned at the lower abdomen, and subsequent de-epithelization. Results have shown that this technique is associated with little associated morbidity or additional operative time. Nosan and colleagues[8] reported only 11% facial concavity after 4.5 years of follow-up using a dermofat graft to correct

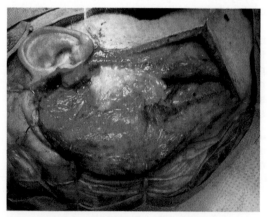

Fig. 1. En bloc abdominal fat graft positioned for volume restoration.

superficial parotid defects. Patients were overcorrected by 10% to 15% to account for resorption.

Curry and colleagues[9] described a method of SMAS plication and dermofat grafting with a 10% to 20% overcorrection after superficial parotidectomy. This method resulted in a statistically significant decrease in facial asymmetry and symptomatic Frey syndrome in 34 patients. SMAS elevation is not always possible, however, after parotidectomy for malignancy.

Regardless of method, most investigators recommend initial volume overcorrection by 10% to 20% for optimal results. Preoperative or postoperative radiation therapy may increase fat reabsorption rate.

Some investigators suggest only performing fat grafting for benign parotid disease, such that the fat grafting does not interfere with tumor surveillance in malignant cases.[9] Abdominal fat grafting after resection of parotid malignancy, however, has not been shown detrimental to clinical or radiologic tumor surveillance.[5] Due to improved imaging techniques and the potential for recurrent tumors to spread deep or longitudinally, radiographic tumor surveillance offers many advantages to clinical evaluation in the monitoring of postparotidectomy patients. The distinctive appearance of fat on MRI allows for easy delineation of the fat graft from normal or pathologic parotid tissue.

Injectable Fillers

Although preferred, volume restoration of the superficial parotid defect may not always be performed primarily. Therefore, techniques for secondary volume restoration may be required. One method of secondary correction is with injectable synthetic dermal fillers to add volume to a concave region. Synthetic dermal fillers are widely used for facial volume loss related to ageing but can also be a beneficial method for patients with postoperative volume deformities. Two dermal fillers, poly-L-lactic acid and calcium hydroxyapatite, bear specific indication by the US Food and Drug Administration for treatment of HIV-associated lipoatrophy in the parotid region, but none has a specific indication for facial asymmetry after parotidectomy.

Poly-L-lactic acid is a biocompatible synthetic polymer that provides volume and incites a local tissue reaction to stimulate proliferation of fibroblasts. It is immunologically inert, safe, and well tolerated. Because of reabsorption over time, the volume correction lasts up to 2 years and a series of several injections is required for optimal results.[10] Partially cross-linked hyaluronic acid dermal fillers are also used for management of facial volume loss in patients suffering from highly active antiretroviral therapy–related lipoatrophy[11] and may also be used for secondary correction of facial asymmetry after superficial parotidectomy.

Acellular Dermal Matrix Placement

AlloDerm (LifeCell, Bridgewater, New Jersey) is one of several acellular matrix grafts derived from human cadaveric dermis that may be used for volume reconstruction of the superficial parotidectomy defect. Advantages of AlloDerm use include the lack of donor site morbidity and minimal additional operative time. AlloDerm is an allograft, however, and is limited by its risk for infection, extrusion, limited volume, and resorption. Govindaraj and colleagues[3] prospectively studied AlloDerm placement compared with controls without any reconstruction and found the objective incidence of Frey syndrome was reduced to 0% in the AlloDerm group compared with 40% for the control group. There was a significantly higher incidence of seromas in the AlloDerm group, however, when compared with the control group (25% vs 9%, respectively). In this study, there was only 1 infection requiring removal of the graft in 32 patients. Sinha and colleagues[12] also found successful reduction of subjective Frey syndrome with AlloDerm placement after superficial parotidectomy. Contrary to the previous study, there were no infections and no increase in seroma rates in the Alloderm group. A meta-analysis by Zeng and colleagues[13] reviewed 5 randomized controlled trials evaluating the use AlloDerm for parotidectomy reconstruction and found an 85% relative risk reduction in objective Frey syndrome without any increase in wound infections or seromas with AlloDerm use compared with controls.

For volume reconstruction with AlloDerm, several pieces are folded to appropriate thickness and carefully secured into position to fill the superficial parotidectomy defect (**Fig. 2**). Overall, this ADM reconstruction is limited by its potential for infection

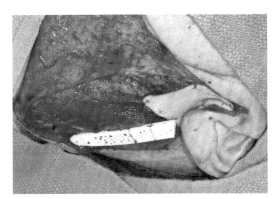

Fig. 2. ADM folded and secured into position of a superficial parotidectomy defect.

and resorption, variable added complexity during possible future reoperation, and added cost.

Local Muscle or Facial Rotational Flaps

Sternocleidomastoid rotational flap

Transposition of the sternocleidomastoid muscle (SCM) to fill the parotidectomy defect was originally described by Jost and colleagues[14] in 1968. The SCM flap can be superiorly or inferiorly based. For a superiorly based flap, the SCM muscle is split into 2 halves along the septum. Then a horizontal incision is used to free the anterior sternal insertion of the SCM muscle. Below this dissection, the accessory spinal nerve is isolated and protected. Finally, the muscle with its cervical fascia is rotated superiorly to fill the defect and sutured to the parotidomasseteric fascia (**Fig. 3**). Inferiorly based flaps are incised at their most superior insertion into the mastoid tip and are mobilized anterosuperiorly into the parotid defect and are anchored to the zygomatic arch and masseter muscle.

The role of the SCM flap in prevention of Frey syndrome and in facial volume reconstruction after superficial or total parotidectomy has been controversial. Kornblut and colleagues[15] found little benefit of the SCM flap in preventing Frey syndrome or facial asymmetry. Casler and Conley[16] compared the SCM flap with SMAS plication and found both methods significantly reduced the incidence of Frey syndrome compared with controls, but there was a trend for better results with SMAS plication. Fasolis and colleagues[7] directly compared SCM flap reconstruction to abdominal fat grafting and found improved cosmetic results with abdominal fat grafting. In this study, 5 of 11 patients receiving SCM flap reconstruction were unhappy with their facial or neck contour defect compared with 3 of 40 patients with abdominal fat grafting. A 2002 prospective randomized controlled trial by Kerawala and colleagues[17] in 2002 found no advantage in patient-perceived or provider-perceived cosmetic outcomes or in the incidence of Frey syndrome in patients reconstructed with an SCM flap compared with controls without any reconstruction. Additionally, there was an increase in facial nerve weakness in the SCM group.

The SCM flap can pose an attractive option because it does not require any additional incisions or significant additional operative time. Due to proximity, however, it is associated with potential injury to the facial, spinal accessory, and greater auricular nerves. Furthermore, because it requires a portion of the SCM, it paradoxically creates a nearby cosmetic deformity with hollowing of neck, resulting in an exchange of one soft tissue concavity for another.

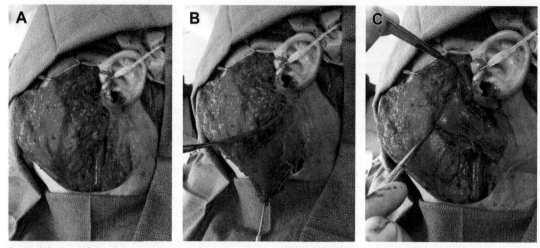

Fig. 3. (*A*) The defect after a superficial parotidectomy is demonstrated. (*B*) A superior based SCM flap is elevated and (*C*) positioned to obliterate the defect.

Temporoparietal fascia rotational flap

The TPF rotational flap has been described to reconstruct the parotid defect. To increase strength and bulk of the otherwise thin TPF flap, it can be elevated with the underlying deep temporalis fascia as a double-layered fascial flap. Ahmed and Kolhe[18] evaluated 24 patients treated with a double-layered TPF flap and found it reduced Frey syndrome to 8% from 43% in controls and all patients had less noticeable contour defects. The benefits of the TPF flap are its thinness and pliability, good vascularity, and inconspicuous donor site (**Fig. 4**). Damage to the superficial temporal vessels during the parotidectomy, however, limits viability of the flap. Further complications include alopecia, injury to the frontal branch of facial nerve, hematoma, and scar extension in the temporal region. Studies have shown success in avoiding Frey syndrome, although due to the thin nature of the flap, less than optimal cosmetic results are obtained while bearing increased operative time.[19]

Superficial muscular aponeurotic system advancement flap

The SMAS consists of fibrofatty muscle interposed between the facial muscles and the skin (**Fig. 5**). Its function is to transmit, distribute, and amplify activity of the facial musculature. The SMAS in the parotid region covers the parotid gland just above the parotid fascia. The SMAS envelops the zygomatic muscles until it reaches the nasolabial groove medially and the platysma muscle inferiorly. In the temporoparietal region, the SMAS is named TPF and the frontal branch of facial nerve and the superficial temporal artery are located within it. When used for parotid reconstruction, the SMAS layer is elevated independently so it can be plicated posteriorly into the defect region. It is sutured to the zygomatic periosteum and to the parotidomasseteric fascia to cover the

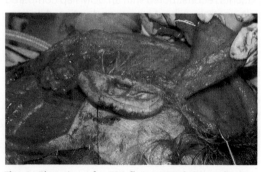

Fig. 4. Elevation of a TPF flap and inferior reflection for coverage of superficial parotidectomy defect.

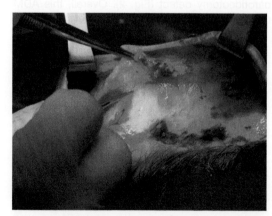

Fig. 5. SMAS flap elevation superficial to the parotidomasseteric fascia. Plication of this layer may be used to fill a posteriorly based parotid defect.

surgical defect. Allison and Rappaport[20] found only 2 cases of Frey syndrome in 112 patients reconstructed with SMAS flap.

The SMAS flap is an attractive option for small, posteriorly based benign disease because it can reconstruct these defects without an overly bulky appearance. Additional operative time is short and uses the same surgical scar as a parotidectomy. The SMAS must be separate, however, from margins of the resection.

TOTAL PAROTIDECTOMY WITH OR WITHOUT NEED FOR SKIN COVERAGE

The facial concavity after total parotidectomy is typically significant. Depending on disease extension and pathology, local skin may be included in the primary resection. The reconstructive surgeon must consider the aggressive or benign nature of the tumor necessitating the resection, patient comorbidities, and anticipated postoperative adjuvant therapy when planning the soft tissue reconstruction. Selected total parotid defects may be conservatively reconstructed with the methods described previously, particularly among patients with multiple comorbidities who could not likely tolerate the stress of prolonged or complicated surgery. Ideally, use of free tissue transfer with and without skin coverage for total parotid defects with or without skin coverage is performed.

Free Tissue Transfer

Originally described for the repair of hemifacial microsomia, microvascular free flap reconstruction for lateral facial volume deficit has been used since 1975.[21,22] Free tissue transfer can correct large contour defects with freedom of orientation and degree of volume augmentation. Additionally, the free tissue provides healthy soft tissues and blood supply to potentially improve wound healing and reduce radiation-induced complications.[23]

The anterolateral thigh (ALT) and radial forearm (RF) flaps are specifically discussed, because these are the authors' preferred options for total parotid reconstruction. Although contour restoration has been described with free muscle flaps (eg, rectus abdominis, latissimus dorsi, and gracilis), long-term results with these flaps are unreliable due to the significant volume regression that invariably follows denervation.

Anterolateral thigh free flap

Since its original description in 1984, the ALT microvascular free flap has become an integral part of head and neck reconstructive surgery.[24] The ALT free flap represents a highly reliable and minimally morbid method for reconstruction of facial defects.[25,26] The ALT free flap is a multilayer composite structure composed of variable amounts of skin, adipose tissue, fascia, and potential harvest of the nerve to vastus lateralis (**Fig. 6**). Its blood supply is derived from the lateral circumflex femoral artery and vein.

Minimal donor site morbidity is a distinct advantage of the ALT free flap. Patients are typically able to fully ambulate immediately after the surgery, with the only long-term sequelae a linear inconspicuous scar and some limited peri-incisional anesthesia. Other benefits of the ALT flap include ease of harvest with the possibility of a 2-team approach, long length (8–16 cm) and large caliber (2–2.5 mm) of the vascular pedicle, and access to the nerve to the vastus lateralis, which can be used as a cable graft of facial nerve segmental defects.

The ALT flap can be harvested with varying degrees of thickness. It can be harvested as a thin cutaneous flap or as a full-thickness fat/fascial flap depending on contour needs. When skin coverage is required, often the best color match is obtained with local skin flaps like the cervicofacial advancement flap over a buried de-epithelialized ALT fee flap for contour (**Fig. 7**). In many individuals, the thigh skin is paler than the chronically sundamaged and darkened or reddened facial skin, making it difficult to obtain an identical facial skin color match with the ALT.

Radial forearm free flap

With a large facial skin defect that cannot be corrected with cervicofacial advancement flap, an RF flap provides a good reconstructive option. The RF flap is based off the radial artery and its vena comitans/cephalic vein and offers many advantages. The chronic sun exposure of the forearm matches the color of the facial skin more closely. The flap contours the face adequately, particularly over the superior cheek (**Fig. 8**). The flap can be de-epithelialized and folded over itself

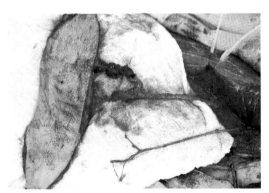

Fig. 6. Harvest of the ALT free flap with simultaneous harvest of the nerve to the vastus lateralis.

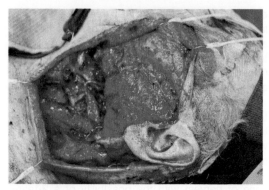

Fig. 7. Buried ALT free flap de-epithelialized for recreation of lateral facial volume and contour.

to fill the concavity of a parotid defect. In the authors' experience, the RF flap is useful for shallow cheek skin defects providing better color match than the ALT flap. For large volume defects, however, the RF flap does not adequately restore facial contour.

RADICAL PAROTIDECTOMY DEFECTS

Radical parotidectomy defects are challenging reconstructions variably involving replacement of skin and/or soft tissue volume and facial reinnervation/reanimation techniques. Up to 20% of malignant parotid tumors require facial nerve sacrifice, leaving patients without crucial facial functions (eg, blink and corneal protection, nasal airflow, and oral competence) in addition to a large soft tissue and skin defect.[27] To address the defect, surgeons must consider patient age, comorbidities, prognosis, goals of treatment, and future adjuvant radiation therapy to create a tailored reconstructive plan. The previous discussion of total parotidectomy reconstruction addresses facial contour/volume reconstruction. Because radical partoidectomy adds facial nerve sacrifice, this section highlights facial reanimation concerns.

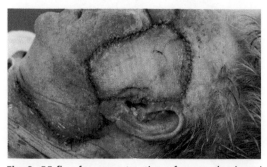

Fig. 8. RF flap for reconstruction of upper cheek and parotidectomy defect. Color match and contour are closely approximated by the RF flap.

Cable Grafting

After a segment of the facial nerve is sacrificed for tumor clearance, segmental interpositional nerve grafting can provide restoration of long-term tone and function.[28] Cable nerve grafting has a long history of success in rehabilitating patients after radical parotidectomy since its original description in 1955.[29] Nevertheless, many controversies regarding facial nerve grafting after radical parotidectomy persist. Areas of controversy include the optimal source for cable nerve grafts, and the effect patient age and postoperative radiation therapy may have on functional outcomes.

Common options for donor cable grafts include the greater auricular nerve or other cervical sensory nerves, sural nerve, and nerve to vastus lateralis if an ALT flap is performed for soft tissue reconstruction. Several investigators support cable nerve grafting using locally available sensory nerves from the cervical plexus. Reddy and colleagues[30] demonstrated 75% success in obtaining House-Brackmann grade 3 facial nerve function (symmetry and tone at rest with obvious dysfunction with motion) at 2 years using cervical plexus sensory nerves as cable grafts. Benefits of using cervical sensory nerves include ease of harvest, appropriate diameter, and extensive arborization of the distal branches allowing for a single graft to be anastomosed to 4 distal facial nerve branches.

The sural nerve is a well-established option for cable grafting facial nerve defects. The sural nerve is sufficiently long, is easily harvested with minimal morbidity, and consists of multiple fascicles with interfascicular bridges that can be anastomosed to up to 3 distal facial nerve branches. Lee and colleagues[31] demonstrated average facial nerve function of House-Brackmann grade 3 or moderate dysfunction after 21 months after sural nerve cable grafting.

Although sensory nerves have been long established for facial nerve reinnervation, recent animal models have suggested there may be improved speed and quality of neural regeneration when using motor nerves for cable grafting after motor nerve resection.[32] Studies suggest that motor nerves have architectural differences, including larger diameter endoneural tubes, allowing a greater number of nerve fibers to cross a nerve defect. In the past, finding an optimal donor nerve for cable grafting has been a major limitation. With increased use of the ALT free flap, however, the nerve to vastus lateralis has been shown a successful option for cable grafting when reconstructing parotid defects. At the time of ALT pedicle dissection, the motor nerve to the vastus lateralis is easily identified and harvested. This nerve is redundant, therefore posing minimal morbidity to the vastus lateralis; provides multiple branches for neural coaptation to multiple distal branches; and bears length equivalent to the sural nerve (**Fig. 9**).[33]

Patient age and the need for postoperative radiation are often considered in the algorithm for facial reanimation following radical parotidectomy. However, Lee and colleagues[31] found facial nerve scores were not affected by patient age or postoperative radiation therapy. Similarly, Reddy and colleagues[30] found no change in functional outcome after cervical sensory nerve cable grafting for facial nerve reinnervation in patients receiving postoperative radiotherapy. However, this study did find a significantly better outcome in patients under the age of 60. Given these findings, our protocol is to perform facial nerve cable grafting for reinervation in all patients when feasible, without regard to age and anticipated postoperative radiation. However, we perform a thorough discussion of anticipated results, as outlined by the previous studies, along with discussion of potential recovery limitations in the setting of advanced age and radiation therapy. In situations of limited recovery or anticipated limited recovery, static suspension or orthodromic temporalis tendon transfer (discussed later) of the midface is performed as a primary or secondary procedure.

Nerve to Masseter

If the proximal facial nerve is unavailable for grafting but distal branches are available, grafting the motor nerve to the masseter muscle to distal facial nerve branches can be a successful option with limited donor site morbidity. The masseteric nerve is the largest motor branch of the trigeminal nerve, with an average diameter of 2 mm. It has a dense population of myelinated fibers, which correspond favorably to the axon counts in the native facial nerve branches. The subzygomatic triangle, defined as the triangle formed by the temporomandibular joint, the zygomatic arch, and the frontal branch of the facial nerve, is a reliable anatomic landmark for rapid, reliable, and minimally invasive identification of the masseteric nerve (**Fig. 10**).[34] Additional benefits of masseter-to-facial nerve transfer are the limited donor site morbidity, synergy with the facial nerve, and potential for effective cerebral adaptation yielding an effortless smile.[35]

It also offers more rapid reinnervation than other cranial nerves commonly used for reinnervation, and with a single coaptation site, it is associated with greater axonal through-growth than other options using 2 coaptation sites. Synergy of the nerve to masseter with the facial nerve allows for an unconscious smile, providing sharp contrast to other motor nerve anastomosis, such as hypoglossal nerve transfers that require pressing the tongue against the teeth or palate to produce a smile.

Static Midface Suspension and Temporalis Tendon Transfer

Although nerve grafting provides the best chance for long-term recovery of facial tone and function, the chance for functional recovery is often unpredictable and the effects are often not noticeable for up to 12 months. Therefore, among patients undergoing radical parotidectomy, reinnervation procedures can be performed in combination with dynamic or static reanimation procedures to provide immediate reconstructive needs for both form and function.

Typically, periorbital procedures addressing lagophthalmos, ectropion, and brow ptosis are required for most patients but are not discussed herein. Midfacial ptosis varies, however, according to degree of facial laxity. Elderly patients with significant facial laxity typically develop significant and debilitating facial ptosis benefiting from combined reinnervation and dynamic or static reanimation efforts. On the other hand, younger

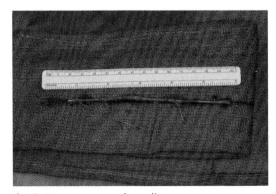

Fig. 9. Nerve to vastus lateralis.

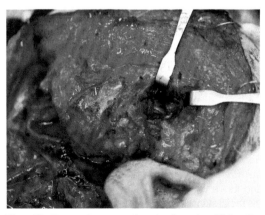

Fig. 10. Nerve to masseter is found within the masseter within the subzygomatic triangle.

patients undergoing radical parotidectomy with limited facial laxity may not develop significant facial ptosis and may be best approached conservatively with static procedures or regional muscle transfer pending the results of nerve reinnervation.

The temporalis tendon transfer provides immediate dynamic reanimation in patients after radical parotidectomy. It provides the potential for both facial symmetry at rest and voluntary facial movement.[36,37] In the setting of parotidectomy, the temporalis muscle insertion on the coronoid process is easily accessible through a transfacial approach and the tendon transfer can be performed without compromising any performed nerve grafting procedures.[38] Although temporalis tendon transfers are not unequivocally successful in restoring movement, they are associated with effective static suspension, providing resting symmetry at a minimum.

Immediate static reanimation via a static sling gives adequate suspension of the alar base and nasolabial fold and provides an adequate alternative to the immediate temporalis tendon transfer when the temporalis tendon transfer cannot be performed or is not ideal. The ability to immediately establish midfacial symmetry improves immediate postoperative appearance, oral competence, and nasal competence.

When dynamic muscle transfers are unavailable because of tumor involvement, static slings may be performed using tensor fascia lata, in conjunction with ALT free flap. The tensor fascia lata has become the authors' preference because of its strength and ease of availability. The fascia lata is directly sutured to the temporalis fascia and attached to the oral commissure, nasolabial fold, and nasal ala.

Free Tissue Transfer for Facial Nerve Reanimation

Although free muscle transfer is embraced as an excellent reanimation technique for facial paralysis, this method is not typically considered as a component of primary reconstruction for radical parotidectomy. The gracilis free flap is commonly used for facial reanimation of the smile. This may be considered an adjunctive procedure after a patient has undergone therapy and has maintained a disease-free state.

SUMMARY

Reconstruction of the parotidectomy defect requires a thorough analysis of the anticipated defect and its varying components. Defects may involve the facial skin, soft tissue volume, or the facial nerve. Although numerous controversies and methods of surgical reconstruction exist in the literature, a reconstructive technique tailored to the patient and specific to the defect can provide optimized results.

REFERENCES

1. Frey L. Le syndrome du nerf auriculo-temporal. Rev Neurol 1923;2:97–104.
2. Ghanem T. Parotid defects. Facial Plast Surg Clin North Am 2009;17(2):263–9.
3. Govindaraj S, Cohen M, Genden EM, et al. The use of acellular dermis in the prevention of Frey's syndrome. Laryngoscope 2001;111(11 Pt 1):1993–8.
4. Vico PG, Delange A, De Vooght A. Autologous fat transfer: an aesthetic and functional refinement for parotidectomy. Surg Res Pract 2014;2014:873453.
5. Conger BT, Gourin CG. Free abdominal fat transfer for reconstruction of the total parotidectomy defect. Laryngoscope 2008;118(7):1186–90.
6. Harada T, Inoue T, Harashina T, et al. Dermis-fat graft after parotidectomy to prevent Frey's syndrome and the concave deformity. Ann Plast Surg 1993; 31(5):450–2.
7. Fasolis M, Zavattero E, Iaquinta C, et al. Dermofat graft after superficial parotidectomy to prevent Frey syndrome and depressed deformity. J Craniofac Surg 2013;24(4):1260–2.
8. Nosan DK, Ochi JW, Davidson TM. Preservation of facial contour during parotidectomy. Otolaryngol Head Neck Surg 1991;104(3):293–8.
9. Curry JM, Fisher KW, Heffelfinger RN, et al. Superficial musculoaponeurotic system elevation and fat graft reconstruction after superficial parotidectomy. Laryngoscope 2008;118(2):210–5.
10. Szczerkowska-Dobosz A, Olszewska B, Lemanska M, et al. Acquired facial lipoatrophy: pathogenesis and therapeutic options. Postepy Dermatol Alergol 2015; 32(2):127–33.
11. Pignatti M, Pedone A, Baccarani A, et al. High-density hyaluronic acid for the treatment of HIV-related facial lipoatrophy. Aesthetic Plast Surg 2012;36(1): 180–5.
12. Sinha UK, Saadat D, Doherty CM, et al. Use of AlloDerm implant to prevent frey syndrome after parotidectomy. Arch Facial Plast Surg 2003;5(1):109–12.
13. Zeng XT, Tang XJ, Wang XJ, et al. AlloDerm implants for prevention of Frey syndrome after parotidectomy: a systematic review and meta-analysis. Mol Med Rep 2012;5(4):974–80.
14. Jost G, Legent F, Baupelot S. Filling of residual depressions after parotidectomy by a sterno-cleido-mastoid strip. Ann Otolaryngol Chir Cervicofac 1968;85(4): 357–60 [in French].
15. Kornblut AD, Westphal P, Miehlke A. The effectiveness of a sternomastoid muscle flap in preventing postparotidectomy occurrence of the Frey syndrome. Acta Otolaryngol 1974;77(5):368–73.

16. Casler JD, Conley J. Sternocleidomastoid muscle transfer and superficial musculoaponeurotic system plication in the prevention of Frey's syndrome. Laryngoscope 1991;101(1 Pt 1):95–100.

17. Kerawala CJ, McAloney N, Stassen LF. Prospective randomised trial of the benefits of a sternocleidomastoid flap after superficial parotidectomy. Br J Oral Maxillofac Surg 2002;40(6):468–72.

18. Ahmed OA, Kolhe PS. Prevention of Frey's syndrome and volume deficit after parotidectomy using the superficial temporal artery fascial flap. Br J Plast Surg 1999;52(4):256–60.

19. Dell'aversana Orabona G, Salzano G, Petrocelli M, et al. Reconstructive techniques of the parotid region. J Craniofac Surg 2014;25(3):998–1002.

20. Allison GR, Rappaport I. Prevention of Frey's syndrome with superficial musculoaponeurotic system interposition. Am J Surg 1993;166(4):407–10.

21. Wells JH, Edgerton MT. Correction of severe hemifacial atrophy with a free dermis-flat from the lower abdomen. Plast Reconstr Surg 1977;59(2):223–30.

22. Baker DC, Shaw WW, Conley J. Reconstruction of radical parotidectomy defects. Am J Surg 1979; 138(4):550–4.

23. Cannady SB, Seth R, Fritz MA, et al. Total parotidectomy defect reconstruction using the buried free flap. Otolaryngol Head Neck Surg 2010;143(5):637–43.

24. Song YG, Chen GZ, Song YL. The free thigh flap: a new free flap concept based on the septocutaneous artery. Br J Plast Surg 1984;37(2):149–59.

25. Knott PD, Seth R, Waters HH, et al. Short-term donor site morbidity: A comparison of the anterolateral thigh and radial forearm fasciocutaneous free flaps. Head Neck 2015. [Epub ahead of print].

26. Collins J, Ayeni O, Thoma A. A systematic review of anterolateral thigh flap donor site morbidity. Can J Plast Surg 2012;20(1):17–23.

27. Theriault C, Fitzpatrick PJ. Malignant parotid tumors. Prognostic factors and optimum treatment. Am J Clin Oncol 1986;9(6):510–6.

28. Malik TH, Kelly G, Ahmed A, et al. A comparison of surgical techniques used in dynamic reanimation of the paralyzed face. Otol Neurotol 2005;26(2):284–91.

29. Conley JJ. Facial nerve grafting in treatment of parotid gland tumors; new technique. AMA Arch Surg 1955;70(3):359–66.

30. Reddy PG, Arden RL, Mathog RH. Facial nerve rehabilitation after radical parotidectomy. Laryngoscope 1999;109(6):894–9.

31. Lee MC, Kim DH, Jeon YR, et al. Functional outcomes of multiple sural nerve grafts for facial nerve defects after tumor-ablative surgery. Arch Plast Surg 2015;42(4):461–8.

32. Moradzadeh A, Borschel GH, Luciano JP, et al. The impact of motor and sensory nerve architecture on nerve regeneration. Exp Neurol 2008;212(2):370–6.

33. Revenaugh PC, Knott D, McBride JM, et al. Motor nerve to the vastus lateralis. Arch Facial Plast Surg 2012;14(5):365–8.

34. Collar RM, Byrne PJ, Boahene KD. The subzygomatic triangle: rapid, minimally invasive identification of the masseteric nerve for facial reanimation. Plast Reconstr Surg 2013;132(1):183–8.

35. Klebuc M. The evolving role of the masseter-to-facial (V-VII) nerve transfer for rehabilitation of the paralyzed face. Ann Chir Plast Esthet 2015;60(5):436–41.

36. Boahene KD. Dynamic muscle transfer in facial reanimation. Facial Plast Surg 2008;24(2):204–10.

37. Fritz M, Rolfes BN. Management of Facial Paralysis due to Extracranial Tumors. Facial Plast Surg 2015; 31(2):110–6.

38. Revenaugh PC, Knott PD, Scharpf J, et al. Simultaneous anterolateral thigh flap and temporalis tendon transfer to optimize facial form and function after radical parotidectomy. Arch Facial Plast Surg 2012; 14(2):104–9.

Septorhinoplasty in the Pediatric Patient

Aditi Bhuskute, MD, Mika Sumiyoshi, MD, Craig Senders, MD*

KEYWORDS

- Pediatric rhinoplasty • Pediatric septoplasty • Nasal surgery • Cleft nose deformity • Cleft lip

KEY POINTS

- The nasal septal cartilage is central to the growth of the midface.
- Animal studies have demonstrated the importance of conservation of periosteum; perichondrium likely does not inhibit growth. Aggressive resection of the perichondrium and periosteum seems to prevent normal growth.
- The quality of clinical studies are far from ideal, but have demonstrated conservative surgery is likely safe.
- Major growth phase of the nose occurs during puberty.
- When possible, delaying surgery until after puberty is optimal; if there are significant functional or social issues conservative surgery before puberty is likely safe.

INTRODUCTION: NATURE OF THE PROBLEM

Nasal surgery in children has been an ongoing topic of discussion in pediatric otolaryngology and facial plastic surgery. Central to this discussion is the effect of surgical manipulation of the nasal structures and the effects of this intervention on the growth and maturation of the nose. Several animal, clinical, and observational studies have attempted to elucidate the effect of intervention on the growing nose throughout the years. These interventions include resection and devascularization to the nasal septum and the growth centers of the nose. Despite the growing body of literature, the topic of pediatric septorhinoplasty and its indications remain an area of continued controversy.

CONTROVERSIES

Pediatric septorhinoplasty continues as an area of controversy. Animal and clinical studies have demonstrated the importance of conservative manipulation on the growing nose. The timing and extent of surgery has been debated. There are certain indications for rhinoplasty where the benefit outweighs the risk of operating on the growing nose.

ANATOMY AND GROWTH

The development and characteristics of the pediatric nose is essential in understanding the effects of septorhinoplasty on its growth. Around the fourth week of gestation, neural crest cells migrate caudally creating nasal placodes. The placodes are then divided into medial and lateral nasal processes. The medial process becomes the anterior septum, philtrum, and premaxilla. The lateral processes form the lateral nasal walls. The differentiation of the muscle, cartilage, and bony elements of the nose occur at 10 weeks gestation.[1]

The septodorsal cartilages are the main supporting structure for the nasal dorsum and consist of the upper lateral cartilages and the nasal septum. The nasal septum in young children extends from the skull base to the nasal floor. Superiorly, the septum is based at the sphenoid at birth. As the perpendicular plate grows and ossifies, the septum in turn is based on the caudal edge of the perpendicular plate by adulthood.[2]

Department of Otolaryngology, University of California, Davis, 2521 Stockton Boulevard, Suite 7200, Sacramento, CA 95817, USA
* Corresponding author. 2521 Stockton Boulevard, Suite 7200, Sacramento, CA 95817.
E-mail address: cwsenders@ucdavis.edu

Facial Plast Surg Clin N Am 24 (2016) 245–253
http://dx.doi.org/10.1016/j.fsc.2016.03.003
1064-7406/16/$ – see front matter © 2016 Elsevier Inc. All rights reserved.

The nasal bones in the neonate are fibrous and connected to the upper lateral cartilages. Interestingly, the upper lateral cartilages extend under nasal bones and attach to the anterior cranial base. As the child grows, the upper lateral cartilages migrate anteriorly from the skull base and are replaced by the ossifying cribriform plate. The degree of migration is not consistent from individual to individual, explaining the varying relationship between the nasal bones and upper lateral cartilages seen in adult rhinoplasty.[2]

Growth of the nasal septum is at its maximum in the newborn and plateaus by the age of 20. In an anatomic study performed by van Loosen and colleagues,[3] the cartilaginous septum shows the greatest velocity growth at the age of 2. Later growth of the nasal septum is owing to ongoing ossification of the septal cartilage at the sphenoethmoid region with concurrent growth and formation of new cartilage.[3]

The nasal septal cartilage seems to be central in the growth of the midface. There are 2 growth zones of the nasal septum. These include the sphenodorsal zone, which extends from the sphenoid septum to the nasal dorsum, and the sphenospinal zone, which extends from the sphenoid to the anterior nasal spine. These 2 areas are thicker owing to mitotic activity and histologic maturation. Growth of the sphenodorsal zone seems to be responsible primarily for the increase in length and height of the nasal dorsum. Growth in the sphenospinal region of the septum drives growth of the premaxilla.[2] Injuries to these pivotal growth centers demonstrate detrimental effects to the maxilla and nasal dorsum.

The maximum growth velocity of the nose in girls seems to vary from 8 to 12 years of age, whereas in boys it is around 13 years of age.[4] The defined completion of nasal growth is a continued controversy. A study by Meng and associates[5] in 1988 demonstrated near completion of growth in girls by the age of 16 and continuing to age 18 in males. However, there have been several other studies that draw varying conclusions on nasal growth, extending it to the age of 20 in females and 25 in males, and even some statistically insignificant growth of the nose in advanced age.[2] Given the debate about when nasal growth is complete, growth after the mid teenage years is not likely clinically significant.

ANIMAL STUDIES

Animal models have been the basis in the understanding of nasal growth and the effects of trauma and surgery. Several models have been developed throughout the years to investigate the effect of septal resection on the growth of the nose and midface in several species of animals. These began as early as the 1850s, where Fick and his colleagues stated that growth of the hard palate was dependent on the nasal septum after investigation in growing dogs, cats, pigs, and goats.[2]

Sarnat and Wexler[6] in the 1960s used aggressive resection of the caudal cartilaginous septum and overlying mucoperichondrium in growing rabbits. This resection resulted in underdevelopment of the snout, saddle deformity, and mandibular prognathism. This type of radical resection of the septum in adult rabbits did not produce the same deformity. Similar studies have been performed in canine pups, baboons, and ferrets demonstrating detrimental effects on midface growth.[7,8]

Although this rather radical approach to septal resection in these studies does not simulate directly the conservative approach taken on pediatric septorhinoplasty, it does give an indication that extensive resection of the mucoperiosteum and cartilage can have detrimental effects on skeletal growth.

Bernstein[7] also performed septal resection preserving the mucoperichondrium. In canines with preserved perichondrium, no change in growth was noted, highlighting the importance of appropriate submucous resection and preservation of mucoperichondrial flaps.[6] In juvenile ferrets, Cupero and colleagues[8] demonstrated no difference in cephalometric analysis when selective submucoperichondrial removal of a small piece of cartilage and vomer was removed. However, these studies are limited by small numbers of study subjects. These animal models again demonstrate the importance of mucoperiosteal preservation in the growing nose.

Instead of resection, the question then arose to removal and replacement of the septal cartilage with cartilage autografts in prevention of growth restriction. In a study by Nolst Trenité and colleagues,[9] septal reimplantation after cutting to the appropriate size was observed. This technique demonstrated growth of the cartilage but did not prevent shortening of the nose or saddling deformity. One benefit demonstrated was prevention of septal perforations. Crushed cartilage did not demonstrate prevention of subsequent deformities with time because it lacks the mechanical strength that intact cartilage has. Reimplanted cartilage has not been found useful in septorhinoplasty in pediatric animal models.[10]

These animal studies demonstrate the essential role of the septum its growth zones in the development of the nose and midface. The evidence from these animal models show that preservation of the mucoperichondrium as well as limited resection and manipulation of the cartilages can affect nasal growth and now play an important role in our conservative approach to pediatric rhinoplasty. Interestingly, these studies are in conflict with clinically observed data in human populations, which will be covered in later sections of this article.

CLINICAL STUDIES

Clinical evidence of the effects of intervention to the nose at a young age is varied. Investigation of these effects on the growth of the nose are difficult owing to the long-term follow-up needed, small sample size, and difficulty of randomized controlled trials. Given this paucity of clinical information, the traditional dogma has been to err on the side of conservative management, given observations of detrimental effects to growth of the midface in animal studies. Several observational studies regarding effects of trauma, nasal abscess, and loss of cartilage to the nasal septum and cartilaginous structures of the nose have been reported.

Detrimental Effects on Growth of the Nose

Grymer and Bosch[11] followed a set of identical twins for a period of 10 years and outlined their facial growth. One had septal destruction after a septal abscess at the age of 7 years. The abscess was drained and homologous septal cartilage from a tissue bank was reimplanted. The patient developed a saddle nose, upward displacement of the anterior maxilla, and diminished vertical development of the nasal cavity as well as retrognathia owing to maxillary retrusion in comparison with his twin without septal destruction.[11] This longitudinal study mimics animal studies with through and through septal resection as well as with Nolst's study on resection and reimplanatation of the septal cartilage and its effects on the midface. In this observation by Grymer and Bosch,[11] as well as in animal studies, it is difficult to ascertain if the growth restriction in the face is owing to effects of the original trauma or the intervention performed.

The insights given by the animal studies as well as observational studies from children with prior trauma or destruction of the nasal septum, a basic guideline for preservation of the mucoperichondrium and conservative cartilage resection was created. This gives clinicians a basis for performing this procedure on children when the clinical indication was present.

Anthropometric Studies

Triglia and colleagues[12] advocated for an external approach in the 1990s, stating preservation of the perichondrium and septum with repositioning showed no change in growth of the nose or need for revision in 24 subjects aged 5 to 14 years. All of his patients had a posttraumatic nasal deformity. His findings were further justified in several anthropometric studies, which are described below.

Crysdale and his partners in Toronto have performed several studies regarding growth of the nose after surgical intervention with anthropometric evaluation. El Hakim and colleagues[13] noted that external septorhinoplasty with use of quadrangular cartilage removal, remodeling, and reimplantation with conservation of the mucoperichondrium in 24 patients ranging from 4.5 to 15.5 years of age, there were no affect to most aspects of nasal and facial growth that were noted on anthropometric measurements with a follow-up of 3.1 years. In a similar study by Bejar and coauthors, 28 patients who underwent external septoplasty ranging from 6 to 15 years of age showed no change in anthropometric measurements from these patients and controls. They did demonstrate a trend toward restricted growth of the nasal dorsum with a follow-up of 3.4 years.[14] Walker and associates[15] also found similar results in a study of 16 children who underwent external rhinoplasty with a 2-year follow-up. This work by Crysdale and his colleagues provides us insight and quantitative evaluation of effects of nasal surgery on children. However, all of these studies are limited by their short follow-up and wide age range.

In a retrospective study in 44 Italian patients by Tasca and Compadretti,[16] an endonasal approach to septoplasty was used. With a mean follow-up of 12.2 years, the investigators found no changes in nasal dorsal length as compared with other North American white subjects. They did, however, find a significant difference in reduction of nasolabial angle in patients who underwent external septoplasty versus endonasal surgery. They, therefore, advocate for endonasal septoplasty to prevent any changes to nasal growth.[16]

These clinical studies describing external and endoscopic septoplasty on the growing nose give us insight into the effects of surgical manipulation of the nasal septum. There are, however, confounding factors in each of these reports. The mean follow-up for each of these observations were 3 years with ages ranging from 5 to 15 years of age. Further investigation of the effects of surgical manipulation of the nose before and after puberty would give insight into the detrimental effects of surgery to the growth zones. In addition, 3-year follow-up for a prepubertal nose would not follow the child until the growth of the nose has been completed.

INDICATIONS AND TIMING FOR PEDIATRIC RHINOPLASTY

The role of the growing nasal septum in midface development noted in clinical observations has led to the delay in surgical intervention. Identification of the differences between the pediatric and adult nose as well as the patterns and zones of growth are invaluable to the pediatric surgeon. The neonatal nose differs from the adult nose in several ways. This includes projection of the nose with a shorter dorsum and columella. The nares are generally rounder and there is a larger nasolabial angle. With growth, the nose as well as the entire face increases in projection and length.[9]

Most authors recommend delay in surgical intervention to the growing nose owing to potential effects to the normal growth. There are, however, several absolute and relative indications to pediatric septorhinoplasty. These include severe nasal trauma, cleft lip nasal deformity, and reconstruction after removal of a nasal lesion such as dermoid or hemangioma. Functional septorhinoplasty has been cited as a relative indication.[9,13,14,17]

Trauma

Obligate mouth breathing has been described historically as a possible cause for facial and dental anomalies including malocclusion and the classic "adenoid facies." Nasal obstruction owing to septal deviation and nasal trauma is also associated with mouth breathing in the pediatric population.

In a multicenter study by D'Ascanio and colleagues,[17] they reported dental anomalies using cephalometric analysis compared with age-matched controls in patients with mouth breathing from nasal trauma and septal deviation. Malocclusion after growth was also noted in neonates with injuries to the nose after 12 years of follow-up by Pentz and colleagues.[18]

Given the data seen in these studies, there is evidence for correction of severe nasal obstruction owing to nasal trauma to prevent abnormalities in facial growth.

Cleft Lip Deformity

Primary rhinoplasty at the time of cleft lip repair is now a common practice among surgeons who repair cleft abnormalities. Primary cleft rhinoplasty has been in practice since the 1970s. Proponents for rhinoplasty at the time of cleft lip repair believe this early restoration of function and symmetry to the noncleft side can minimize cleft nasal deformity as the child grows.[19] Early techniques often led to scarring, stenosis, and unacceptable

results; however, recently developed techniques have shown a vast improvement of nasal outcomes with growth. This improved symmetry has been noted to be maintained into adulthood and also reduced the number of revisions and changes needed during definitive rhinoplasty after maturity is reached.[20–22]

Primary cleft rhinoplasty can be divided into deformities related to unilateral cleft lip nasal deformity and bilateral cleft lip nasal deformity. Differences in the unilateral cleft lip nasal deformity from the normal pediatric nose include a shorter columella on the cleft side, with movement of the columella to the noncleft side. In addition, the alar base is displaced laterally, posteriorly, and inferiorly on the cleft side. With respect to nasal anatomy, the alar dome is flat and laterally displaced with a caudally displaced lateral crus of the lower lateral cartilage, resulting in a hooding deformity. In the bilateral cleft lip nasal deformity, the columella is short, with a wide base bilaterally. The alar domes are poorly defined and separated, often producing an amorphous tip.[23–25] Goals of primary cleft rhinoplasty include repositioning of the lower lateral cartilages, creation of symmetry at the alar base, and closure of the nasal floor.

In the unilateral cleft lip nasal deformity, the cleft side medial and lateral crura are released from the overlying soft tissue envelope. The medial crura is lengthened and the lateral crura is shortened by repositioning. This correction is then suspended with sutures and nasal conformers[22] (**Fig. 1**). In the bilateral cleft lip nasal deformity, the lower lateral cartilages are again freed from the skin envelope. However, the alar domes are sutured together to narrow the alar base, and the dorsal nasal skin is repositioned caudally for tip projection. In addition, many surgeons have used nasal conformers to aid in reshaping the lower lateral cartilages over the last 15 years. Surgery on the nasal bones or nasal septum is not performed during primary rhinoplasty, but during definitive rhinoplasty after skeletal maturity.[19–23]

Congenital Nasal Defects

Midline congenital lesions of the nose including nasal encephaloceles, gliomas, and dermoid cysts are congenital malformations of the ectopic neuroectoderm. The failure of the fonticulus frontalis fusion or foramen cecum to obliterate can cause these lesions to have extensions into the skull base and the frontal brain. Proliferation of the entrapped epithelium produces a dermoid, which is an epithelial-lined sac. A glioma occurs when brain tissue is isolated extracranially. If there is

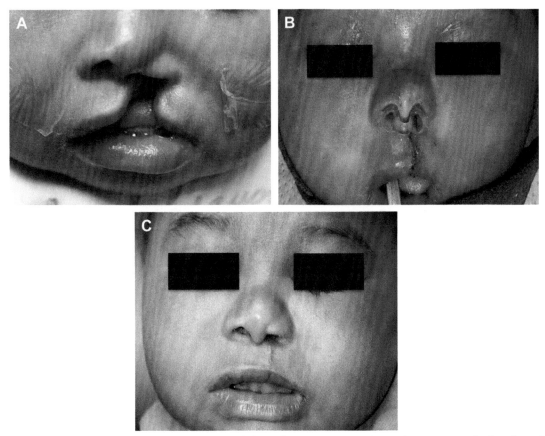

Fig. 1. (*A*) A 6-month-old girl with unilateral cleft lip deformity, preoperative evaluation. Note the hooding of the ala on the clef side as well as the deviation of the nasal tip to the noncleft side. (*B*) A 6-month-old girl with unilateral cleft lip deformity immediately postoperatively. Note the corrected symmetry of the nasal ala and movement of the tip to midline. Nasal conformers have been placed to keep the symmetry between the nostrils and mold the lower lateral cartilages while they heal. (*C*) Four months postoperative result of primary rhinoplasty performed at the time of the unilateral cleft lip repair.

herniation of dura and brain tissue, this results in an encephalocele.

These midline malformations can occur in at the nasal dorsum, nasal tip and columella. Preoperative radiographic imaging, includes a computed tomography scan and an MRI if intracranial extension is suspected on computed tomography imaging.

Many authors have advocated early excision, as early as 6 months of age, to decrease the risk of local infection and intracranial complication.[26] Nasal lesions can be approached through an open rhinoplasty approach or a direct excision with a vertical excision in limited, smaller lesions. A combination of these 2 approaches is may also be appropriate in many cases because it provides optimum exposure. After incisions are made, the nasal skin/soft tissue envelope is elevated from the lesion. The tract of the lesion is chased to its origin, generally diving between the upper lateral cartilages and nasal bones and originating at the top of the quadrangular cartilage. The lesions is removed en bloc; complete excision is important to avoid recurrence. Lesions with an intracranial component require a combined approach with an external and intracranial approach for complete excision and are best performed by a pediatric craniofacial team.

The nasal lesions can create a defect in both the subcutaneous soft tissue as well as a deficiency in the skin. Our approach has been to perform local tissue advancement to fill the subcutaneous and skin defect and to perform a definitive rhinoplasty at full growth (**Fig. 2**).

Hemangioma

The majority of hemangiomas arise in the head and neck; 15% of these involve the nose and 5% occur at the nasal tip.[27] Often, during the proliferative phase of the hemangioma, it can expand and

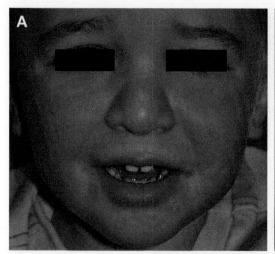
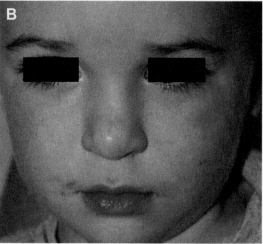

Fig. 2. (*A*) Preoperative photo of a 2 year-old-male with nasal dermoid. Note the fullness in the vault of the nasal dorsum. (*B*) Postoperative examination 6 weeks after excision of nasal dermoid. Nasal dermoid was removed through an elliptical incision, which included the draining pit and closed primarily with rotation of subcutaneous underlying soft tissue to fill defect.

cause outward distraction of the nasal cartilages causing a bulbous tip, often described as "Cyrano" or "Pinocchio" nose. These changes can also cause nasal obstruction.

In the past, options for treatment have included corticosteroids, interferon, and laser or surgical excision. Oral propranolol has changed dramatically the treatment of hemangiomas since its therapeutic benefit was first described in 2008 and this is currently the first-line treatment. Most reports describe a very high response rate to propranolol, although some authors have found that hemangiomas of the nasal region respond slightly less than other facial hemangiomas.[28] Surgical therapy remains an option for those who are nonresponders to beta-blockers or those with significant redundancy of skin and residual fibrofatty tissue after propranolol treatment.

We offer early surgical resection when it becomes clear that will be significant deformity after involution. The incisions follow the nasal subunits and the incisions are made between the nasal tip and the ala. The lesion is excised using bipolar cautery and sharp dissection between the hemangioma and the skin. Excess skin, if present is excised and draped back over the nasal cartilage framework (**Fig. 3**).

Functional Septorhinoplasty

The optimal timing for a functional septorhinoplasty in children is controversial. Traditionally, a more conservative approach waiting until age 16 to 18 years has been used by most surgeons to avoid the potential impact on nasal and midface growth. Arguments against delaying surgery exist, including functional and developmental consequences for the child.

In children, a balance between improving the form and function of the nose and promoting the continued development nose and face must be sought. There are 2 distinct postnatal growth spurts, one at age 2 to 5 years and again during puberty. Completion of facial growth occurs at 16 to 18 in girls and 18 to 20 in boys. If surgery is performed between or before the growth spurts, the iatrogenic growth restriction and distortion can be concealed until after the final growth spurt.

The consequence of conservative management in patients with nasal obstruction have been studied. In a cephalometric study comparing 98 children, D'Ascanio and colleagues[17] reported that obligate mouth-breathing children owing to nasal septal deviations have facial and dental anomalies compared with nose-breathing controls. It was found that the mouth-breathing children had increased upper and lower anterior facial height, greater gonial angle, and retrognathic position of the maxilla and mandible compared with the controls. The mouth-breathers also were more likely to have class II malocclusion than their nose-breathing counterparts, who demonstrated normal occlusion.

Several clinical situations exist where early surgical intervention is favored or necessary owing to functional or social indications. No consensus guidelines exist for indications for pediatric septorhinoplasty. In our practice, we have performed nasal surgeries in the following cases

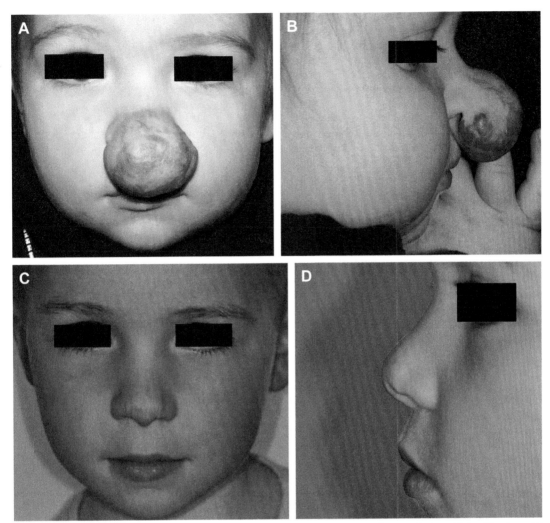

Fig. 3. (*A*) Preoperative photo of 2-year-old boy with nasal tip hemangioma after involution. (*B*) Profile view of 2-year-old boy with nasal tip hemangioma. (*C*) Postoperative examination 4 years after excision of nasal tip hemangioma. Excess skin and fibrofatty subcutaneous tissue was excised with incisions between nasal subunits, nasal tip and ala. (*D*) Postoperative profile view 4 years after excision of nasal tip hemangioma.

before the full growth of the nose: septal abscess, malignancies, benign tumors, deformities like cleft lip nasal deformity, congenital midline nasal lesions, severe nasal obstruction resulting in sleep apnea, chronic mouth breathing, and malocclusion.

As in other surgical procedures, informed consent is paramount in pediatric septorhinoplasty. Consent includes all of the components of an adult septorhinoplasty with a discussion of the expected benefits of early surgical correction and weighing the risk of restriction in nasal growth, unpredictable postoperative deformation as well as the possibility of the need for revision surgery in the future.

We utilize both a closed and open approach for septorhinoplasty. Clinical judgement regarding the need for an open approach should be evaluated on case-by-case basis, recognizing that an open approach may change the nasolabial angle.

Careful elevation and preservation of the mucoperichondrial flap should be attempted. If possible, unilateral elevation is preferred to provide stability to the remaining the septum. However, bilateral elevation has not been shown to interfere with normal growth.[6] As described in the previous section, there are 2 growth centers in the nasal septum, the sphenodorsal zone and sphenospinal zone.[2] Disruption of these zones can cause underdevelopment in the vertical height and sagittal projection of the nose. Most authors agree that younger children are more susceptible to growth restriction with disruption of these growth zones than older, adolescent children. Keeping this in mind, a conservative septoplasty preserving these regions is important. Most authors have also advocated straightening portions of cartilages that have been trimmed and reinserting with or without use of an absorbable plate or mesh.[29]

The T-bar is formed by the septal and upper lateral cartilage and disruption of the T-bar structure of the dorsoseptal cartilage should be avoided. Hump resection and spreader grafts can disrupt the T-bar structure and cause irregularities of the dorsum, and thus should be avoided until near complete facial growth. If a bony pyramid deformity exists, limited osteotomies may mobilize displaced nasal bones and align the nasal dorsum without causing growth disturbances.[30]

SUMMARY

The evaluation and treatment of pediatric nose differs that from adults. Pediatric septorhinoplasty remains as an area of controversy. Understanding the risk of early intervention and applying a conservative approach to the pediatric septorhinoplasty is important when treating the pediatric nose. Pediatric septorhinoplasty should focus on restoring the natural anatomy and function and promoting normal development of the nose. A thorough informed consent should be discussed with both patient and parent and the possibility of a late secondary surgery should be discussed. There is a need for long-term follow-up and evaluation of prepubertal and pubertal pediatric rhinoplasty and its effect on nasal and facial growth.

REFERENCES

1. Hengerer AS, Oas RE. Congenital anomalies of the nose: their embryology, diagnosis, and management (SIPAC). Alexandria (VA): American Academy of Otolaryngology; 1987.
2. Verwoerd CD, Verwoerd-Verhoef HL. Rhinosurgery in children: developmental and surgical aspects of the growing nose. GMS Curr Top Otorhinolaryngol Head Neck Surg 2010;9: Doc05.
3. van Loosen J, Van Zanten GA, Howard CV, et al. Growth characteristics of the human nasal septum. Rhinology 1996;34.78–82.
4. Van der Heijden P, Korsten-meijer AG, Van der Laan BF, et al. Nasal growth and maturation age in adolescents. Arch Otolaryngol Head Neck Surg 2008;134:1288–93.
5. Meng HP, Goorhuis J, Kapila S, et al. Growth changes in the nasal profile from 7 to 18 years of age. Am J Orthod Dentofacial Orthop 1988;94: 317–26.
6. Sarnat BG, Wexler MR. Growth of the face and jaws after resection of the septal cartilage in the rabbit. Am J Anat 1966;118:755–67.
7. Bernstein L. Early submucous resection of nasal septal cartilage. Arch Otolaryngol 1973;97(3): 273–8.
8. Cupero TM, Middleton CE, Silva AB. Effects of functional septoplasty on the facial growth of ferrets. Arch Otolaryngol Head Neck Surg 2001;127: 1403–5.
9. Nolst Trenité GJ, Verwoerd CDA, Verwoerd-Verhoef HL. Reimplantation of autologous septal cartilage in the growing nasal septum. I. Influence of resection and reimplantation upon nasal growth: an experimental study in rabbits. Rhinology 1987; 25:225–36.
10. Verwoerd-Verhoef HL, Meeuwis CA, van der Heul RO, et al. Histologic evaluation of crushed cartilage grafts in the growing nasal septum of young rabbits. ORL J Otorhinolaryngol Relat Spec 1991;53:305–9.
11. Grymer LF, Bosch C. The nasal septum and the development of the midface. A longitudinal study of a pair of monozygotic twins. Rhinology 1997;35:6–10.
12. Triglia JM, Connoni M, Pech A. Septorhinoplasty in children: benefits of the external approach. J Otolaryngol 1990;19:274–8.
13. El-Hakim H, Crysdale WS, Abdollei M, et al. A study of anthropometric measures before and after external septoplasty in children. Arch Otolaryngol Head Neck Surg 2001;127:1362–6.
14. Bejar I, Farkas LG, Messner AH, et al. Nasal growth after external septoplasty in children. Arch Otolaryngol Head Neck Surg 1996;122: 816–21.
15. Walker PJ, Crysdale WS, Farkas LG. External septorhinoplasty in children: outcome and effect on growth of septal excision and reimplantation. Arch Otolaryngol Head Neck Surg 1993;119: 984–9.
16. Tasca I, Compadretti GC. Nasal growth after pediatric septoplasty at long-term follow-up. Am J Rhinol Allergy 2011;25:e7–12.
17. D'Ascanio L, Lancione C, Pompa G, et al. Craniofacial growth in children with nasal septum deviation: a cephalometric comparative study. Int J Pediatr Otorhinolaryngol 2010;74: 1180–3.

18. Pentz S, Pirsig W, Lenders H. Long-term results of neonates with nasal deviation: a prospective study over 12 years. Int J Pediatr Otorhinolaryngol 1994; 28:183–91.
19. Sykes JM. The importance of primary rhinoplasty at the time of initial unilateral cleft lip repair. Arch Facial Plast Surg 2010;12(1):53–5.
20. Millard DR Jr, Morovic CG. Primary unilateral cleft nose correction: a 10 year follow up. Plast Reconstr Surg 1998;102(5):1331–8.
21. McComb HK. Primary repair of the bilateral cleft lip nose: a long-term follow up. Plast Reconstr Surg 2009;124(5):1610–5.
22. Salyer KE. Primary correction of the unilateral cleft lip nose: a 15 year experience. Plast Reconstr Surg 1986;77:558.
23. Lee TS, Schwartz GM, Tatum SA. Rhinoplasty for cleft and hemangioma-related nasal deformities. Curr Opin Otolaryngol Head Neck Surg 2010; 18(6):526–35.
24. Wright RJ, Murakami CS, Ambro BT. Pediatric nasal injuries and management. Facial Plast Surg 2011; 27:483–90.
25. Shandilya M, Herder CD, Dennis SCR, et al. Pediatric Rhinoplasty in an academic setting. Facial Plast Surg 2007;23:245–57.
26. Bloom DC, Carvalho DS, Dory C, et al. Imaging and surgical approach of nasal dermoids. Int J Pediatr Otorhinolaryngol 2002;62:111–22.
27. Ben-Amitai D, Halachmi S, Zvulunov A, et al. Hemangiomas of the nasal tip treated with propranolol. Dermatology 2012;225:371–5.
28. Bagazgoitia L, Torrelo A, Gutierrez JC, et al. Propranolol for infantile hemangiomas. Pediatr Dermatol 2011;28:108–14.
29. Boenisch M, Nolst Trenité GJ. Reconstructive septal surgery. Facial Plast Surg 2006;22(4): 249–54.
30. Lawrence R. Pediatric septoplasty: a review of literature. Int J Pediatr Otorhinolaryngol 2012;76:1078–81.

Controversies in the Management of Patients with Cleft Lip and Palate

 CrossMark

Regina E. Rodman, MD[a], Sherard Tatum, MD[b],*

KEYWORDS

- Cleft lip • Cleft palate • Cleft nasal deformity • Rhinoplasty • Nasoalveolar molding
- Presurgical infant orthopedics

KEY POINTS

- Nasoalveolar molding (NAM) is a form of presurgical infant orthopedics (PSIO) whose goal is to reduce the severity of the cleft deformity and improve surgical outcomes. The data on efficacy and benefit of NAM are mixed.
- Those in favor of NAM report improved nasal symmetry and appearance, reduced overall costs, psychosocial benefit to family, and decreased need for early nasal revision.
- Those in opposition to NAM argue NAM causes increased caregiver burden, poor patient compliance, increased costs in the short term, relapse of nasal symmetry in the first year, and no conclusive data of improved outcomes.

INTRODUCTION

Cleft lip and palate is one of the most common congenital craniofacial disorders. Patients born with a cleft deformity might experience problems with feeding, speech, and hearing, as well psychological stresses and issues with social well-being secondary to their aesthetic deformity. To fully address the needs of the cleft patient, a multidisciplinary team approach is required. Complete care of the cleft patient is a challenging task, with new techniques and technologies developing all the time. This article focuses on the new developments in the management of cleft lip and palate patients and the controversies surrounding such technique.

PRESURGICAL INFANT ORTHOPEDICS

For many years, surgeons have been attempting to reduce the severity of the deformity before the surgical repair to achieve a better outcome. The field of PSIO emerged based on this need. Reports of attempts to retract the premaxilla in bilateral cleft cases date back to the sixteenth century. Since then, multiple treatments have been developed in an attempt to reduce the deformity before definitive primary lip surgery, including maxillary plates, the Latham appliance, lip taping, elastic bands, lip adhesion, and NAM (**Figs. 1** and **2**). Infant orthopedics (IO) was first introduced by McNeil in the 1950s[1] and further developed over the following decades. A device that was screwed into the lateral arch segments and activated with pins through the premaxilla was developed by Georgiade and colleagues[2,3] in the 1960s. The Latham device, developed in the 1980s, is another device that expanded the lateral alveolar cleft segments and deprojected the maxilla by activating a screw mechanism.[4,5]

NASOALVEOLAR MOLDING

In the late 1990s, Grayson and Cutting described a presurgical appliance that added additional nasal

Disclosure: The authors have nothing to disclose.
[a] Facial Plastics and Craniofacial Surgery, SUNY Upstate, 750 East Adams Street, Syracuse, NY 13207, USA;
[b] Division of Facial Plastic Surgery, Cleft and Craniofacial Center, Upstate Medical University, 750 East Adams Street, Syracuse, NY 13210, USA
* Corresponding author.
E-mail address: tatums@upstate.edu

Facial Plast Surg Clin N Am 24 (2016) 255–264
http://dx.doi.org/10.1016/j.fsc.2016.03.004

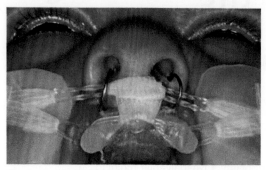

Fig. 1. Taping for bilateral cleft lip and palate. The taping is similar to the UCLP case except each retention tape inserts on the retention button on its respective side. Differential force can be placed on each tape to address any premaxillary deviation. A prolabial tape can be added to facilitate nonsurgical columella elongation. A cross-cheek tape can be added to provide additional force for premaxillary retraction. (*From* Goudy SL, Tollefson TT. Complete cleft care: cleft and velopharyngeal insufficiency treatment in children. New York: Thieme; 2014; with permission.)

molding prongs.[6–8] The NAM technique uses acrylic nasal stents attached to the vestibular shield of an oral molding plate to mold the nasal alar cartilages into more normal form and position during the presurgical period. This technique is based on the technique of molding auricular deformities in the neonate described by Matsuo and colleagues.[9] This technique nonsurgically improves congenital deformities by taking advantage of the plasticity of infant cartilage thought to be the result of increased levels of circulating maternal estrogen during the first 6 months of life. In addition, NAM attempts to lengthen the columella through the application of tissue expansion principles. The

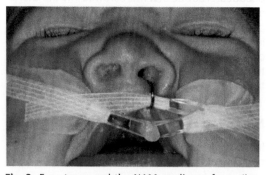

Fig. 2. Face tapes and the NAM appliance for unilateral cleft lip and palate. Base tapes are applied to the cheeks. The appliance is then inserted and the retention tapes are secured to the retention button. Greater tension can be placed on the side with the cleft to favor alveolar cleft closure. (*From* Goudy SL, Tollefson TT. Complete cleft care: cleft and velopharyngeal insufficiency treatment in children. New York: Thieme; 2014; with permission.)

columellar improvement is achieved by gradual elongation of the nasal stents and application of tissue-expanding elastic forces applied to the prolabium.[8,10] The process begins as soon as possible after birth; a custom-made alveolar mold is worn full time with weekly or biweekly adjustments until the alveolar cleft is narrowed to 5 mm or less, achieving the goals of bringing the lip segments together, reducing the alar base width, and relaxing tension on the splayed alar rim. A nasal stent extending from the intraoral plate to the cleft nostril is then added to elevate the alar rim into a more symmetric and convex position.[11]

A recent survey of all surgeons in the American Cleft Palate-Craniofacial Association and the Canadian Society of Plastic Surgeons revealed that 71% of cleft surgeons use some form of presurgical orthopedics at least occasionally and that NAM is used at least occasionally by 38% and greater than half the time by 25% of surgeons.[12] This increase in use in the past 20 years raises the question, Is NAM effective? The purpose of this article is to review the data for and against the use of NAM.

BENEFITS OF NASOALVEOLAR MOLDING
Psychosocial Benefit to Caregivers

Proponents of NAM claim several benefits, including improved aesthetic outcome, reduced overall costs, and a psychosocial benefit to the family. To evaluate the psychosocial effects of NAM, a prospective, multicenter longitudinal study was performed examining 118 caregivers at 6 different cleft treatment centers in the United States.[13] The patients were in 2 groups: those who underwent NAM plus traditional care and those who underwent traditional care only. Although the first year was demanding for all caregivers, NAM onset and the child's lip surgery were particularly stressful times. Qualitative and quantitative results, however, indicated caregivers of NAM-treated infants experienced more rapid declines in anxiety and depressive symptoms and better coping skills over time than caregivers whose infants had traditional care.[14] This is believed to be because the frequent visits for NAM adjustments reduce caregiver anxiety and lead to a sense of empowerment. These changes arise as a caregiver develops increased skill in managing the NAM appliance, observes improvement in the baby's appearance, and receives support and counseling from weekly visits to the cleft team.[13]

Clinical Benefits of Nasoalveolar Molding

When evaluating the clinical effects of NAM, they can be broken down into maxillary growth, dentition and occlusion, facial appearance, nasal symmetry, nasal growth, and speech. It has been shown in a randomized controlled clinical trial that non-NAM forms of PSIO offer no measurable advantage or disadvantage in terms of facial growth, facial appearance, maxillary arch dimensions, or occlusion relative to infants treated without PSIO.[15–21] NAM was not studied, however, in these trials. Proponents of NAM argue that it does have a significant effect on maxillary arch and occlusion. Keçik and Enacar[22] evaluated the effects of presurgical NAM (PNAM) therapy on nasal and alveolar tissues in patients with unilateral cleft lip and palate. They examined the impressions of 22 patients before and after NAM therapy and found a decrease in cleft width and arch length and a significant increase in arch circumference on the affected side.[22] A study from India by Sabarinath and colleagues[23] examined pre-NAM and post-NAM study models of 10 unilateral cleft lip-palate infants. Results from this study showed that NAM was effective in reducing the severity of the initial cleft deformity mainly at the anterior portion of the maxillary arch, because it increased the arch perimeter and intertuberosity distance while decreasing the width of the alveolar cleft and anterior arch length and width.[23]

It is suggested that the primary shortfall of all PSIO techniques other than NAM is that they neglect to address the nasal cartilage deformity during the period of cartilage plasticity.[13] The main difference of NAM from traditional PSIO is the reshaping of the nasal cartilage and providing aesthetic benefits in terms of nasal tip and alar symmetry.[6,24–27]

Effect of Nasoalveolar Molding on Nasal Appearance in Unilateral Cleft Lip-Palate

The effect of NAM on nasal appearance is the focus of multiple studies.[6,22,25–35] The few studies with the longest follow-up and evidence level II and level III are described. Barillas and colleagues[29] retrospectively reviewed the results of patients 9 years after NAM and measured nasal symmetry using nasal impressions in stone cast; 15 patients with unilateral cleft lip and palate who had NAM were compared with a group of 10 unilateral cleft lip and palate patients who had not undergone NAM either because of age of presentation or parental preference (**Fig. 3**). They found that nasal symmetry, including ala projection, dome height, alar groove position, and nasal bridge deviation, was improved by NAM but that columellar deviation was equivalent to non-NAM treatment.[29]

Bennun and colleagues[28] performed a prospective controlled trial of unilateral cleft lip and palate patients. They compared 44 patients managed with an occlusal prosthesis plus NAM to 47 patients

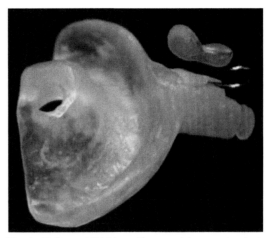

Fig. 3. Unilateral NAM appliance, with retention button and nasal stent. (*From* Goudy SL, Tollefson TT. Complete cleft care: cleft and velopharyngeal insufficiency treatment in children. New York: Thieme; 2014; with permission.)

who had an occlusal prosthesis alone as well as 48 noncleft controls. The results at 6 years showed the nasoalveolar group exhibited greater nasal tip protrusion, columellar length, and columellar width compared with the non-NAM group, and tip protrusion was similar to that of noncleft controls. Both the NAM and non-NAM groups had greater nasal width than the noncleft controls.[28]

Liou and colleagues[30] examined the progressive changes of NAM by evaluating 25 patients with unilateral cleft lip-palate. They photographically compared preoperative and postoperative and cleft and noncleft nostril appearance. They found an improvement in the ratio of cleft to noncleft nostril height, dome height, columellar length, nasal base width, and nostril width. This improvement was seen after NAM and further improved by cheiloplasty. This improvement partially relapsed after 1 year but remained greater than baseline and then remained stable at 2-year and 3-year evaluations.[30]

Another retrospective study on unilateral cleft lip-palate by Chang and colleagues[32] compared primary rhinoplasty alone, NAM alone, NAM plus primary rhinoplasty, and NAM plus primary rhinoplasty with overcorrection. Photography taken 5 years after surgery showed no difference in nostril height, nostril width, nostril area, or nostril height–to–nostril width ratio. There was a significant difference seen in the NAM groups showing improved symmetry in the medial nostril height and nasal sill height.[32]

Effect of Nasoalveolar Molding on Nasal Appearance in Bilateral Cleft Lip-Palate

These studies all focus on unilateral cleft lip-palate. Fewer studies have been done evaluating bilateral cleft lip-palate. Bilateral cleft lip-palate has a lower incidence compared with unilateral cleft lip-palate (**Fig. 4**). The incidence of cleft lip-palate is 1 to 2 per 1000 live births, depending on ethnicity,[36] and bilateral clefts are only 15% to 36% of those.[37,38] The bilateral cleft presents a different set of challenges, although the same presurgical appliance is used. In the bilateral cleft, the alar cartilages have failed to migrate up to the nasal tip and elongate the columella. The alar cartilages are positioned along the alar margins and are stretched over the cleft as flaring alae.[39] In addition, the premaxilla is suspended from the tip of the nasal septum and is often protruded and widely separate from the lateral alveolar segments. The first goal of NAM in these cases must be to move the premaxillary segment posteriorly and medially while preparing the lateral alveolar segments to come in contact with the premaxilla. Several months of appliance adjustments are often required. Delaying repair until 5 months is not uncommon.[40] In addition to orthopedic retraction of premaxilla and molding of the posterior lateral alveolar ridges to an appropriate width to accept the premaxilla, the other goal of NAM in bilateral clefts is columella elongation.[41]

The few studies that focus specifically on bilateral cleft lip-palate show similar trends to the studies of NAM in unilateral clefts: improved nasal symmetry and facial appearance. But long-term studies and controlled trials are lacking. Suri and colleagues[42] compared 29 bilateral cleft lip-palate patients who underwent NAM with 17 patients who had IO only and found significant improvement in columellar length and alignment of alveolar segments compared with those who underwent IO only. Measurements were taken at the time of primary lip repair, but there was no long-term follow-up.[42] Spengler and colleagues[43] found that NAM created a statistically significant reduction of premaxillary protrusion and deviation. Extraoral measurements revealed that there was a significant increase in the bialar width and nostril height as well as increase in the columellar length, width, and deviation. This study included 9 patients, and measurements were compared before and after NAM treatment with no control group.[43]

Garfinkle and colleagues[44] studied 77 nonsyndromic patients with bilateral cleft lip-cleft palate, all of whom underwent NAM and compared them with age-matched controls. Nasal tip protrusion, alar base width, alar width, columella length, and columella width were measured at 5 time points spanning 12.5 years. The nasal tip protrusion, alar base width, alar width, columella length, and columella width were not statistically different from those of the noncleft, age-matched control group at age 12.5 years.[44]

Two long-term studies have evaluated the efficacy of NAM. Liou and colleagues[45] examined basilar photographs of 22 bilateral cleft lip-cleft palate infants before and after NAM, 1 week after cheiloplasty, and yearly for 3 years. The results revealed that the columella was significantly lengthened after NAM and was further improved after primary cheiloplasty. There was a relative relapse in columella length, however, because of the differential growth between the columella and the rest of the nose in the first and second years postoperatively.[45] Again there was no control group in this study. Lee and colleagues[46] performed a retrospective review of 26 consecutive patients with bilateral cleft lip-cleft palate, comparing 13 patients who had a cleft lip repair and nasal correction with banked fork flaps to 13 patients who had nonsurgical columellar elongation with NAM followed by cleft lip closure and primary nasal correction. There was also a group of 13 age-matched controls. Columellar length was measured at presentation and at 3 years of age. The number of nasal operations was recorded to 9 years. The Kruskal-Wallis and Tukey-Kramer tests were used for statistical analysis. The NAM group had significantly greater columellar length than that of the forked flap group and was similar to age-matched controls at 3 years. Furthermore, the NAM group had a significantly reduced need for secondary nasal surgery.[46]

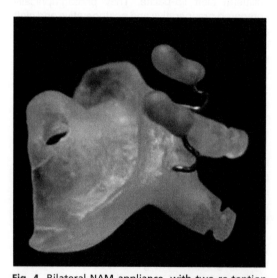

Fig. 4. Bilateral NAM appliance, with two re-tention buttons and two nasal stents. Note the two nasal stents will be connected following addition of the horizontal columella band. (*From* Goudy SL, Tollefson TT. Complete cleft care: cleft and velopharyngeal insufficiency treatment in children. New York: Thieme; 2014; with permission.)

Effect of Nasoalveolar Molding on Speech Development

The effect of presurgical orthopedics on speech development has shown inconclusive results. Suzuki and colleagues[47] evaluated 17 patients with unilateral and bilateral cleft lip-palate. Analysis of tongue movements was by ultrasound and speech therapist analyzed articulation approximately 4 years after palate repair. They found that infants with cleft palate could not create negative pressure in the oral cavity, even with the presurgical orthopedics. Continuous use of the orthopedics up to the time of palatoplasty seemed effective for the postoperative articulatory, inhibiting irregular movements of the tongue, and possibly preventing "palatalized articulation."[47]

Karling and colleagues[48] studied 84 patients with unilateral cleft lip and 19 patients with bilateral cleft lip, divided into those treated with presurgical orthopedics and those who were not, and compared them to a group of 40 noncleft controls. All subjects were recorded and judged by professional listeners. No significant differences in articulation or resonance were found between the subgroups of unilateral cleft patients; however, the mean ages at time of evaluation varied from 10.6 for the group who had PSIO and 17.6 years for the group who did not. The results also indicated that the bilateral cleft patients had poorer speech and needed more speech therapy than the unilateral cleft patients. All cleft patients were found to have poorer speech than the noncleft subjects despite considerable speech therapy and complementary surgical treatment.[48]

In a prospective randomized clinical trial (Dutchcleft), patients with complete unilateral cleft lip-palate were followed-up longitudinally at 2 years, 2.5 years, 3 years, and 6 years. One group of 6 infants was treated with IO in the first year of life; the other group of 6 did not receive this treatment. Phonological skills, such as number of acquired consonants, order of phonological development, use of phonological processes, and occurrence of nasal escape, were evaluated. At age 3, the children in the IO group had acquired more initial consonants, suggesting children treated with IO during their first year of life followed a more normal path of phonological development between 2 years and 3 years of age.[49] The trial also examined receptive language skills and expressive language skills. Children treated with IO during their first year of life produced longer sentences than non-IO children at the ages of 2.5 and 3 years. At 6 years of age, however, both groups presented similar expressive language skills. Hence, IO treatment did not have long-lasting effects on language development.[50]

Possible Reduced Overall Costs with Nasoalveolar Molding

Another argument for using NAM is that it reduces overall costs, because the patients have less need for alveolar bone graft[51,52] and fewer revision nasal surgeries later in life[53] Two studies have looked at the cost of NAM plus surgery versus surgery alone and the likelihood of needing an alveolar bone graft later in life. One found that patients treated with NAM and gingivoperiosteoplasty reduced the need for bone grafting later in life, and the overall cost was therefore reduced.[51] The same conclusion was found when examining exclusively bilateral cleft lip and palate patients.[52] When comparing the rate of revision nasal surgery in patients treated with NAM plus surgery and surgery alone, they found that NAM significantly reduced the risk of undergoing revision surgery. Based on the risk reduction, they concluded that NAM can reduce the number of early secondary nasal revision surgeries and, therefore, reduce the overall cost of care.[53]

IN OPPOSITION TO NASOALVEOLAR MOLDING
Poor Caregiver Compliance with Nasoalveolar Molding

Opponents of NAM argue that it is complex and expensive and offers no lasting clinical benefit. One of the biggest drawbacks of the NAM appliance is parental compliance.[40,54] In addition to bringing patients to the office for weekly adjustments, parents and caregivers assume the responsibility of daily care for the appliance. The responsibility of cleaning, taping, and maintaining the appliance is a large task considering these families are under psychological stress, having just undergone the birth of a child with a significant orofacial defect. Compliance issues were of great concern, with an estimated incidence of 30% for broken appointments and an estimated incidence of 26% for removal of the NAM appliance by the tongue, according to 1 study.[54] Parents tend to think that the appliance is the cause of the infant's fussiness and remove the appliance. Often, a parent feels guilty for not having the appliance in place and does not report this to the team until the next visit; several weeks without the appliance in place may go by.[40] Another study had a dropout rate of 32.5% due to skin irritations or lack of parental support.[55] It was demonstrated in 1 study that in the few cases of parents not complying well with instructions, the patients did not show significant changes in nasal esthetics.[27] This emphasizes the variability that can occur depending on caregiver compliance.

Increased Short-Term Costs with Nasoalveolar Molding

Although data are still evolving on the long-term costs and possible cost savings attributed to NAM, the treatment does cost more in the short term. A cost analysis was performed by Severens and colleagues[56] and found that there was significant cost associated with presurgical orthopedic treatment both directly and indirectly. The non-PSIO treatment group had a significantly different mean medical cost US $304 compared with US $852 for PSIO treatment. Mean travel costs and indirect nonmedical costs were US $128 and US $231 for PSIO and US $79 and US $130 for non-PSIO, respectively. Furthermore, presurgical treatment did not reduce the operating time, with the durations of the surgical lip closure procedures an average of 57.2 minutes for PSIO and 56.4 minutes for non-PSIO.[56]

Effect of Nasoalveolar Molding on Facial Growth

One of the major concerns of presurgical orthopedics, including NAM, is an adverse effect on maxillary growth. Yu and colleagues[57] reported a study with mixed results of NAM. They examined 15 infants with unilateral cleft lip-cleft palate treated by NAM therapy, and the control group consisted of 15 infants with non-presurgically treated unilateral cleft lip-palate. They showed a trend toward morphologic improvement in maxillary alveoli, having reduced the cleft gap, corrected the maxillary midline, and improved the sagittal length of the maxilla. The alveolar height decreased significantly, however, after the treatment, which indicated that the traction force of the appliance could have obstructive effects on the vertical growth of the alveolar bone.[57]

No Clinical Benefit with Nasoalveolar Molding

Although there are some studies that indicate a positive trending effect with NAM, there are many studies with mixed or negative results. Clark and colleagues[33] retrospectively compared 20 patients who underwent primary lip repair after NAM to 5 patients who underwent primary lip repair alone. Neither group had primary nasal repair at time of surgery, and analysis was performed at 5 years and 6 years, respectively. Study patients showed no difference in the measures of philtrum, lip scar, nasal anatomy, dental arch, nasal measurements, lip measurements, and maxillary arch analysis.[33]

Opponents of NAM argue that studies show no significant effects on maxillary growth, dentition, or occlusion. Lee and colleagues[58] assessed the

effects of NAM and gingivoperiosteoplasty in 20 unilateral cleft lip-palate patients and found that midface growth in sagittal or vertical planes (up to the ages of 9–13 years) were not affected by presurgical alveolar molding and gingivoperiosteoplasty. Adali and colleagues[59] studied the effect of NAM on arch circumference and arch form in 75 unilateral cleft lip palate patients and found that presurgical orthopedics produced no statistically significant mean change in any arch form variable when compared with the non-PSO group. Lip repair produced greater change in arch form than did presurgical orthopedics, reducing the mean alveolar cleft width by 4.45 mm compared with 0.69 mm by NAM.[59]

Clark and colleagues[33] performed a study on 20 infants treated with NAM to 5 infants without NAM. The evaluators were blinded to which patients received NAM and reviewed their facial morphology, dental arch configuration, and occlusion. Clinically, the improvement in the NAM group was most evident in nasal and lip anatomy. There were no statistically significant differences, however, between the 2 groups on each of the measurements on 3-D facial images and dental models.[33]

Mishra and colleagues[60] found that children with NAM did have significant lengthening of the columella, but that nostril height, nostril width, and alar perimeter were not changed in a statistically significant way. Furthermore, patients of unilateral cleft lip had more reduction in alveolar gap than bilateral group.[60]

Other opponents of NAM argue that the changes brought by NAM relapse after a short period. Liou and colleagues'[30] study showed that after the primary cheiloplasty, the nasal asymmetry significantly relapsed in the first year postoperatively. They recommend surgically overcorrecting and continuing a nasal conformer after surgery.[30] Similarly, a study by Pai and colleagues[34] found relapse in nasal symmetry after 1 year. The study by Chang and colleagues[32] suggested that NAM alone could not provide nostril symmetry in the long term. They also advocated for surgical overcorrection and an additional 6 months of nasal splint appliance after surgery.[32] Because many of the studies on NAM measure the effect at the time of lip repair, it is unclear what the long-term outcomes are and what percentage of the initial changes will relapse. Although this technique of NAM plus surgical overcorrection and/or postoperative nasal conformers may be effective, there is no control group and no evidence that surgical overcorrection alone or postoperative nasal conformers alone may achieve the same outcome in the long term. A study by Yeow and colleagues[61] showed improvement in long-term outcomes, measured at age 5 years and 8 years, with postoperative nasal splints alone. Improvement was seen in nostril symmetry, alar cartilage slump, alar base level, and columella tilt compared with the surgery-only group.[61]

At this time, it is unclear if there are negative effects associated with NAM treatment. Studies report side effects of pressure ulcer,[60] cheek skin rashes, thrush, and alveolar arch irritations,[40] with tissue irritation at an estimated incidence greater than 10%.[54] Although most side effects reported are minor, practitioners should be cautious about the possible negative consequences of therapy.

ISSUES WITH REVIEW ARTICLES AND META-ANALYSIS

Several review articles[11,41,62] have been written about this topic and although there seems to be a trend towards a positive effect, the data have been largely inconclusive. The difficulty in studying cleft outcomes comes from small sample sizes given the low prevalence of clefts in the general population, and long-term follow-up is complicated by care migration. A multicenter comparison is difficult because of variations in nasal measurements between patients of different ethnic descents.

The Eurocleft and Americleft studies attempted to pool data to come up with some conclusions but also produced mixed results. The Eurocleft study was a longitudinal cohort study between 5 different cleft centers in Northern Europe that examined patient results at 9 years, 12 years, and 15 years of follow-up. They examined many different aspects of cleft care, including nasolabial appearance. In this study, they found that the 2 centers with less favorable ratings had a more complex treatment program, including presurgical orthopedics.[63] They also cited difficulty, however, with the rating system, such as low interexaminer agreement and variability in the quality of the photographs. The Americleft study compared data from 4 North American cleft lip and palate centers at patients ages 6 and 12. In this study, they found no significant differences in patient appearance despite differences in protocols, including presurgical orthopedics.[64] This study had better interexaminer agreement but was also limited by the consistency of the photography.

There is poor agreement between studies, with some showing positive results, whereas others show negative or mixed results. This may in part be attributed to variations in protocol and technique of NAM application. Between studies, there is variation in timing, duration, adjustments, and differences in appliances. Before NAM is applied, there is divergence in pretreatment protocols, with some institutions using taping and others using NAM as the first intervention. Regarding timing, studies varied in when the patients first obtained the NAM appliance, beginning as early as 7 days old and up to 12 weeks of age. This relatively advanced age might have altered the results of these patients because the cartilages lose postnatal malleability during this time. Duration of device use varies between studies with time frames ranging from 2 months to 8 months. There is no standard protocol for adjustments, and the frequency of adjustment also varies. It is unclear if patients who had weekly visits and adjustments have better outcomes than those who had less frequent appointments. Furthermore, there are likely differences in the appliance used as well as variation in the skill and technique of the dentist and orthodontist. Finally, there may be a selection bias in many studies because the inadequate reporting of indications and the process of selection for NAM.[62]

After undergoing NAM, there are further variations in the surgical repair. Just as the duration of NAM varies, so does the timing of the lip repair. There are many techniques used for lip repair,[65] and the chosen technique varies by institution and is likely dependent on each surgeon's skill and experience. Surgery is a part of every patient's treatment, but with diverse methods of surgery, it is impossible to separate the effect of surgery from the effect of NAM. Some studies have tried to control for this by retrospectively comparing patients who underwent surgery by the same surgeon before and after using NAM in the practice. A sample of patients taken over a long period of time, however, may be confounded by the learning curve of the practitioner. This may influence the effect of the treatment instead of the treatment itself. Many of the studies reviewed claim improvement at the time of primary lip repair, based on pre-NAM and post-NAM treatment measurements without a control group. Although these studies show a trend towards a positive effect, only a patient-controlled study can show that NAM alone is responsible for the improved outcome.

The outcomes of cleft surgery are also not well defined. Although it is largely agreed on that the goals of NAM are improvement in the cleft nasal deformity and improvement in the alveolar gap, the specific measurements used to define these are diverse. Additionally, the methods used to measure these outcomes are mixed. Some measure the anesthetized infant, others measure photographs, and others measure molds. It is difficult to standardize the margin of error between methods, but it is clear that a small discrepancy may have a large effect. The outcomes of these studies are measured in millimeters and even a small lapse of accuracy might have a significant impact on the statistics of a study.

Finally, the literature lacks long-term follow-up. It has been demonstrated in several studies that there is some relapse of the nasal cartilages in the first year. Studies with measurements taken only before and after NAM treatment do not fully illustrate the effect of NAM throughout the child's development.

SUMMARY

What is the answer to the question, Is NAM effective? It is impossible to give an absolute answer due to the many variables in NAM protocols, methods of data collection, and varied results. Furthermore, there is no consistent set of measurements used by all surgeons. Different landmarks were measured in each study, and with such small subjects, any variability in measurements could have a large impact on the outcome. In these trials, NAM was compared with the non-cleft side or to normal controls. Although these studies suggest improved outcomes, the literature lacks a high-quality randomized controlled trial comparing NAM to other methods.

REFERENCES

1. McNeil CK. Orthodontic procedures in the treatment of congenital cleft palate. Dent Rec (London) 1950; 70(5):126–32.
2. Georgiade N, Mladick RA, Thorne FL. Positioning of the premaxilla in bilateral cleft lips by oral pinning and traction. Plast Reconstr Surg 1968;41(3):240–3.
3. Georgiade NG, Latham RA. Maxillary arch alignment in the bilateral cleft lip and palate infant, using pinned coaxial screw appliance. Plast Reconstr Surg 1975; 56(1):52–60.
4. Millard DR, Latham RA. Improved primary surgical and dental treatment of clefts. Plast Reconstr Surg 1990;86(5):856–71.
5. Latham RA. Orthopedic advancement of the cleft maxillary segment: a preliminary report. Cleft Palate J 1980;17(3):227–33.
6. Grayson BH, Cutting CB. Presurgical nasoalveolar orthopedic molding in primary correction of the nose, lip, and alveolus of infants born with unilateral and bilateral clefts. Cleft Palate Craniofac J 2001;38(3):193–8.
7. Grayson BH, Santiago PE, Brecht LE, et al. Presurgical nasoalveolar molding in infants with cleft lip and palate. Cleft Palate Craniofac J 1999;36(6): 486–98.
8. Cutting C, Grayson B, Brecht L, et al. Presurgical columellar elongation and primary retrograde nasal reconstruction in one-stage bilateral cleft lip and nose repair. Plast Reconstr Surg 1998;101(3):630–9.
9. Matsuo K, Hirose T, Tomono T, et al. Nonsurgical correction of congenital auricular deformities in the early neonate: a preliminary report. Plast Reconstr Surg 1984;73(1):38–51.
10. Grayson BH, Cutting C, Wood R. Preoperative columella lengthening in bilateral cleft lip and palate. Plast Reconstr Surg 1993;92(7):1422–3.
11. Abbott MM, Meara JG. Nasoalveolar molding in cleft care: is it efficacious? Plast Reconstr Surg 2012; 130(3):659–66.
12. Sitzman TJ, Girotto JA, Marcus JR. Current surgical practices in cleft care: unilateral cleft lip repair. Plast Reconstr Surg 2008;121(5):261e–70e.
13. Grayson BH, Garfinkle JS. Early cleft management: the case for nasoalveolar molding. Am J Orthod Dentofacial Orthop 2014;145(2):134–42.
14. Sischo L, Clouston SAP, Phillips C, et al. Caregiver responses to early cleft palate care: a mixed method approach. Health Psychol 2015;35(5):474–82.
15. Prahl C, Prahl-Andersen B, Van't Hof MA, et al. Presurgical orthopedics and satisfaction in motherhood: a randomized clinical trial (Dutchcleft). Cleft Palate Craniofac J 2008;45(3):284–8.
16. Prahl C, Kuijpers-Jagtman AM, Van 't Hof MA, et al. Infant orthopedics in UCLP: effect on feeding, weight, and length: a randomized clinical trial (Dutchcleft). Cleft Palate Craniofac J 2005;42(2):171–7.
17. Bongaarts CAM, van 't Hof MA, Prahl-Andersen B, et al. Infant orthopedics has no effect on maxillary arch dimensions in the deciduous dentition of children with complete unilateral cleft lip and palate (Dutchcleft). Cleft Palate Craniofac J 2006;43(6): 665–72.
18. Bongaarts CAM, Prahl-Andersen B, Bronkhorst EM, et al. Infant orthopedics and facial growth in complete unilateral cleft lip and palate until six years of age (Dutchcleft). Cleft Palate Craniofac J 2009; 46(6):654–63.
19. Bongaarts CAM, Kuijpers-Jagtman AM, van 't Hof MA, et al. The effect of infant orthopedics on the occlusion of the deciduous dentition in children with complete unilateral cleft lip and palate (Dutchcleft). Cleft Palate Craniofac J 2004;41(6):633–41.
20. Masarei AG, Wade A, Mars M, et al. A randomized control trial investigating the effect of presurgical orthopedics on feeding in infants with cleft lip and/or palate. Cleft Palate Craniofac J 2007;44(2):182–93.
21. Noverraz RLM, Disse MA, Ongkosuwito EM, et al. Transverse dental arch relationship at 9 and 12 years in children with unilateral cleft lip and palate treated with infant orthopedics: a randomized clinical trial (DUTCHCLEFT). Clin Oral Investig 2015;19(9): 2255–65.
22. Keçik D, Enacar A. Effects of nasoalveolar molding therapy on nasal and alveolar morphology in unilateral cleft lip and palate. J Craniofac Surg 2009; 20(6):2075–80.

23. Sabarinath VP, Thombare P, Hazarey PV, et al. Changes in maxillary alveolar morphology with nasoalveolar molding. J Clin Pediatr Dent 2010;35(2): 207–12.

24. Maull DJ, Grayson BH, Cutting CB, et al. Long-term effects of nasoalveolar molding on three-dimensional nasal shape in unilateral clefts. Cleft Palate Craniofac J 1999;36(5):391–7.

25. Suri S, Tompson BD. A modified muscle-activated maxillary orthopedic appliance for presurgical nasoalveolar molding in infants with unilateral cleft lip and palate. Cleft Palate Craniofac J 2004;41(3): 225–9.

26. Singh GD, Levy-Bercowski D, Santiago PE. Three-dimensional nasal changes following nasoalveolar molding in patients with unilateral cleft lip and palate: geometric morphometrics. Cleft Palate Craniofac J 2005;42(4):403–9.

27. Punga R, Sharma SM. Presurgical orthopaedic nasoalveolar molding in cleft lip and palate infants: a comparative evaluation of cases done with and without nasal stents. J Maxillofac Oral Surg 2013;12(3):273–88.

28. Bennun RD, Perandones C, Sepliarsky VA, et al. Nonsurgical correction of nasal deformity in unilateral complete cleft lip: a 6-year follow-up. Plast Reconstr Surg 1999;104(3):616–30.

29. Barillas I, Dec W, Warren SM, et al. Nasoalveolar molding improves long-term nasal symmetry in complete unilateral cleft lip-cleft palate patients. Plast Reconstr Surg 2009;123(3):1002–6.

30. Liou EJ-W, Subramanian M, Chen PKT, et al. The progressive changes of nasal symmetry and growth after nasoalveolar molding: a three-year follow-up study. Plast Reconstr Surg 2004;114(4):858–64.

31. Uzel A, Alparslan ZN. Long-term effects of presurgical infant orthopedics in patients with cleft lip and palate: a systematic review. Cleft Palate Craniofac J 2011;48(5):587–95.

32. Chang C-S, Por YC, Liou EJ-W, et al. Long-term comparison of four techniques for obtaining nasal symmetry in unilateral complete cleft lip patients: a single surgeon's experience. Plast Reconstr Surg 2010;126(4):1276–84.

33. Clark SL, Teichgraeber JF, Fleshman RG, et al. Long-term treatment outcome of presurgical nasoalveolar molding in patients with unilateral cleft lip and palate. J Craniofac Surg 2011;22(1):333–6.

34. Pai BC-J, Ko EW-C, Huang C-S, et al. Symmetry of the nose after presurgical nasoalveolar molding in infants with unilateral cleft lip and palate: a preliminary study. Cleft Palate Craniofac J 2005;42(6):658–63.

35. Nakamura N, Sasaguri M, Nozoe E, et al. Postoperative nasal forms after presurgical nasoalveolar molding followed by medial-upward advancement of nasolabial components with vestibular expansion for children with unilateral complete cleft lip and palate. J Oral Maxillofac Surg 2009;67(10):2222–31.

36. Vanderas AP. Incidence of cleft lip, cleft palate, and cleft lip and palate among races: a review. Cleft Palate J 1987;24(3):216–25.

37. Cooper ME, Stone RA, Liu Y, et al. Descriptive epidemiology of nonsyndromic cleft lip with or without cleft palate in Shanghai, China, from 1980 to 1989. Cleft Palate Craniofac J 2000;37(3):274–80.

38. Hagberg C, Larson O, Milerad J. Incidence of cleft lip and palate and risks of additional malformations. Cleft Palate Craniofac J 1998;35(1):40–5.

39. Santiago PE, Schuster LA, Levy-Bercowski D. Management of the alveolar cleft. Clin Plast Surg 2014; 41(2):219–32.

40. Tollefson TT, Gere RR. Presurgical cleft lip management: nasal alveolar molding. Facial Plast Surg 2007;23(2):113–22.

41. Niranjane PP, Kamble RH, Diagavane SP, et al. Current status of presurgical infant orthopaedic treatment for cleft lip and palate patients: a critical review. Indian J Plast Surg 2014;47(3):293–302.

42. Suri S, Disthaporn S, Atenafu EG, et al. Presurgical presentation of columellar features, nostril anatomy, and alveolar alignment in bilateral cleft lip and palate after infant orthopedics with and without nasoalveolar molding. Cleft Palate Craniofac J 2012;49(3): 314–24.

43. Spengler AL, Chavarria C, Teichgraeber JF, et al. Presurgical nasoalveolar molding therapy for the treatment of bilateral cleft lip and palate: a preliminary study. Cleft Palate Craniofac J 2006;43(3):321–8.

44. Garfinkle JS, King TW, Grayson BH, et al. A 12-year anthropometric evaluation of the nose in bilateral cleft lip-cleft palate patients following nasoalveolar molding and cutting bilateral cleft lip and nose reconstruction. Plast Reconstr Surg 2011;127(4): 1659–67.

45. Liou EJ-W, Subramanian M, Chen PKT. Progressive changes of columella length and nasal growth after nasoalveolar molding in bilateral cleft patients: a 3-year follow-up study. Plast Reconstr Surg 2007; 119(2):642–8.

46. Lee CTH, Garfinkle JS, Warren SM, et al. Nasoalveolar molding improves appearance of children with bilateral cleft lip-cleft palate. Plast Reconstr Surg 2008;122(4):1131–7.

47. Suzuki K, Yamazaki Y, Sezaki K, et al. The effect of preoperative use of an orthopedic plate on articulatory function in children with cleft lip and palate. Cleft Palate Craniofac J 2006;43(4):406–14.

48. Karling J, Larson O, Leanderson R, et al. Speech in unilateral and bilateral cleft palate patients from Stockholm. Cleft Palate Craniofac J 1993;30(1):73–7.

49. Konst EM, Rietveld T, Peters HFM, et al. Phonological development of toddlers with unilateral cleft lip and palate who were treated with and without infant orthopedics: a randomized clinical trial. Cleft Palate Craniofac J 2003;40(1):32–9.

50. Konst EM, Rietveld T, Peters HFM, et al. Language skills of young children with unilateral cleft lip and palate following infant orthopedics: a randomized clinical trial. Cleft Palate Craniofac J 2003;40(4): 356–62.

51. Pfeifer TM, Grayson BH, Cutting CB. Nasoalveolar molding and gingivoperiosteoplasty versus alveolar bone graft: an outcome analysis of costs in the treatment of unilateral cleft alveolus. Cleft Palate Craniofac J 2002;39(1):26–9.

52. Dec W, Shetye PR, Davidson EH, et al. Presurgical nasoalveolar molding and primary gingivoperiosteoplasty reduce the need for bone grafting in patients with bilateral clefts. J Craniofac Surg 2013;24(1): 186–90.

53. Patel PA, Rubin MS, Clouston S, et al. Comparative study of early secondary nasal revisions and costs in patients with clefts treated with and without nasoalveolar molding. J Craniofac Surg 2015;26(4): 1229–33.

54. Levy-Bercowski D, Abreu A, DeLeon E, et al. Complications and solutions in presurgical nasoalveolar molding therapy. Cleft Palate Craniofac J 2009;46(5): 521–8.

55. Rau A, Ritschl LM, Mücke T, et al. Nasoalveolar molding in cleft care–experience in 40 patients from a single centre in Germany. PLoS One 2015; 10(no. 3):e0118103.

56. Severens JL, Prahl C, Kuijpers-Jagtman AM, et al. Short-term cost-effectiveness analysis of presurgical orthopedic treatment in children with complete unilateral cleft lip and palate. Cleft Palate Craniofac J 1998;35(3):222–6.

57. Yu Q, Gong X, Shen G. CAD presurgical nasoalveolar molding effects on the maxillary morphology in infants with UCLP. Oral Surg Oral Med Oral Pathol Oral Radiol 2013;116(4):418–26.

58. Lee CTH, Grayson BH, Cutting CB, et al. Prepubertal midface growth in unilateral cleft lip and palate following alveolar molding and gingivoperiosteoplasty. Cleft Palate Craniofac J 2004;41(4):375–80.

59. Adali N, Mars M, Petrie A, et al. Presurgical orthopedics has no effect on archform in unilateral cleft lip and palate. Cleft Palate Craniofac J 2012;49(1):5–13.

60. Mishra B, Singh AK, Zaidi J, et al. Presurgical nasoalveolar molding for correction of cleft lip nasal deformity: experience from northern India. Eplasty 2010;10:e55.

61. Yeow VK, Chen PK, Chen YR, et al. The use of nasal splints in the primary management of unilateral cleft nasal deformity. Plast Reconstr Surg 1999;103(5): 1347–54.

62. van der Heijden P, Dijkstra PU, Stellingsma C, et al. Limited evidence for the effect of presurgical nasoalveolar molding in unilateral cleft on nasal symmetry: a call for unified research. Plast Reconstr Surg 2013; 131(1):62e–71e.

63. Brattström V, Mølsted K, Prahl-Andersen B, et al. The Eurocleft study: intercenter study of treatment outcome in patients with complete cleft lip and palate. Part 2: craniofacial form and nasolabial appearance. Cleft Palate Craniofac J 2005;42(1):69–77.

64. Mercado A, Russell K, Hathaway R, et al. The Americleft study: an inter-center study of treatment outcomes for patients with unilateral cleft lip and palate part 4. Nasolabial aesthetics. Cleft Palate Craniofac J 2011;48(3):259–64.

65. Demke JC, Tatum SA. Analysis and evolution of rotation principles in unilateral cleft lip repair. J Plast Reconstr Aesthet Surg 2011;64(3):313–8.

Evidence-based Medicine in Facial Plastic Surgery
Current State and Future Directions

Raj Dedhia, MD[a], Tsung-Yen Hsieh, MD[a],
Travis T. Tollefson, MD, MPH[b], Lisa E. Ishii, MD, MHS[c],*

KEYWORDS

- Evidence-based medicine • Level of evidence • Grades of recommendation
- Patient-reported outcomes • Clinician-reported outcomes

KEY POINTS

- Evidence-based medicine involves application of the best available evidence while attending to patient preferences.
- Choosing the appropriate levels of evidence hierarchy depends on the type of study: treatment, prognosis, diagnosis, and economic/decision analysis.
- Clinical practice guideline recommendations are based on assessments of the quality of evidence and strength of recommendation.
- Outcome measures are essential to evidence-based medicine, and consist of (1) patient-reported outcomes, (2) clinical efficacy outcomes, and (3) actuarial or financial outcomes.
- Inconsistent patient characteristics and poorly defined outcome measures pose major challenges to performing meta-analyses and, ultimately, implementing existing evidence to individual patient care.

INTRODUCTION

The current state of evidence-based medicine (EBM) encompasses the evaluation and application of best available evidence, incorporation of clinical experience, and emphasis on patient preference and values. Anecdotally, surgeons exiting a national lecture on EBM were concerned with the possibility that EBM leads to more narrowed treatment options, less emphasis on individualized care, and an algorithmic approach to patients. Others complain about the stifling of innovative treatment options and emphasis on levels of evidence (LOEs).[1] This article describes the value of EBM to surgeons, relating clinical applications and future quality improvement opportunities.

Although the modern outcomes movement in EBM has been attributed to concepts explored and developed by Dr David Sackett in the 1970s and 1980s,[2–5] early evidence of this idea can be found historically. Examples include Nurse Florence Nightingale, Dr Eugen Bleuler, and Dr Ernest Codman, who promoted mindful observation, meticulous data collection, and thorough analysis

[a] Department of Otolaryngology–Head and Neck Surgery, UC Davis Medical Center, 2521 Stockton Boulevard, Suite 7200, Sacramento, CA 95817, USA; [b] Facial Plastic and Reconstructive Surgery, Department of Otolaryngology–Head and Neck Surgery, UC Davis Medical Center, 2521 Stockton Boulevard, Suite 7200, Sacramento, CA 95817, USA; [c] Department of Otolaryngology–Head & Neck Surgery, Johns Hopkins School of Medicine, Baltimore, MD 21287, USA
* Corresponding author.
E-mail address: Learnes2@jhmi.edu

Facial Plast Surg Clin N Am 24 (2016) 265–274
http://dx.doi.org/10.1016/j.fsc.2016.03.005
1064-7406/16/$ – see front matter © 2016 Elsevier Inc. All rights reserved.

as means to improve outcomes in clinical practice.[6–8] In 1981, Dr David Sackett[3] published a series of articles emphasizing the importance of critical analysis of published research in medical literature. This series highlighted use of epidemiology in conjunction with best available evidence applied in the clinical settings.[2–5] This concept was later developed and coined as EBM by Dr Gordon Guyatt in the early 1990s.[4]

The foundation of EBM is based on the core principles of assessment and application of best available evidence to guide clinical practice while attending to the informed patients' preferences and values.[9] Incorporating these two fundamental, interrelated principles in medical decisions bridges the gap between EBM and preference-based medicine, which calls for patient-centered research. Facial plastic and reconstructive surgery requires a conscientious blending of patient preference and values, while ensuring best outcomes. For example, success after rhinoplasty includes both patient-reported and clinician-derived outcome measures, which incorporate patient satisfaction, surgeon perception, and objective measures (eg, photograph analysis).[10]

Sackett and colleagues[5] explained EBM as a "bottom up approach that integrates the best external evidence with individual clinical expertise and patients' choice." Since its inception, EBM methodology has advanced through technology and international, multidisciplinary collaborations. This progress enables clinicians to critically examine external evidence from systematic research and apply it to clinical practice. EBM is integral to the policy changes of health care reform in the United States, the goals of which include enhancing quality, reducing cost, and improving patient satisfaction (a noble, potentially difficult goal).

This article discusses principles essential to EBM, examines resources commonly used in EBM practice, and emphasizes strengths while identifying limitations of EBM in relation to facial plastic and reconstructive surgery.

LEVELS OF EVIDENCE

Critical to the practice of EBM is identifying and implementing the highest level of evidence (LOE) to answer clinical questions. LOEs are a hierarchical ranking system that provides a framework for physicians and patients to find the best evidence.

The Canadian Task Force on the Periodic Health Examination first described LOE in 1979.[11] The task force's goal was to provide recommendations on preventive health interventions. To this effect, they rated the available evidence to determine the effectiveness of a given intervention and used that rating when providing recommendations for the annual physical examinations. Notably, they placed randomized controlled trials (RCTs) at the highest LOE, emphasizing the importance of reducing error caused by bias and confounding factors.[12]

Sackett[13] and other participants of the American College of Chest Physicians Conference on Antithrombotic Therapy expanded the definition of LOE in 1986. The basis of their undertaking was to establish a classification system that allowed recommendations to be based on rigorous, controlled studies whenever possible. They particularly subdivided RCTs by the qualitative degree of type I (false-positive) and type II (false-negative) errors shown by the study.[13] Most LOE rating scales ow in use are based on the University of Oxford Centre for Evidence Based Medicine (**Table 1**), which was further modified in 2000 and 2009.[14]

As EBM became increasingly accepted, surgical and other procedure-based specialties argued that applicable research questions did not lend themselves to RCTs and advocated modified LOE definitions. There are 4 types of studies that are relevant in choosing the appropriate LOE hierarchy: treatment, prognosis, diagnosis, and economic/decision analysis.[15]

Therapeutic studies lend themselves to rigorous RCTs. The researcher determines the intervention and the predetermined outcome measure. Therefore, placing high-quality RCTs at the top of the rating scale is appropriate. However, prognostic studies are more common in surgery, in which randomization is difficult. RCTs in surgery are difficult in application but also in the ensuring of ethical

Table 1 Oxford Centre for Evidence-Based Medicine evidence rating scale	
LOE	**Description**
I	Systematic review of randomized trials or n-of-1 trials
II	Randomized trial or observational study with dramatic effect
III	Nonrandomized controlled cohort/ follow-up study
IV	Case series, case-control studies, or historically controlled studies
V	Mechanism-based reasoning

Adapted from OCEBM Levels of Evidence Working Group. The Oxford levels of evidence 2. Oxford Centre for Evidence-Based Medicine. Available at: http://www.cebm.net/index.aspx?o55653. Accessed September 25, 2015.

equivalency between surgical treatments. Thus, prospective cohort studies or a systematic review of similar studies are often the highest LOE for prognostic studies. To this effect, the American Society of Plastic Surgeons (ASPS) separate LOE rating scales for therapeutic, diagnostic, and prognostic studies (**Tables 2–4**).[16]

Within facial plastic and reconstructive surgery, there has been a trend toward higher LOEs over the past 2 decades. Xu and colleagues[17] reviewed the LOEs for all facial plastic surgery articles in *The Laryngoscope*, *Archives of Facial Plastic Surgery*, *Otolaryngology–Head and Neck Surgery*, *Journal of Plastic Surgery*, and *Plastic and Reconstructive Surgery* between 1999 and 2008. There was a statistically significant increase in the proportion of level 2 and 3 evidence articles with a concomitant decline in proportion of level 4 and 5 evidence. Publications with level 1 evidence remained rare over that 10-year span.[17]

Although the quality of a study's design is reflected in the LOE, practice recommendations are not directly proportional. The strength of recommendations is discussed later. Systematic reviews and meta-analyses provide higher-level evidence, but are only as strong as the study design of the included reviews. In addition, the surgeon evaluating the available evidence must consider the following: ability to generalize the studies to the patient, risk-benefit analysis of treatment, evaluation of alternative treatments, and patient values.[14]

STRENGTH OF RECOMMENDATION AND CLINICAL PRACTICE GUIDELINES

In their 2011 report, "Clinical Practice Guidelines We Can Trust," the Institute of Medicine defined clinical practice guidelines as "recommendations intended to optimize patient care that are informed by a systematic review of evidence and an assessment of the benefits and harms of alternative care options."[18] Therefore, generating guidelines requires a method to rate the quality of evidence (eg, LOEs) and grade the strength of recommendations.

Like LOEs, multiple grading systems exist for recommendations, which has led to inconsistent methodologies by guideline developers.[19] In an effort to generate consistency, the Grading of Recommendations Assessment, Development and Evaluation (GRADE) Working Group has developed a rigorous and transparent method for both rating the quality of evidence and grading the strength of recommendations.

The GRADE method uses a quality-of-evidence scale, which consists of 4 categories: high quality, moderate quality, low quality, and very low quality. RCTs start off as high quality. The RCT is downgraded because of criteria such as limitations, inconsistency of results, indirectness of evidence, imprecision, and reporting bias.[19] Similarly, observational studies, which begin as low quality, may be upgraded based on a large magnitude of effect, dose-response gradient, or if all possible biases would decrease the apparent treatment effect.[19]

Grading recommendations using GRADE incorporates the LOE with the degree of uncertainty about the desired and undesired effects of the intervention, patient values, and whether the intervention would lead to appropriate use of resources.[19] There are 4 categories, using strong and weak grades either for or against an intervention.

The GRADE framework has now been adopted widely by multiple major organizations, including the World Health Organization, Cochrane Collaboration, and Centers for Disease Control and Prevention. The American Academy of Pediatrics uses a classification scheme using their own rating system for quality of evidence, which, when combined with benefit-harm analysis, provides strong recommendation, recommendation, option, or no recommendation for each intervention.[20] This grading system has been adopted

---

Table 2
ASPS scales for rating LOEs and grading recommendations: evidence rating scale for therapeutic studies

LOE	Description
I	High-quality, multicenter or single-center, randomized controlled trial with adequate power; or systematic review of these studies
II	Lesser-quality, randomized controlled trial; prospective cohort study; or systematic review of these studies
III	Retrospective comparative study; case-control study; or systematic review of these studies
IV	Case series with pretest/posttest; or only posttest
V	Expert opinion; case report or clinical example; or evidence based on physiology, bench research, or first principles

Adapted from American Society of Plastic Surgeons. Evidence rating scales. Available at: http://www.plasticsurgery.org/Documents/medical-professionals/health-policy/evidence-practice/ASPS-Rating-Scale-March-2011.pdf. Accessed September 30, 2015.

Table 3
ASPS scales for rating LOEs and grading recommendations: evidence rating scale for diagnostic studies

LOE	Description
I	High-quality, multicenter or single-center, cohort study validating a diagnostic test (with gold standard as reference) in a series of consecutive patients; or a systematic review of these studies
II	Exploratory cohort study developing diagnostic criteria (with gold standard as reference) in a series of consecutive patients; or a systematic review of these studies
III	Diagnostic study in nonconsecutive patients (without consistently applied gold standard as reference); or a systematic review of these studies
IV	Case-control study; or any of the above diagnostic studies in the absence of a universally accepted gold standard
V	Expert opinion developed via consensus process; case report or clinical example; or evidence based on physiology, bench research, or first principles

Adapted from American Society of Plastic Surgeons. Evidence rating scales. Available at: http://www.plasticsurgery.org/Documents/medical-professionals/health-policy/evidence-practice/ASPS-Rating-Scale-March-2011.pdf. Accessed September 30, 2015.

by the American Academy of Otolaryngology–Head and Neck Surgery for their clinical practice guidelines.

OUTCOMES MEASURES

An important aspect of EBM is demonstration of the value of a given intervention through outcomes-based research. This aspect becomes increasingly important with the current health care transformation from a fee-for-service to value-based reimbursement system.

Outcomes studies can be categorized as (1) patient-reported outcomes, (2) clinical efficacy outcomes, and (3) actuarial or financial outcomes.[21] Clinical efficacy outcomes can be further divided into clinician-reported outcome measures and objective outcome measures.[22]

The gold standard for patient-reported outcomes remains validated quality-of-life (QOL) instruments, either disease specific or global. The most widely used global QOL instrument in the world is the Medical Outcome Study Short Form 36-Item Health Survey.[23] The benefit of these global surveys is that they allow comparison of patient-reported outcomes in individuals with different health conditions or even healthy patients. However, they may fail to detect differences in QOL in patients with certain diseases by failing to ask relevant disease-specific questions that affect QOL.[23] This consideration is particularly important in facial plastic surgery, in which functional, aesthetic, and emotional aspects of health are variably affected by any given intervention.

Patient-reported, disease-specific instruments may be more sensitive to changes in QOL for a

Table 4
ASPS scales for rating LOEs and grading recommendations: evidence rating scale for prognostic/risk studies

LOE	Description
I	High-quality, multicenter or single-center, prospective cohort or comparative study with adequate power; or a systematic review of these studies
II	Lesser-quality prospective cohort or comparative study; retrospective cohort or comparative study; untreated controls from a randomized controlled trial; or a systematic review of these studies
III	Case-control study; or systematic review of these studies
IV	Case series with pretest/posttest; or only posttest
V	Expert opinion developed via consensus process; case report or clinical example; or evidence based on physiology, bench research, or first principles

Adapted from American Society of Plastic Surgeons. Evidence rating scales. Available at: http://www.plasticsurgery.org/Documents/medical-professionals/health-policy/evidence-practice/ASPS-Rating-Scale-March-2011.pdf. Accessed September 30, 2015.

given intervention. In facial plastic and reconstructive surgery, these have been used with various interventions, including scar treatment, facial reanimation, rhinoplasty, and facial rejuvenation procedures.[24] Although these specific QOL instruments often detect small but clinically significant changes before and after an intervention, their development requires rigorous tests of validity, reliability, and responsiveness, which can take years.[24]

Clinical efficacy outcomes research ranges from case studies to RCTs. Through clinician-reported scales or objective tools, clinical efficacy studies attempt to objectively measure effectiveness of given interventions.[24] Although many disease processes lack a gold standard for objective outcome measures, a recent increase in well-designed instruments may lend itself to the development of a gold standard objective measure.[22] Another challenge for clinical efficacy outcomes research is the lack of rigorous reliability testing or use of limited resources, limiting their universal use and acceptance.[24]

Facial reanimation studies serve as an excellent example of the application of all 3 mentioned outcome measures and are discussed later.

OUTCOME MEASURES IN FACIAL REANIMATION

Increasing options for treating dysfunction of the facial nerve (from otologic, oncologic, or idiopathic causes) provides a field of study in facial plastic and reconstructive surgery that allows for expansion of outcome measures.[25] Rhee and McMullin[24] in 2008 surveyed the existing literature for outcome measures in facial plastic surgery and found 12 grading scales for facial nerve function, 4 global scales, and 8 regional scales.

The House-Brackmann Facial Nerve Grading System (HBFNGS) was introduced in 1983 and is one of the most commonly used scales of global facial nerve function (**Table 5**). The scale ranges from normal (House-Brackmann grade I) to total paralysis (House-Brackmann grade VI) based on symmetry at rest and in motion of each facial horizontal third and the presence of synkinesis, contracture, and hemifacial spasm. It became a widely accepted tool because of its ease of use, sensitivity, and established reliability.[26] Although accurate for normal or total facial paralysis, studies found that, for differential function along different branches of the facial nerve, a single HBFNGS score did not fully capture facial function and did not correlate with the worst functioning region.[26,27]

This system led to the development of scales that focus more on regional assessment. The Sunnybrook Facial Grading System (SFGS) scores facial symmetry at rest and with voluntary movement, as well as degree of synkinesis (**Fig. 1**).[28] Resting symmetry is scored in 3 individual regions: eye, nasolabial fold, and mouth. Symmetry with

Table 5 HBFNGS	
Grade	Defined by
I	Normal facial function in all areas
II	Slight weakness noticeable only on close inspection. At rest: normal symmetry of forehead, ability to close eye with minimal effort and slight asymmetry, ability to move corners of mouth with maximal effort and slight asymmetry. No synkinesis, contracture, or hemifacial spasm
III	Obvious but not disfiguring difference between 2 sides, no functional impairment; noticeable but not severe synkinesis, contracture, and/or hemifacial spasm. At rest: normal symmetry and tone. Motion: slight to no movement of forehead, ability to close eye with maximal effort and obvious asymmetry, ability to move corners of mouth with maximal effort and obvious asymmetry. Patients who have obvious but not disfiguring synkinesis, contracture, and/or hemifacial spasm are grade III regardless of degree of motor activity
IV	Obvious weakness and/or disfiguring asymmetry. At rest: normal symmetry and tone. Motion: no movement of forehead; inability to close eye completely with maximal effort. Patients with synkinesis, mass action, and/or hemifacial spasm severe enough to interfere with function are grade IV regardless of motor activity
V	Only barely perceptible motion. At rest: possible asymmetry with droop of corner of mouth and decreased or absent nasal labial fold. Motion: no movement of forehead, incomplete closure of eye and only slight movement of lid with maximal effort, slight movement of corner of mouth. Synkinesis, contracture, and hemifacial spasm usually absent
VI	Loss of tone; asymmetry; no motion; no synkinesis, contracture, or hemifacial spasm

Resting Symmetry

Compared to normal side

Eye (choose one only)	
normal	0
narrow	1
wide	1
eyelid surgery	1
Cheek (naso-lablal fild)	
normal	0
absent	2
less pronounced	1
more pronounced	1
Mouth	
normal	0
corner dropped	1
corner pulled up/out	1
Total	☐
Resting symmetry score — Total X 5	☐

Patient's name

Dx

Date

Symmetry of Voluntary Movement / Synkinesis

Degree of muscle EXCURSION compared to normal side | **Rate the degree of INVOLUNTARY MUSCLE CONTRACTION associated with each expression**

Standard Expressions	Unable to initiate movement/no movement (Gross Asymmetry)	Initiates slight movement (Severe Asymmetry)	Initiated movement with mild excursion (Moderate Asymmetry)	Movement almost complete (Mild Asymmetry)	Movement complete (Normal Symmetry)		NONE: No synkinesis or mass movement	MILD: Slight synkinesis	MODERATE: Obvious but not disfiguring synkinesis	SEVERE: Disfiguring synkinesis/ Gross mass movement of several muscles	
Forehead Wrinkle (FRO)	1	2	3	4	5	☐	0	1	2	3	☐
Gentle eye closure (OCS)	1	2	3	4	5	☐	0	1	2	3	☐
Open mouth smile (ZYG/RIS)	1	2	3	4	5	☐	0	1	2	3	☐
Snarl (LLA/LLS)	1	2	3	4	5	☐	0	1	2	3	☐
Lip Pucker (OOS/OOI)	1	2	3	4	5	☐	0	1	2	3	☐
					Total	☐					
Voluntary movement score:					Total X 4	☐	Synkinesis score:			Total	☐

Vol mov't score ☐ – Resting symmetry score ☐ – Synk score ☐ = Composite score ☐

Fig. 1. SFGS. (*From* Ross BG, Fradet G, Nedzelski JM. Development of a sensitive clinical facial grading system. Otolaryngol Head Neck Surg 1996:114(3);380–6; with permission.)

voluntary motion is based on muscle groups and consists of the following actions: brow lift, eye closure, open-mouth smile, snarl, and lip pucker. Combined with a synkinesis score, the SFGS provides a composite score that is a continuous variable and thereby captures differences in facial function caused by regional variations. On validation testing, SFGS is at least comparable in inter-rater repeatability and was found to be superior in inter-rater reliability to HBFNGS.[28]

Patient-reported outcomes of treating facial nerve dysfunction have gained attention. Synkinesis has been found to be one of the most bothersome symptoms of facial nerve dysfunction, and affects eating, drinking, and facial expression.[29] The Synkinesis Assessment Questionnaire (Fig. 2) was developed to measure the bothersome effects of synkinesis during various facial activities by the patient, and therefore the effects on QOL.[29] The synkinesis assessment questionnaire has been validated and shown to be a reliable instrument in assessing synkinesis and to detect differences in the outcomes of facial reanimation treatments.[29]

Of particular interest, researchers have begun evaluating the outcome of surgical reconstruction, not by comparing with normal but by measuring the perception of lay and expert observers.[30] This novel idea theorizes that the repair should be adequate to allow a layperson to perceive normal, even if the perfect outcome is not achieved. Perception of a range of normal may allow less risky interventions to be performed, avoiding complications and maximizing value.

Eye-tracking technology has led to the recent development of creative objective outcomes

Synkinesis Assessment Questionnaire (SAQ)

Date:

Please answer the following questions regarding facial function, on a scale from 1 to 5, according to the following scale:

1 = seldom or not at all
2 = occasionally, or very mildly
3 = sometimes, or mildly
4 = most of the time or moderately
5 = all the time or severely

	Question	Score
1	When I smile, my eye closes	
2	When I speak, my eye closes	
3	When I whistle or pucker my lips, my eye closes	
4	When I smile, my neck tightens	
5	When I close my eyes, my face gets tight	
6	When I close my eyes, the corner of my mouth moves	
7	When I close my eyes, my neck tightens	
8	When I eat, my eye waters	
9	*When I smile, my lower lips are matched in position*	
10	When I move my face, my chin develops a dimpled area	

Total Synkinesis Score: Sum of Scores 1 to 9 / 45 X 100

Fig. 2. Original synkinesis assessment questionnaire, with question 9 removed from final questionnaire. (*Adapted from* Mehta RP, WernickRobinson M, Hadlock TA. Validation of the synkinesis assessment questionnaire. Laryngoscope 2007;117(5):924; with permission.)

research in facial paralysis. To objectively measure social perception, Dey and colleagues[30] recorded eye-movement patterns of naive observers looking at paralyzed faces before and after facial reanimation and compared with normal controls. They found deviation in eye fixation from the central triangle in paralyzed faces compared with normal, with natural redistribution after facial reanimation surgery (**Fig. 3**).

The examples given earlier show that researchers use a wide variety of outcome measures to determine the effectiveness of their interventions. The next level of research involves combining studies using similar outcomes measures in meta-analyses and systematic reviews.

CHALLENGES OF EVIDENCE-BASED MEDICINE IN FACIAL PLASTIC SURGERY

Navigating the available evidence in facial plastic and reconstructive surgery is increasingly difficult. Systematic reviews and meta-analyses provide a rigorous assembling of available evidence and reduce the effect of chance by increasing statistical power. They offer a synthesis of existing evidence in examining the safety and efficacy of medical interventions, playing an instrumental role in the development of clinical practice guidelines.[31] Identifying the objective of a systematic

review frequently involves defining a specific clinical question. PICO(S) (population, intervention, comparison, outcome [and study design]) is often used as a guide to formulate key elements of the study,[32] which is particularly challenging in facial plastic and reconstructive surgery because of limitations such as inconsistent patient characteristics, study design, and outcome measures.

An archetypal example of this is the current state of literature regarding antibiotic prophylaxis in facial fractures. Many patient-specific and fracture-specific variables that affect postoperative infection rates are omitted from studies of antibiotic prophylaxis. Some studies lack stratification of patient factors that play a large role in postoperative healing and infection rates, including immunocompromised states, malabsorption, smoking status, oral hygiene, and diabetes.[33–36] The inability to stratify patients by those factors would potentially limit a meta-analysis from detecting a difference in infection rates (outcome) for various prophylactic antibiotic regimens (intervention). Categorization of open and closed fractures is also critical, but not always performed; open fractures have higher infection rates and may require antibiotics.[37,38]

Mundinger and colleagues[39] performed a systematic review of 44 studies on the routine use of antibiotics in facial fractures. They sought

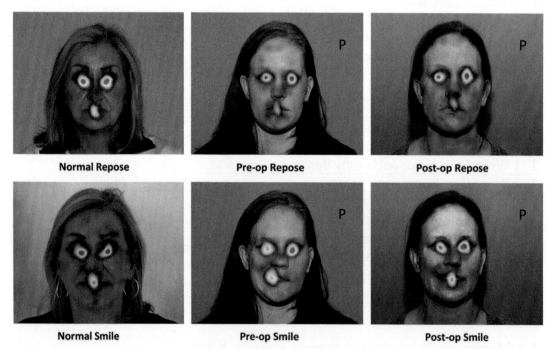

Normal Repose   **Pre-op Repose**   **Post-op Repose**

Normal Smile   **Pre-op Smile**   **Post-op Smile**

Fig. 3. Heat maps of visual fixation show the deviation in eye fixation from the central triangle in paralyzed faces (Pre-op) compared with normal, and with natural redistribution after (Post-op) facial reanimation surgery. (*From* Dey JK, Ishii LE, Byrne PJ, et al. Seeing is believing: objectively evaluating the impact of facial reanimation surgery on social perception. Laryngoscope 2014;124(11):2491; with permission.)

additional covariates that would alter the use of antibiotic prophylaxis in facial fracture treatment. Collectively, these studies supported the use of antibiotics preoperatively only in comminuted mandible fractures, perioperative antibiotics in all facial fractures, and no postoperative antibiotics. In contrast with this systematic review, a survey of expert opinions at the Advanced Orbital Surgery Symposium showed antibiotic use in the preoperative, perioperative, and postoperative periods at the following rates: upper face fractures 47.1%, 94.1%, 70.6%; midface fractures 47.1%, 100%, 70.6%; and mandible fractures 68.8%, 94.1%, 64.7%, respectively.[39]

The incongruence can in part be explained by surgeons having to treat individual patients with complex medical history or wounds and is not represented by the patients in the literature, which represents the argument of many surgeons who recognize the ultimate challenge of implementing EBM in clinical practice. Future goals must drive clinicians to extend the current evidence by including multidisciplinary, multi-institutional, and well-defined outcomes.

REFERENCES

1. Tollefson TT. A place for innovation and rigorous surgical research in evidence-based medicine. Curr Opin Otolaryngol Head Neck Surg 2014;22(4):253–4.
2. Sackett DL, Haynes RB, Gibson ES, et al. Randomized clinical trial of strategies for improving medication compliance in primary hypertension. Lancet 1975;1(7918):1205–7.
3. How to read clinical journals: I. Why to read them and how to start reading them critically. Can Med Assoc J 1981;124(5):555–8.
4. Evidence-Based Medicine Working Group. Evidence-based medicine. A new approach to teaching the practice of medicine. JAMA 1992;268(17):2420–5.
5. Sackett DL, Rosenberg WM, Gray JA, et al. Evidence based medicine: what it is and what it isn't. BMJ 1996;312:71–2.
6. Aravind M, Chung KC. Evidence-based medicine and hospital reform: tracing origins back to Florence Nightingale. Plast Reconstr Surg 2010;125:403–9.
7. Kaska SC, Weinstein JN. Historical perspective. Ernest Amory Codman, 1869–1940. A pioneer of evidence-based medicine: the end result idea. Spine (Phila Pa 1976) 1998;23:629–33.
8. Stam J, Vermeulen M. Eugen Bleuler (1857-1939), an early pioneer of evidence based medicine. J Neurol Neurosurg Psychiatr 2013;84(6):594–5.
9. Guyatt GH, Haynes RB, Jaeschke RZ, et al. Users' guides to the medical literature: XXV. Evidence-based medicine: principles for applying the users' guides to patient care. Evidence-Based Medicine Working Group. JAMA 2000;284(10):1290–6.
10. Lee MK, Most SP. Evidence-based medicine: rhinoplasty. Facial Plast Surg Clin North Am 2015;23(3):303–12.
11. The periodic health examination. Canadian Task Force on the Periodic Health Examination. Can Med Assoc J 1979;121:1193–254.
12. Burns PB, Rohrich RJ, Chung KC. The levels of evidence and their role in evidence-based medicine. Plast Reconstr Surg 2011;128(1):305–10.
13. Sackett DL. Rules of evidence and clinical recommendations on the use of antithrombotic agents. Chest 1986;89(2 Suppl):2S–3S.
14. J Howick, I Chalmers, P Glasziou, et al. Explanation of the 2011 Oxford Centre for Evidence-Based Medicine (OCEBM) levels of evidence (background document). Oxford Centre for Evidence-Based Medicine. Available at: http://www.cebm.net/index.aspx?o=5653. Accessed September 30, 2015.
15. Devries JG, Berlet GC. Understanding levels of evidence for scientific communication. Foot Ankle Spec 2010;3(4):205–9.
16. American Society of Plastic Surgeons Evidence Rating Scales. Available at: http://www.plasticsurgery.org/Documents/medical-professionals/health-policy/evidence-practice/ASPS-Rating-Scale-March-2011.pdf. Accessed September 30, 2015.
17. Xu CC, Côté DW, Chowdhury RH, et al. Trends in level of evidence in facial plastic surgery research. Plast Reconstr Surg 2011;127(4):1499–504.
18. Consensus report, Institute of Medicine. Clinical practice guidelines we can trust. 2011. Available at: http://www.iom.edu/Reports/2011/Clinical-Practice-Guidelines-We-Can-Trust.aspx. Accessed on October 15, 2015.
19. Guyatt GH, Oxman AD, Vist GE, et al. GRADE: an emerging consensus on rating quality of evidence and strength of recommendations. BMJ 2008;336(7650):924–6.
20. Classifying recommendations for clinical practice guidelines. Pediatrics 2004;114(3):874–7.
21. Luce EA. Outcome studies and practice guidelines in plastic surgery. Plast Reconstr Surg 1999;104(4):1187–90.
22. Rhee JS, McMullin BT. Measuring outcomes in facial plastic surgery: a decade of progress. Curr Opin Otolaryngol Head Neck Surg 2008;16(4):387–93.
23. Pusic AL, Lemaine V, Klassen AF, et al. Patient-reported outcome measures in plastic surgery: use and interpretation in evidence-based medicine. Plast Reconstr Surg 2011;127(3):1361–7.
24. Rhee JS, McMullin BT. Outcome measures in facial plastic surgery: patient-reported and clinical

efficacy measures. Arch Facial Plast Surg 2008; 10(3):194–207.

25. Teng J, Christophel JJ. Early practice focus: evidence-based practice in facial plastic surgery. Facial Plast Surg Clin North Am 2015;23(3):393–405.

26. Yen TL, Driscoll CL, Lalwani AK. Significance of House-Brackmann facial nerve grading global score in the setting of differential facial nerve function. Otol Neurotol 2003;24(1):118–22.

27. Reitzen SD, Babb JS, Lalwani AK. Significance and reliability of the House-Brackmann grading system for regional facial nerve function. Otolaryngol Head Neck Surg 2009;140(2):154–8.

28. Kanerva M, Poussa T, Pitkäranta A. Sunnybrook and House-Brackmann facial grading systems: intrarater repeatability and interrater agreement. Otolaryngology Head Neck Surg 2006;135(6):865–71.

29. Mehta RP, WernickRobinson M, Hadlock TA. Validation of the Synkinesis Assessment Questionnaire. Laryngoscope 2007;117(5):923–6.

30. Dey JK, Ishii LE, Byrne PJ, et al. Seeing is believing: objectively evaluating the impact of facial reanimation surgery on social perception. Laryngoscope 2014;124(11):2489–97.

31. Liberati A, Altman DG, Tetzlaff J, et al. The PRISMA statement for reporting systematic reviews and meta-analyses of studies that evaluate health care interventions: explanation and elaboration. J Clin Epidemiol 2009;62(10):e1–34.

32. Hassouneh B, Brenner MJ. Systematic review and meta-analysis in facial plastic surgery. Facial Plast Surg Clin North Am 2015;23(3):273–83.

33. Zix J, Schaller B, Iizuka T, et al. The role of postoperative prophylactic antibiotics in the treatment of facial fractures: a randomized, double blind, placebo-controlled pilot clinical study. Part 1: orbital fractures in 62 patients. Br J Oral Maxillofac Surg 2013;51(4):332–6.

34. Schaller B, Soong PL, Zix J, et al. The role of postoperative prophylactic antibiotics in the treatment of facial fractures: a randomized, double blind, placebo-controlled pilot clinical study. Part 2: Mandibular fractures in 59 patients. Br J Oral Maxillofac Surg 2013;51(8):803–7.

35. Soong PL, Schaller B, Zix J, et al. The role of postoperative prophylactic antibiotics in the treatment of facial fractures: a randomized, double-blind, placebo-controlled pilot clinical study. Part 3: Le Fort and zygomatic fractures in 94 patients. Br J Oral Maxillofac Surg 2014;52(4):329–33.

36. Mottini M, Wolf R, Soong PL, et al. The role of postoperative antibiotics in facial fractures: comparing the efficacy of a 1-day versus a prolonged regimen. J Trauma Acute Care Surg 2014;76(3):720–4.

37. Aderhold L, Jung H, Frenkel G. Untersuchungen über den werteiner Antibiotika Prophylaxe bei Kiefer-Gesichtsverletzungen. Eine prospective Studie. Dtsch Zahnarztl Z 1983;38:402.

38. Lauder A, Jalisi S, Spiegel J, et al. Antibiotic prophylaxis in the management of complex midface and frontal sinus trauma. Laryngoscope 2010;120(10): 1940–5.

39. Mundinger GS, Borsuk DE, Okhah Z, et al. Antibiotics and facial fractures: evidence-based recommendations compared with experience-based practice. Craniomaxillofac Trauma Reconstr 2015; 8(1):64–78.

Controversies in Contemporary Facial Reanimation

Leslie Kim, MD, MPH, Patrick J. Byrne, MD, MBA*

KEYWORDS

- Facial reanimation • Facial paralysis • Facial palsy • Dynamic reanimation • Nerve transfers
- Free gracilis muscle transfer

KEY POINTS

- Determining the cause, pattern, and duration of facial palsy is critical. Timely intervention is perhaps the most important factor that influences outcome after facial reanimation.
- Smile reanimation options include regional muscle transfer, neurotization, and free muscle transfer. The selection of a donor nerve for the last two is highly individualized.
- Dual innervation by the masseteric nerve and cross-facial nerve graft may optimize both strength and spontaneity of movement when free muscle transfer is used.
- Analysis of clinical outcomes in facial nerve reconstruction remains limited because of the lack of universal evaluation methods and standardized outcome measures.

 Video content accompanies this article at http://www.facialplastic.theclinics.com

INTRODUCTION

Facial palsy (FP) is a devastating condition with profound functional, aesthetic, and psychosocial implications. Injury to the facial nerve disrupts the complex association between facial expression and emotion, thereby compromising social interactions and adversely affecting quality of life.[1,2] FP can result in a myriad of aesthetic and functional sequelae, including facial asymmetry, paralytic lagophthalmos and subsequent exposure keratopathy, eyelid retraction and ectropion, nasal obstruction secondary to nasal valve collapse, impaired oral competence, and articulation deficits. Ultimate outcomes following facial nerve insult are widely heterogeneous, ranging from full return of normal function to complete flaccid facial paralysis, with varying degrees of static and kinetic hypoactivity, hyperactivity, and synkinesis in between. There are numerous causes of FP. The most common cause is Bell palsy, followed by benign or malignant tumors, iatrogenic injury, Varicella-zoster virus–associated FP, trauma, and congenital palsy.[3] The treatment of FP is equally as diverse and requires a thoughtful, highly individualized approach based on the cause, pattern, and time course of FP.

OVERVIEW OF FACIAL REANIMATION

Although the complexity of facial expression and intricate synergy of facial mimetic muscles are difficult to fully restore, the ultimate goal of FP treatment is to reestablish facial symmetry and movement. Static techniques and nonsurgical procedures lack true reanimation, although they are a useful adjunct in many patients to improve facial resting appearance. In order to identify the appropriate techniques for dynamic reanimation, it is essential to have a thorough understanding of

Disclosure: No commercial or financial conflicts of interest and no funding sources.
Division of Facial Plastic & Reconstructive Surgery, Department of Otolaryngology-Head and Neck Surgery, Johns Hopkins Medicine, 601 North Caroline Street, 6th Floor, Baltimore, MD 21287-0910, USA
* Corresponding author.
E-mail address: PBYRNE2@jhmi.edu

the mechanism and extent of facial nerve injury, the duration of palsy, and viability of facial musculature. Equally as important are patient factors, such as age, overall health, motivation, and goals for rehabilitation. A holistic approach with attention to both the paralyzed and nonparalyzed sides of the face tends to yield more effective results.[4]

Classification of Facial Palsy

Outcomes following facial nerve insult are widely heterogeneous, ranging from full return of normal function to complete flaccid facial paralysis, with varying degrees of static and kinetic hypoactivity, hyperactivity, and synkinesis in between. *Complete flaccid FP* results in loss of symmetry at rest, paralytic lagophthalmos, nasal obstruction, oral incompetence, and loss of dynamic facial movement. In *nonflaccid FP*, symptoms are dictated by the specific pattern of dysfunction with varying degrees of mass movement and synkinesis occurring on the affected side and compensatory hyperactivity on the healthy side. Lack of a meaningful smile can also occur in severe nonflaccid palsy.[5] It is important to identify the type of facial paralysis as it intimately affects management.

Reversible Versus Irreversible Facial Palsy

One of the most critical assessments in FP management is determining whether the FP is reversible or irreversible. Although *reanimation* (via regional or free muscle transfer) is possible even in cases of irreversible paralysis, *reinnervation* is not. Thus, the clock starts ticking from the day of onset of facial paralysis. Facial nerve biopsies from patients with long-term FP show that the size and number of nerve axons decline even during the first 3 months.[6] Facial muscles with *reversible* palsy have viable muscle fibers with intact motor units that will respond to ingrowing axons. When the time from injury to reinnervation exceeds more than 18 to 24 months, facial paralysis becomes *irreversible;* denervated muscles develop nonfunctional motor end plates and irreversible atrophy, eliminating any chance of successful reinnervation.[7]

Key Principles in Dynamic Facial Reanimation

The facial nucleus and nerve provide tone, volitional movement, and emotional animation that cannot be adequately replaced. Where feasible, *primary facial nerve repair* provides the best outcomes. When tension-free primary repair is not possible but the proximal facial nerve remains intact and available, a *nerve interposition graft* (most commonly with the greater auricular or sural

nerve) is the next best choice.[8] However, when the proximal facial nerve stump is not available because of damage of its intracranial and/or intratemporal segments, *neurotization or nerve transfer* using a new motor nerve is an option. Neurotization procedures seek to repurpose an alternative neural source to restore existing facial mimetic muscles and are indicated when the native muscles remain amenable to reinnervation. The most commonly used nerve substitutes are the contralateral facial nerve, motor nerve to the masseter muscle, and the hypoglossal nerve.

Methods that reinnervate native facial muscles in a timely matter are preferred if possible, as no other skeletal muscle can adequately simulate the complex morphology and organization of facial mimetic muscles. However, when native muscles are congenitally absent or are irreversibly paralyzed because of prolonged denervation, *regional muscle transfer* (ie, temporalis tendon transfer) or *free muscle transfer* (ie, microvascular gracilis muscle transfer) can be used to replace muscle function in dynamic reanimation. Static suspension techniques, nonsurgical procedures such as chemodenervation, and physical therapy are useful adjuvant and, sometimes, primary treatment options for some patients.

The duration of facial muscle denervation and timeliness of intervention are perhaps the most important factors that determine the ultimate success of any reinnervation procedure.[7,9] Patient age has also been shown to be an important factor influencing outcomes, with elderly age associated with poorer results.[8–10] The age-related decline in neural regeneration is well established and thought to be multifactorial, secondary to myelin sheath deterioration, axonal atrophy, decline in nerve conduction, and slower rate of axonal regeneration.[11]

CONTROVERSIES IN CONTEMPORARY FACIAL REANIMATION

The management of FP is challenging because of the wide variability in cause and presentation and the diversity of available treatment options. Contemporary facial reanimation is particularly charged with debate in the following areas (summary in **Table 1**):

Patient evaluation
- How should FP be graded and outcomes assessed?

Timing of intervention
- At what point in the time course of FP is reanimation surgery appropriate, particularly in

cases of complete facial paralysis whereby the facial nerve is anatomically intact?

Smile reanimation
- What is the optimal approach for smile reanimation? What is the best donor nerve for neurotization or free muscle transfer procedures and why? When is regional muscle transfer a better choice than free muscle transfer? What is the role for reanimation surgery in incomplete, nonflaccid FP?

An evidence-based discussion regarding these controversial questions is presented.

CONTROVERSIES IN PATIENT EVALUATION

A thorough history should elicit the cause of FP, onset and duration, clinical symptoms, patient concerns, and goals of care. Comprehensive physical examination should then be performed in a zonal fashion to systematically assess facial function.[12] Photographs and video recordings are essential for documenting facial appearance at rest and during a full range of volitional movements (repetitive blink, brow elevation, light-effort and full-effort eye closure, lip pucker, light-effort and full-effort smile, and lower lip depression). These photographs and video recordings should be obtained on presentation and at every follow-up visit.

Facial Palsy Grading Scales

The measurement of facial nerve function through a robust grading system is essential for evaluating and communicating the course of FP and outcomes after intervention.[13] However, the development of a universal grading system is challenged by the complexity of facial nerve dysfunction and the inherent subjectivity of describing facial expression. Consensus among facial nerve specialists regarding appropriate clinician-graded and patient-reported scales is lacking.[14]

The ideal facial nerve grading system should be relatively quick and convenient, reproducible with low interobserver variability, include measures of both static and dynamic components of facial muscle function, and incorporate secondary defects of facial nerve dysfunction, such as synkinesis.[15] Introduced in 1983 and officially endorsed by the American Academy of Otolaryngology–Head and Neck Surgery (AAO-HNS), the Facial Nerve Grading System 1.0 or more commonly known as the House-Brackmann (HB) scale[16] (**Table 2**) has been the standard for facial nerve disorders. It is a 6-point grading scale originally intended solely for reporting the degree of FP following

vestibular schwannoma resection. As it has been applied to a variety of other conditions that result in FP, the major criticisms of the HB scale have been its lack of sensitivity in tracking zonal changes and in distinguishing subtle differences in facial nerve recovery as well as poor interobserver reliability.[15]

Newer scales have been developed as a result; the most commonly used one is the Sunnybrook scale (**Table 3**).[17] Published in 1996, it is a weighted system that provides a composite score based on the evaluation of resting symmetry, degree of voluntary excursion, as well as synkinesis. Although it is susceptible to the same interobserver variability as the HB scale, the Sunnybrook system provides a continuous scale that is more sensitive to finer differences in facial nerve function. In 2009, the Facial Nerve Disorders Committee of the AAO-HNS published a revised version of the HB scale called the Facial Nerve Grading System 2.0 (**Table 4**),[18] with the goal of preserving the simplicity of the original while incorporating the valuable features of the newer grading scales. This new system includes regional scoring of facial movements and accounts for synkinesis but maintains agreement comparable with the original scale.[18]

A recently validated electronic facial paralysis assessment tool (eFACE) is a 16-item clinician-graded digital instrument that allows for the assessment of static, dynamic, and synkinesis parameters on continuous scales.[19] It consists of a database-linked graphical user interface designed for rapid administration using a touch-screen device. In this smart-phone and tablet-dominated age, the eFACE software is a promising new tool, still being studied to define its ease, reproducibility, and application in clinical practice. A digital and database-amenable format, if globally accepted, would be tremendous in permitting easy communication among providers and patients and in allowing comparison of different treatments across studies.

In addition to clinician-graded scales for facial function, standardized patient-graded assessments of symptom severity and quality of life are necessary to track the burden of disease as well as response to interventions. The Facial Disability Index[20] and the Facial Clinimetric Evaluation[21] are validated for use in FP and are highly recommended for tracking patient experience and response to interventions over time.

CONTROVERSIES IN TIMING OF DYNAMIC REANIMATION

When the facial nerve is interrupted, there is no question that immediate or early nerve repair is

Table 1
Summary of controversies in contemporary facial reanimation

Controversial Topics	Summary Points
Patient evaluation: Evaluating patients with FP is challenging because of the wide variability in cause, presentation, and treatment options.	
FP grading scales	• A universal facial nerve grading scale would allow the effective comparison of outcomes from different management strategies. There is currently a lack of consensus among facial nerve specialists. • The *HB* (FNGS 1.0) and *Sunnybrook scales* are the most commonly used. A revised *FNGS 2.0* was recently published by the AAO-HNS. New digital instruments are of interest. • *Best practice:* Consistent use of one or more clinician-graded and patient-reported scales is recommended until consensus is reached.
Timing of dynamic reanimation: When the facial nerve is interrupted, there is no question that immediate or early nerve repair is recommended. Timing is not so clear in cases of complete facial paralysis whereby the facial nerve is thought to be anatomically intact, such as after vestibular schwannoma extirpation.	
Timing of intervention	• The chance of potential spontaneous recovery must be weighed against the risk that delayed innervation might result in a poorer outcome. Prognostic factors for spontaneous recovery are lacking. • *Rate of recovery* during the first year after injury has recently been shown to predict long-term recovery. • *Best practice:* If patients with an anatomically intact facial nerve and HB grade V to VI do not improve at least one HB grade after 6 months of observation, consider early reinnervation to limit the degenerative effects of muscle denervation.
Smile reanimation: Dynamic smile reanimation may be achieved through reinnervation of native facial musculature (in reversible paralysis) via nerve transfer procedures or replacement of facial mimetic muscles (in irreversible paralysis) with regional or free muscle transfers.	
Nerve transfers: selection of a donor nerve	• *CFNG:* Only a donor is capable of producing a truly spontaneous/emotional smile. Limitations are the time-sensitive nature (denervation ≤6 mo), 2 coaptations, relatively weak motor donor, and donor sensory deficits. • *Masseteric nerve:* Many advantages include limited donor morbidity, proximity and similar diameter to the facial nerve, single coaptation, rich motor donor, rapid recovery, and ease of cortical adaptation. Its main limitation is that the smile that evolves may be effortless but not truly spontaneous and requires motor retraining therapy. • *Hypoglossal nerve:* It is used less often given the potential for significant hemiglossal dysfunction, despite evolution in techniques. • *Babysitter procedure/dual innervation:* CFNG with masseteric nerve or mini-hypoglossal nerve innervation may provide both improvements in resting tone as well as in smile excursion. • *Best practice:* The choice is highly individualized. The desire for spontaneous/emotional smile and the preference to avoid postoperative motor training favors CFNG innervation. Masseteric innervation may be more suitable for older patients, those who do not want to undergo 2 stages, and those who could benefit from its motor strength, such as patients with a heavy face, significant rest asymmetry, or powerful smile on their normal side. Dual innervation may be optimal in select patients.

Regional muscle transfer vs free muscle transfer	• Limited literature directly compares T3 vs free muscle transfer. Evidence suggests that free muscle transfer achieves greater oral commissure excursion; but it is a complex procedure that requires an inpatient stay, risks adding undesirable bulk to the face, and results in a delay of many months prior to dynamic movement. Conversely, T3 is a reliable, quick, outpatient procedure with short postoperative recovery, immediate improvement in symmetry, and early dynamic movement. • *Best practice:* This choice is best determined with the patients' age, comorbidities, motivation, and goals of care in mind.
Free muscle transfers: selection of a donor nerve	• Advantages/disadvantages of each donor nerve choice described earlier also apply. Additional relevant topics include the following: • *1- vs 2-stage CFNG:* The literature is conflicted but the classic 2-stage procedure currently prevails; it theoretically avoids denervation atrophy of the gracilis in the face while awaiting neural regeneration across the CFNG. • *Masseteric vs CFNG:* Several recent studies show better oral commissure excursion with free gracilis powered by the masseteric nerve compared with the CFNG, in both children and adults. • *Dual innervation:* It is increasingly popular, but questions remain regarding the number of stages and the ideal coaptation pattern. • *Best practice:* Free muscle transfer (gracilis) is the current criterion standard in dynamic smile reanimation. Although CFNG has long been considered the ideal donor nerve, masseteric innervation and dual innervation are becoming increasingly popular, the latter for optimizing both strength and spontaneity.
Reanimation in incomplete palsy	• Some patients with nonflaccid FP recover with facial tone at rest but diminished/absent excursion with movement. The presence of some degree of nerve function complicates intervention. • Neurotization procedures should be used when additional innervation is thought to result in more muscle fiber recruitment. • If additional innervation is not expected to recruit more facial mimetic motion, functional muscle transfer is a better option. Clinically, these patients are those who have recovered with varying degrees of hyperactivity and synkinesis. • *Best practice:* The optimal approach is to functionally upgrade tone and movement without sacrificing any existing function.

Abbreviations: AAO-HNS, American Academy of Otolaryngology-Head and Neck Surgery; CFNG, cross-facial nerve graft; FNGS, Facial Nerve Grading System; HB, House-Brackmann; T3, temporalis tendon transfer.

Table 2
Facial nerve grading system 1.0/House-Brackmann scale

Grade	Gross	Resting Tone	Forehead	Eye Closure	Mouth
I					
Normal function	Normal	Normal	Normal	Normal	Normal
II					
Mild dysfunction	Slight weakness	Normal	Moderate to good movement	Complete with minimal effort	Slight asymmetry
III					
Moderate dysfunction	Obvious difference, noticeable synkinesis	Normal	Slight to moderate movement	Complete with full effort	Slightly weak with maximal effort
IV					
Moderately severe dysfunction	Disfiguring asymmetry	Normal	None	Incomplete	Asymmetric with maximal effort
V					
Severe dysfunction	Barely perceptible motion	Asymmetric	None	Incomplete	Slight movement
VI					
Total paralysis	No movement	Asymmetric	None	Incomplete	No movement

From House JW, Brackmann DE. Facial nerve grading system. Otolaryngol Head Neck Surg 1985;93:146; with permission.

recommended, ideally with tension-free primary repair or interposition grafting. The timing is not so clear in cases of complete facial paralysis whereby the facial nerve is thought to be anatomically in continuity, a scenario that is unfortunately not uncommon after cerebellopontine angle (CPA) tumor extirpation. If there is a potential for recovery, a period of observation of 1 year has been traditionally recommended. However, this approach delays the timely intervention in the subset of patients who ultimately do not recover spontaneously or satisfactorily. Identifying patients who will ultimately benefit from early intervention is desirable but challenging as no patient, tumor, or intraoperative factors have yet been found to be reliably prognostic of a poor outcome.[22]

In a review of 281 patients with an anatomically intact facial nerve following vestibular schwannoma resection, Rivas and colleagues[23] found that the rate of recovery during the first year could be used to predict long-term facial nerve recovery. Their predictive model using rate of functional improvement as the sole independent variable was found to anticipate poor outcomes in patients with initial HB grades V to VI as soon as 7 months after surgery, with 97% sensitivity and 97%

specificity. Therefore, they suggest that after resection of a vestibular schwannoma, if a patient with an anatomically intact facial nerve and an HB grade V to VI shows no improvement of at least one HB grade after 6 months of observation, early reinnervation should be considered to limit the degenerative effects of muscle denervation. Rivas and colleagues[23] also observed that lack of intraoperative electromyographic facial nerve stimulation at the brainstem after tumor resection had a strong correlation with poor functional outcome. However, when present, the nerve stimulation response threshold failed to correlate with facial nerve function.

In a follow-up study using the rate of recovery during the first 6 months after CPA tumor resection as the sole predictor of outcome, patients with postoperative FP (with an anatomically intact facial nerve) were prospectively stratified into an observation group and an intervention group.[24] The observation group was composed of patients who were expected to spontaneously regain satisfactory facial function. The intervention group consisted of patients who showed no clinical signs of recovery by 6 months postoperatively and were offered nerve transfer using the masseteric or

Table 3
Sunnybrook facial nerve grading system

Resting Symmetry (Compared with Normal Side)		Symmetry of Voluntary Movement (Compared with Normal Side)						Synkinesis			
		Expression	No Movement	Slight Movement	Mild Excursion	Almost Complete Movement	Complete Movement	None	Mild	Moderate	Severe
Eye											
Normal	0	Forehead wrinkle	1	2	3	4	5	0	1	2	3
Narrow	1										
Wide	1	Gentle eye closure	1	2	3	4	5	0	1	2	3
Eyelid surgery	1										
Cheek (NLF)											
Normal	0	Open mouth smile	1	2	3	4	5	0	1	2	3
Absent	2										
Less pronounced	1	Snarl	1	2	3	4	5	0	1	2	3
More pronounced	1										
Mouth											
Normal	0	Lip pucker	1	2	3	4	5	0	1	2	3
Corner drooped	1										
Corner pulled up/out	1										
Total ____		Total ____						Total ____			
Total × 5 = Resting symmetry score		Total × 4 = voluntary movement score						Total × 1 = synkinesis score			

COMPOSITE SCORE = Voluntary movement score – resting symmetry score – synkinesis score.

Abbreviation: NLF, nasolabial fold.

From Ross BG, Fradet G, Nedzelski JM. Development of a sensitive clinical facial grading system. Otolaryngol Head Neck Surg 1996;114:382; with permission.

Table 4
Facial nerve grading system 2.0

Score	Region			
	Brow	Eye	NLF	Oral
1	Normal	Normal	Normal	Normal
2	Slight weakness >75% of normal	Slight weakness >75% of normal Complete closure with mild effort	Slight weakness >75% of normal	Slight weakness >75% of normal
3	Obvious weakness >50% of normal	Obvious weakness >50% of normal Complete closure with maximal effort	Obvious weakness >50% of normal Resting symmetry	Obvious weakness >50% of normal Resting symmetry
4	Asymmetry at rest <50% of normal	Asymmetry at rest <50% of normal Cannot close completely	Asymmetry at rest <50% of normal	Asymmetry at rest <50% of normal
5	Trace movement	Trace movement	Trace movement	Trace movement
6	No movement	No movement	No movement	No movement

Score	Degree of Secondary Movement
0	None
1	Slight synkinesis; minimal contracture
2	Obvious synkinesis; mild to moderate contracture
3	Disfiguring synkinesis; severe contracture

Grade	Total Score (Sum for Each Region and Secondary Movement)
I	4
II	5–9
III	10–14
IV	15–19
V	20–23
VI	24

Abbreviation: NLF, nasolabial fold.
From Vrabec JT, Backous DD, Djalilian HR, et al. Facial nerve grading system 2.0. Otolaryngol Head Neck Surg 2009;140:447; with permission.

hypoglossal nerve. Overall, early facial reanimation surgery decreased the total duration of paralysis. Masseteric nerve grafting resulted in earlier recovery compared with hypoglossal nerve grafting (5.6 vs 10.8 months). In patients who underwent nerve grafting, there was a 0% risk of premature intervention; direct facial nerve stimulation at the time of surgery yielded no electromyographic response and facial muscle contraction in all of these patients. Of note, 8 patients who demonstrated no signs of recovery by 6 months postoperatively but declined surgery demonstrated, at best, an HB grade V recovery after a mean follow-up of 20 months. This finding provides some insight into the natural course of the anatomically intact but injured facial nerve, when early facial nerve function is poor.

Timing of intervention has also been shown to be critical in patients with vestibular schwannoma who present with preoperative FP. Ozmen and colleagues[25] retrospectively reviewed 194 patients who underwent interposition grafting in the internal auditory canal at the time of vestibular schwannoma resection and found that duration of preoperative facial nerve deficit was the only significant predictor of prognosis; the most critical time for recovery to HB grades III and IV function was preoperative deficit of 6 months or less. When suboptimal recovery of the repaired facial nerve is expected, such as in the setting of prolonged preoperative FP, a masseteric nerve or hypoglossal nerve interposition graft can be coapted to a distal buccal branch for signal upgrading, leaving the facial nerve intact.[22]

The specific timing considerations for neural transfer techniques are discussed in a later section.

CONTROVERSIES IN DYNAMIC SMILE REANIMATION

Dynamic facial reanimation seeks to restore 2 critical functions: eyelid reanimation and smile reconstruction. Although treatment options for periocular reanimation are complex, they are less fraught with controversy and the goals are simple: to maximize corneal protection and improve periocular symmetry. The authors, therefore, focus on dynamic smile reanimation in the remainder of this article.

Depending on the time course and pattern of FP, dynamic smile reanimation may be achieved through *reinnervation* of native facial musculature (in *reversible* paralysis) via nerve transfer procedures or *replacement* of facial mimetic muscles (in *irreversible* paralysis) with regional or free muscle transfers.

Selection of a Donor Nerve for Direct Reinnervation

When the ipsilateral facial nucleus and proximal facial nerve are not available, neurotization procedures are used to repurpose an alternative neural source to restore facial mimetic muscles that remain amenable to reinnervation. The most commonly used donor nerves in facial reanimation are the contralateral facial nerve, masseteric nerve, and hypoglossal nerve. The accessory, phrenic, and C4 and C7 root nerves have also been used.[9] Each donor nerve varies with respect to its donor deficit and morbidity, axonal density and motor power, and synergy with facial expression to allow for cortical readaptation in function.

Contralateral facial nerve (cross-facial nerve graft)

Originally developed by Scaramella[26] and Smith[27] working independently in the early 1970s, the cross-facial nerve graft (CFNG) has long been considered the criterion standard donor nerve source (**Box 1, Fig. 1**). By synchronizing the transmission of neural impulses from the contralateral, intact facial nerve to similar branches of the affected facial nerve through the use of an interposition nerve graft (most commonly, the sural nerve or greater auricular nerve), the CFNG is the only procedure that is capable of producing a truly spontaneous/emotional smile in addition to improving resting tone.

However, there are several limitations. First, to use this as a stand-alone technique, the denervation time must be less than 6 months. This requirement is based on the premise that axons regenerating at 1 to 2 mm/d will take up to 6 to 9 months to cross a 15- to 20-cm CFNG. Because muscles denervated for 1 year start developing nonfunctional motor end plates and irreversible atrophy, a denervation interval of greater than 6 months results in suboptimal reinnervation. CFNGs are also noted to be relatively weak motor donors[28] and neural input from the contralateral facial nerve must cross 2 sites of coaptation. Only 20% to 50% of axons generally cross a nerve graft,[29] which can be problematic for the CFNG, as the axonal load has been shown to correlate with functional outcome.[30] Despite using the largest donor nerve that does not produce a functional deficit on the unaffected side, muscle excursion achieved with the CFNG can sometimes be limited, particularly in older patients who have decreased potential for neural regeneration.[31] If a donor buccal branch from the intact side is not carefully selected, facial weakness in the normal side as well as problematic blink-triggered activation or ocular synkinesis can result. Lastly, permanent sensory deficits secondary to the donor nerve harvest are not trivial.

Masseteric nerve (cranial nerve V to VII) transfer

In 1978, Spira[32] first reported the use of the motor nerve to the masseter muscle for facial reanimation (**Box 2, Figs. 2** and **3**).[32] It was initially popularized for reinnervation of free muscle transfers and, over the past decade, has increasingly become the technique of choice for direct neurotization.[33]

First, there is limited donor site morbidity. Functional loss from partial denervation of the masseter muscle is minimal as the masseter and temporalis muscles work together in mastication and only the descending branch is divided, leaving the more proximal branches intact. The main trunk of the masseteric nerve is typically identified 3 cm anterior to the tragus and 1 cm below the zygomatic arch, and the descending branch consistently courses obliquely towards the oral commissure between the deep and middle layers of the muscle.[34,35] The subzygomatic triangle using the zygomatic arch, temporomandibular joint, and the frontal branch of the facial nerve provides a rapid method for identifying the nerve with minimal dissection.[36]

Because of its proximity and similar diameter to the facial nerve, the masseteric nerve can be directly anastomosed to the facial nerve without the use of an interposition graft.[37] It is a rich source of myelinated motor fibers; although the absolute count depends on the method of

---

Box 1
Surgical pearls for cross-facial nerve grafting

Nerve selection

- The most commonly used donor nerve is the sural nerve because of its ease of access, modest donor site morbidity, and favorable length (25–35 cm).
- The medial antebrachial cutaneous nerve has a branching pattern that should be considered for immediate reconstruction of the main facial nerve trunk and pes anserinus after their resection (ie, in radical parotidectomy).

Sural nerve harvest

- The authors find stair-step incisions to be efficient and favorable. A single incision is possible with endoscopic assistance.
- Use of a tendon stripper and long thin malleables are very helpful in the dissection.
- Mark the inferior end for orientation; this end should be coapted to the donor facial nerve on the nonparalyzed side.

Identification of the donor facial nerve

- The donor branches of interest are generally at the midpoint of a line between the tragus and the oral commissure, approximately 2 cm below the zygoma.
- The ideal nerve activates the zygomatic muscle complex, elevating the oral commissure and defining the nasolabial fold. As long as 1 to 2 additional branches that also innervate the zygomatic complex are identified, use the largest branch for the donor (number of axons predicts outcome).

Subcutaneous tunnel

- A subcutaneous tunnel is extended from the selected buccal branch on the intact side to the pretragal region on the contralateral paralyzed side (see **Fig. 1**). A small gingivolabial incision helps connect the two sides.
- If the CFNG is being used to innervate a free muscle transfer, it can be banked within a gingivolabial incision for later coaptation to the obturator nerve. A polypropylene (Prolene) stitch can facilitate its later identification.
- The use of a tendon stripper or a plastic drain with a trocar (where the sural nerve is sutured to the end) is very helpful for creating the subcutaneous tunnel.

Neurorrhaphy

- Two to 3 epineural 9-0 nylon sutures are used to perform a meticulous microneural anastomosis. Some surgeons wrap the coaptation in a dural regeneration matrix (Durepair) and secure it with a fibrin sealant (Evicel) to thwart loss of axons into surrounding tissues. Others prefer sutures alone, as the data on benefit are inconclusive.
- If only one dominant buccal branch on the nonparalyzed side is identified, neurorrhaphy can be performed end-to-side after partial axotomy in the donor nerve.

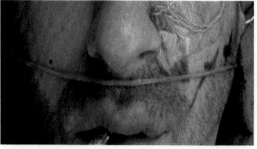

Fig. 1. Anticipated subcutaneous course of the sural nerve graft (*asterisk*).

histomorphometric analysis, Coombs and colleagues[38] showed that the masseteric nerve contains 1542 myelinated fibers compared with 834 fibers in a buccal branch. Also given the close proximity, rapid tone and motion recovery are expected within 3 to 6 months postoperatively.

Lastly, studies suggest a connectedness between the trigeminal and facial nuclei and nerves that seems to contribute to the ease of cerebral adaptation after CN V to VII transfer.[39–41] This finding may be partly explained by the fact that in 40% of adults, natural masseter contraction occurs during normal smile.[42] Most patients

---

Box 2
Surgical pearls for masseteric nerve transfer

Nerve identification

- The main trunk of the masseteric nerve is typically identified 3 cm anterior to the tragus and 1 cm below the zygomatic arch. The descending branch consistently courses obliquely towards the oral commissure between the deep and middle layers of the muscle. The proximal branches can usually be spared.

- The subzygomatic triangle using the zygomatic arch, temporomandibular joint, and the frontal branch of the facial nerve provides a rapid method for identifying the nerve with minimal dissection (see **Fig. 2**).

- It is helpful to have an assistant retract the masseter muscle fibers with 2 small Cummings retractors as dissection proceeds deeper into the muscle. A nerve stimulator can be used to assist in the location of the nerve.

- Once the nerve is located, a right angle retractor is used to place a vessel loop around the nerve. Gentle traction is used to dissect approximately 1.5 to 2.0 cm of the nerve before it begins dividing into multiple small branches (see **Fig. 3**).

Neurorrhaphy

- Transect the masseteric nerve as distally as possible under the operating microscope. If there is concern that the nerve will retract after transection, it can be partially transected and a 9-0 nylon epineural stitch placed at the midpoint of its distal end.

- Two to 3 epineural 9-0 nylon sutures are used to perform a meticulous microneural anastomosis. Some surgeons wrap the coaptation in a dural regeneration matrix (Durepair) and secure it with a fibrin sealant (Evicel) to thwart loss of axons into surrounding tissues. Others prefer sutures alone, as the data on benefit are inconclusive.

---

following masseteric nerve transfer seem to be able to develop an effortless smile without clenching their teeth. Klebuc[41] reported 75% of patients following masseteric nerve transfer developed an effortless smile without teeth clenching after 2 or more years of follow-up. In another study whereby the masseteric nerve was used as the donor for gracilis free muscle transfer, Manktelow and colleagues[43] found that 59% of patients could smile effortlessly without conscious effort and 85% of patients could smile without teeth clenching.

The main disadvantage of the masseteric nerve transfer is that although the smile that frequently evolves is effortless or reflexive, it is not truly spontaneous or emotionally mediated and often requires a significant amount of patient motivation for facial neuromuscular retraining therapy. Minor donor complications, such as slight weakness with mastication, masseteric atrophy with resultant cosmetic deformity, and facial twitching with mastication, have been reported, although none seem to produce any quality-of-life implications.[44]

Hypoglossal nerve (CN XII–VII) transfer

Popularized by Conley and Baker[45] in 1979, classic hypoglossal nerve transfer is no longer in favor because of significant donor morbidity; hemiglossal dysfunction results in difficulties with speech, swallowing, and mastication.[46] As a result, hypoglossal nerve transfer techniques have evolved. Incising the hypoglossal nerve distal to the descendens hypoglossi and bridging the gap between the facial and hypoglossal nerves using an interpositional jump graft has been shown to preserve tongue function in 87% of patients; however, weaker facial response and longer recovery times have also been seen.[47] Another modification is to split the hypoglossal nerve longitudinally. Terzis and Konofaos[9] describe a mini-hypoglossal transfer whereby the nerve is split longitudinally and only the superior 40% is used. Despite these modifications in nerve transfer technique, the hypoglossal nerve is not as popular today because of the potential for significant donor morbidity and mass movement. Facial spasms can be frequently seen with tongue movement, which is often constant and involuntary.

Dual innervation/babysitter procedures

If reinnervation with a CFNG is desired, the preceding duration of denervation is critical. In intermediate-duration FP of 6 to 24 months, the time it takes for reinnervation of the paralyzed facial muscles to occur by the CFNG is too great. The babysitter procedure first described by Terzis in 1988 can be used to rapidly salvage the facial muscle targets and prevent atrophy and fibrosis, until motor fibers from the contralateral facial nerve

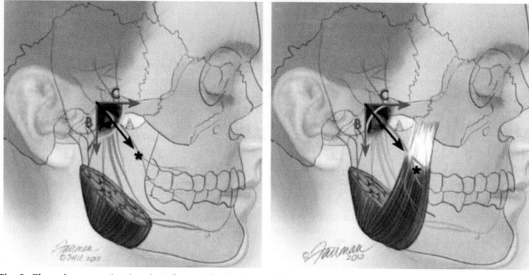

Fig. 2. The subzygomatic triangle is formed by the frontal branch of the facial nerve (A), a vertical line through the anterior border of the temporomandibular joint (B), and the inferior border of the zygomatic arch (C). The masseteric nerve (*asterisk*) is identified near the apex of the triangle. (*From* Collar RM, Byrne PJ, Boahene KDO. The subzygomatic triangle: rapid, minimally invasive identification of the masseteric nerve for facial reanimation. Plast Reconstr Surg 2013;132:185; with permission.)

arrive through the CFNG. This procedure has been shown to have superior outcomes in patients with intermediate-duration FP.[48] Mini-hypoglossal nerve transfers were largely described with this technique over the past 2 decades, but the authors favor the use of the masseteric nerve for many of the advantages described earlier. Dual innervation using the masseteric nerve and CFNG coapted to buccal branches has been described in a couple of recent case series with improvement in resting tone and excellent oral commissure excursion.[49,50] Bianchi and colleagues[50] report that in their single-stage dual-innervation experience,

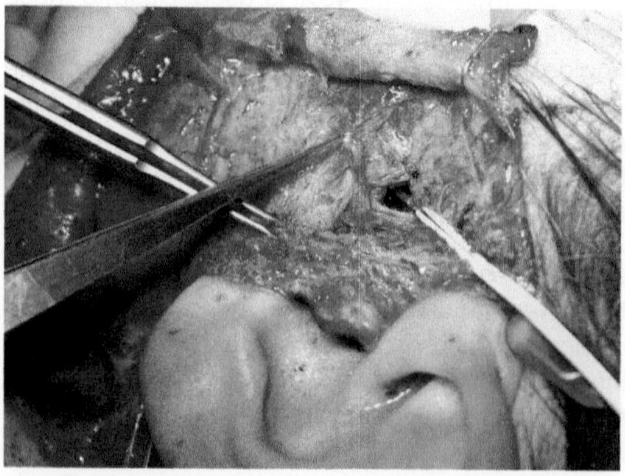

voluntary contraction with teeth clenching were noted an average of 2 to 4 months postoperatively and spontaneous smile achieved at 7 to 13 months.

Selection of Reanimation Procedure in Cases of Long-Standing Paralysis

In cases of long-standing, irreversible paralysis, reinnervation of native facial musculature is no longer an option. The clinician may still offer effective treatment options to restore symmetry and a dynamic smile. The choice comes down to either regional muscle transfer or free muscle transfer.

Regional muscle transfer techniques

Regional muscle transfers have been practiced for more than 50 years; but increasingly consistent functional and aesthetic results have made free muscle transfer the current criterion standard in dynamic smile reanimation, particularly in children. Despite this, contiguous muscle transfer is an excellent option among adults and should remain in the armamentarium of facial reanimation surgeons.

The direction and strength of the transferred muscles determine the quality and symmetry of dynamic reanimation. Temporalis muscle transfer is used for dynamic smile reanimation, with masseter muscle transfer occasionally used in complement to restrain the strong upward pull of the temporalis. The anterior belly of the digastric muscle can be transferred to the lower lip as an

Fig. 3. A vessel loop has been placed around the masseteric nerve. The frontal branch of the facial nerve (*asterisk*) marks the inferior and anterior border of the subzygomatic triangle.

antagonistic counterbalance to the strong upward pull of normally innervated musculature (ie, in isolated marginal mandibular nerve paralysis) or the strong upward pull following temporalis muscle transfer.[51]

Temporalis muscle transfer is the most commonly performed regional muscle transfer (**Box 3**, **Figs. 4–6**). The classic antidromic technique described by Gilles in the 1930s[52] involved transposition of the temporalis muscle over the zygomatic arch. Because of the resulting contour deformities with bulging over the zygomatic arch and temporal hollowing, orthodromic techniques came into favor. McLaughlin[53] originally described orthodromic temporalis tendon transfer (T3) with fascia lata extension grafts in 1953, but it was not popularized until 2007 when Byrne and colleagues[54] described their successful experience with this procedure in 7 patients. In 1997, Labbé and Huault[55] reported their technique on lengthening temporalis myoplasty whereby the entire muscle is mobilized from the temporalis fossa, resecured at a lower level within the fossa, and the fascial portion advanced to the upper lip and oral commissure. Boahene and colleagues[56] later described a minimally invasive method for T3 whereby the entire procedure is performed through a single incision made externally at the nasolabial fold or transorally via a buccal sulcus incision.

T3 techniques attempt to transfer the tendon to the perioral muscles, which require lengthening of the muscle from its anatomic neutral position. As a result, variable amounts of overcorrection of the smile occur in the resting state. Fascia lata extension grafts have been used to decrease the amount of overcorrection at rest, but the addition of a static graft may lead to uncontrolled relaxation and failure of the smile over time.[55] The authors have found that the use of intraoperative transcutaneous electrical stimulation (ie, using a train-of-4 monitor) is a valuable tool for determining the ideal tension to optimize excursion of transferred temporalis tendon units in smile restoration.[57]

Regional muscle transfer versus free muscle transfer

There are variable reports on the degree of oral commissure excursion attainable with the T3. Labbé and Huault[55] reported up to 15 mm of excursion from their lengthening temporalis myoplasty, whereas Byrne and colleagues[54] reported

---

Box 3
Surgical pearls for temporalis tendon transfer

Preoperative markings

- Markings of the desired vector of pull should be made with patients awake and upright in the preoperative area.
- Photographs and a video recording should be obtained and displayed in the operating room as a constant reference of patients' contralateral vector of smile.

Temporalis tendon dissection

- The temporalis tendon inserts on the medial aspect of the coronoid process and extends inferiorly toward the buccinator line. Dissecting the tendon to its inferior extent increases the length of the tendon that can be mobilized (see **Fig. 4**).
- The tendon can be exposed through a limited melolabial fold incision or transoral gingivobuccal incision. The authors tend to use the external approach when patients have a well-defined melolabial crease.
- Before detaching the coronoid using a reciprocating saw, a Kocher clamp is placed to prevent retraction.

Transposition and insertion

- With a Kocher clamp on the detached tendon, the temporalis muscle may be stimulated through surface electrodes using a train-of-4 muscle stimulator while varying traction tension on the tendon (see **Fig. 5**). This stimulation assists in determining the ideal tension of the tendon, and the tendon is sutured to the modiolus at that length.
- When excessive traction tension is required to reach the modiolus or there is significant pull of the philtrum away from the paralyzed side, a fascia lata extender graft is used. The fascia lata is secured to the temporalis tendon and tunneled into the upper and lower lips across the midpoint to the contralateral side (see **Fig. 6**). Small stab incisions can be made along the lip to secure the graft without bunching.

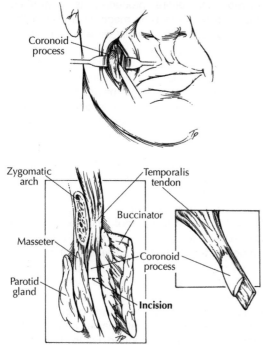

Fig. 4. Dissecting the temporalis tendon in a subperiosteal fashion from its inferior extent increases the length of the tendon that can be mobilized. The coronoid process is then divided in an oblique manner, leaving as much of the tendon attached to the coronoid as possible. (*From* Boahene KD, Farrag TY, Ishii L, et al. Minimally invasive temporalis tendon transposition. Arch Facial Plast Surg 2011;13:10; with permission.)

a range of excursion from 1.6 mm to 8.5 mm (mean 4.2 mm) in 7 patients. To the authors' knowledge, only one study directly compares the results of T3 with free muscle transfer (gracilis, pectoralis

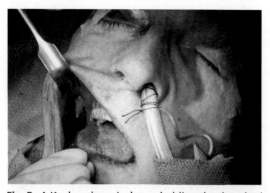

Fig. 5. A Kocher clamp is shown holding the detached tendon in a transoral approach. The temporalis muscle may be stimulated through surface electrodes using a train-of-4 muscle stimulator while varying traction tension on the tendon (not pictured).

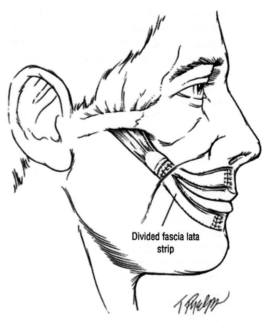

Fig. 6. A split fascia lata extender graft is secured to the temporalis tendon and tunneled into the upper and lower lips across the midpoint to the contralateral side. (*From* Boahene KD, Farrag TY, Ishii L, et al. Minimally invasive temporalis tendon transposition. Arch Facial Plast Surg 2011;13:11; with permission.)

minor, or latissimus dorsi). Erni and colleagues[58] found that although there were no differences found at rest, the range of oral commissure excursion was statistically significantly better after free muscle transfer (5.0 mm) than after T3 (1.7 mm).

Differences in surgical technique and surgeon experience may play some role; but further objective comparisons between T3 and free muscle transfer are warranted to assist in decision-making, particularly in middle-aged to older adults. Both procedures each provide significant improvement and high patient satisfaction.[54,55,59,60] However, they differ greatly. The T3 can be performed relatively quickly as an outpatient procedure. No additional bulk is added to the face. Postoperative recovery is short; symmetry is improved immediately, and dynamic movement can be seen very early (**Fig. 7**). However, the degree of movement seen is, on average, less than that obtained with free gracilis muscle transfer.[58] On the other hand, free muscle transfer is a much more complicated procedure, requires an inpatient stay for monitoring, may add undesirable bulk to the hemi-face, and results in a delay of many months before dynamic movement. But the degree of movement seen is typically greater than after regional muscle transfer. This decision is often challenging, and the authors engage patients

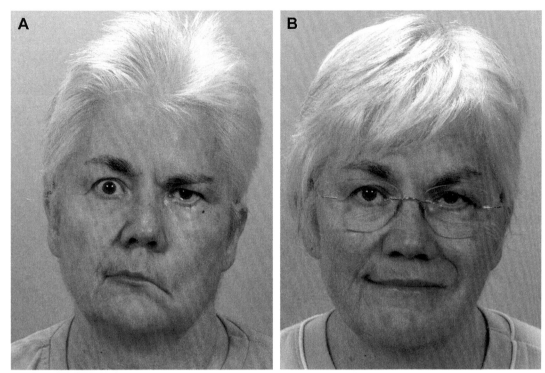

Fig. 7. A 57-year-old woman with complete left facial paralysis following vestibular schwannoma resection underwent T3 and brow-lift. Preoperative at repose (*A*) and 6-month postoperative (*B*) results.

to choose based on their age, comorbidities, motivation, and goals of care.

Free Muscle Transfer: Selection of a Donor Nerve for Reinnervation

Increasingly consistent functional and aesthetic results have made free muscle transfer the current gold standard in dynamic reanimation of irreversible paralysis, particularly in children. Although techniques vary, all have a common need for a donor muscle and a nerve to motorized the muscle. The gracilis muscle is the most commonly used donor muscle because of its ease of harvest, minimal donor morbidity, adequate length, excellent contractility, and ability to thin and reduce in bulk. Other donor muscles described include the pectoralis minor, latissimus dorsi, rectus abdominis, and extensor digitorum brevis muscles.

Free muscle transfer: masseteric innervation

Harii and colleagues[61] first reported free functional gracilis muscle transfer in 1976,[61] and it was advanced by Zuker and colleagues[59,62] for the management of patients with Möbius syndrome (**Box 4**, **Fig. 8**, Videos 1 and 2). Reconstruction can be performed in either 1 or 2 stages, depending on the innervation source. The single-stage free gracilis muscle transfer is most commonly

powered by the masseteric nerve. The major advantage, as previously described, is its tendency to produce a powerful and relatively quick result in a single procedure. The main disadvantage is the need for retraining to achieve effortless expression. This retraining can be particularly problematic for certain patients, such as young children or adults who are unable to participate in therapy.

Free muscle transfer: cross-facial nerve graft innervation, 1- versus 2-stage

The 2-stage protocol requires neural regeneration across a CFNG before subsequent muscle transfer with the goal of producing spontaneous, emotion-elicited facial movement. Most facial nerve surgeons prefer to perform free muscle transfer with CFNG in 2 stages to avoid denervation atrophy of the free muscle in the face while awaiting axons to regenerate across the CFNG. Although a seemingly sound theory, animal studies as well as clinical studies comparing 1-stage and 2-stage surgery have actually yielded conflicting results.

Kumar and Hassan[63] compared 15 patients who underwent the classic 2-stage technique for CFNG and free gracilis muscle transfer and 10 patients who underwent a single-stage technique.

Box 4
Surgical pearls for free gracilis muscle transfer

Preoperative markings

- Markings of the desired vector of pull, desired anchor points, proposed nasolabial crease, and approximate dimensions of the flap should be made with patients awake and upright in the preoperative area.

- Photographs and a video recording should be obtained and displayed in the operating room as a constant reference of patients' contralateral vector of smile.

Free gracilis muscle harvest

- The contralateral leg is typically used.

- With the leg in abduction, the adductor longus tendon is palpable as a firm cord, even in an obese individual. A line extending from the tendon to the medial femoral condyle is drawn. The incision is designed 2 fingerbreadths posterior/medial to this line.

- The gracilis muscle is identified and retracted medially to expose the neurovascular pedicle that runs in between the adductor longus and adductor magnus muscles. The nerve stimulator can be used to confirm identification of the obturator nerve before circumferential dissection of the muscle and the neurovascular pedicle.

- It is helpful to leave a layer of subcutaneous fat as well as fascia on the muscle to facilitate a glide plane in the face.

- It is critical to mark the resting tension of the muscle by placing sutures at 2-cm intervals for the length of the flap before flap harvest.

Thinning the flap

- Approximately one-third of the width and height of the gracilis is harvested based on the preoperative measurements and desired pedicle position (see **Fig. 8**). The ultimate desired weight is between 16 g and 20 g.

- The obturator nerve is intermittently stimulated to ensure the most contractile portion of the muscle is being harvested.

- Intraoperative laser angiography using the SPY Elite system also helps to ensure that the harvested muscle is well perfused in situ (see Video 1). The SPY Elite system (NOVODAQ Technologies, Inc., Bonita Springs, FL, USA) can be used a second time after microvascular anastomosis in the face to further thin the flap if needed (see Video 2).

- The proximal and distal cuts are best made using a gastrointestinal anastomosis stapler or a Harmonic scalpel. If the latter is used, oversewing the muscle ends with a running suture can facilitate inset.

Flap inset

- Precise placement of anchoring sutures at the proposed nasolabial crease is required. The authors use three or four 2-0 polydioxanone sutures. A lighted facelift retractor is helpful in placing these sutures through a facelift incision.

- After microneurovascular anastomoses, the distal end of the muscle is inset into the periosteum of the zygoma and/or temporalis fascia. The 2-cm distance between suture markers should be preserved to ensure adequate muscle power.

- If necessary, portions of the SMAS and buccal fat can be judiciously excised to prevent bulkiness after flap inset.

Abbreviation: SMAS, superficial muscular aponeurotic system.

Although there were fewer complications with the single-stage method with reduction of rehabilitation by 10 months, the 2-staged method yielded better symmetry at rest. On the other hand, Biglioli and colleagues[64] reviewed their experience with free latissimus dorsi transfer using the thoracodorsal nerve as a cross-facial nerve graft anastomosed to the contralateral, intact facial nerve and found that clinical results were similar to those obtained with the classic 2-staged technique. In a rabbit model comparing 1- versus 2-stage free rectus femoris muscle transfer with CFNG, no significant difference between groups was seen in terms of rectus nerve morphometry,

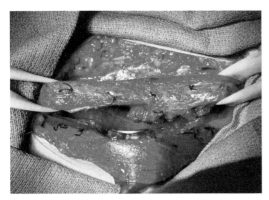

Fig. 8. The gracilis muscle is divided in situ, and approximately one-third of the muscle is harvested. Sutures are placed at 2-cm intervals along the length of the muscle to mark its resting tension.

muscle reinnervation, or tetanic force production.[65] Although the benefits of 1-stage surgery include less number of surgical procedures, shorter recovery time, and associated economic implications, the 2-staged CFNG is more predictable and currently prevails.

Free muscle transfer: masseteric versus cross-facial nerve graft innervation

The choice of donor nerve to power a free gracilis muscle transfer is highly individualized. The desire for a spontaneous, emotional smile and the preference to avoid postoperative motor training often motivates individuals and experts to select CFNG innervation (patient example in **Fig. 9**, Video 3). Given that increasing age is associated with reduced neural regeneration potential, some experts recommend the 1-stage approach with masseteric innervation for adults greater than 30 years old and the 2-staged approach with CFNG innervation for all children aged 18 years and younger.[66] Masseteric innervation may also be particularly suitable for patients who cannot or do not want to undergo 2 surgical stages or patients who could benefit from its motor strength, such as those with a heavy face, significant rest asymmetry, or those who have a very powerful smile on their normal side (patient example in **Fig. 10**, Video 4).[43] In cases of bilateral facial paralysis, as in Möbius syndrome, the gracilis muscle transfer is typically performed in a single stage

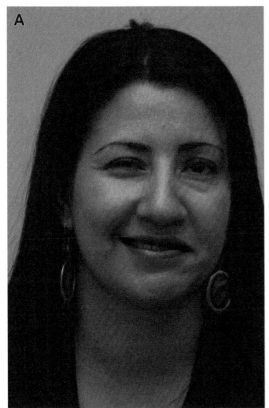

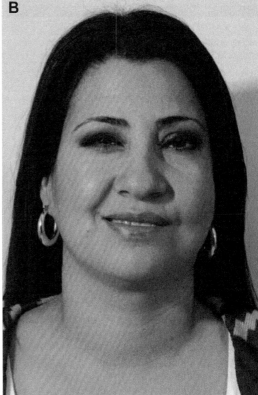

Fig. 9. A 32-year-old woman with incomplete, irreversible left facial paralysis following facial schwannoma resection (with primary cable grafting) underwent CFNG followed by free gracilis muscle transfer 14 months later. Preoperative (*A*) and 2-year postoperative (*B*) results.

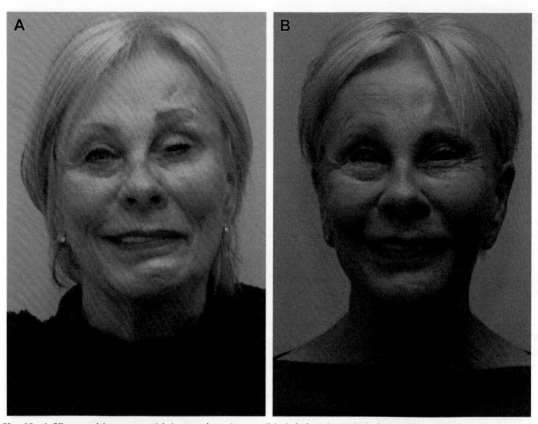

Fig. 10. A 65-year-old woman with incomplete, irreversible left facial paralysis following vestibular schwannoma resection underwent free gracilis muscle transfer with masseteric nerve innervation. Preoperative (*A*) and 2-year postoperative (*B*) results.

driven by the masseteric nerve (or alternative motor nerve if CN V is not available).

Several recent studies show better oral commissure excursion following free gracilis muscle transfer innervated with the masseteric nerve compared with the CFNG, in both children and adults. In a study of 166 free muscle transfers in children, Bae and colleagues[67] reported an increased amount of oral commissure excursion in the gracilis powered by the masseteric nerve group (average 14.2 mm) compared with gracilis powered by the CFNG group (7.9 mm), with oral commissure excursion in the masseteric nerve group nearly identical to the unaffected side of the face (15.2 mm). Similar findings of increased oral commissure excursion were found in other studies,[29,60,68] although Bhama and colleagues[60] noted that although there was greater excursion in those innervated by the masseteric nerve, those innervated by the CFNG had better postoperative symmetry during smile.

The greater degree of excursion is likely explained by the increased axonal counts in the masseteric nerve compared with the CFNG.[29,34,38] In a combined histomorphometric and clinical study, Snyder-Warwick and colleagues[29] showed more than a 3-fold greater number of axons in the masseteric nerve (5289 fibers per square millimeter) compared with the downstream CFNG (1647 fibers per square millimeter). In their study of 91 pediatric patients, greater oral commissure contraction and excursion was seen with the masseteric nerve (8.1 ± 4.0 mm) compared with the 2-stage technique with CFNG (4.1 ± 2.9 mm). They suggest that based on animal studies, force deficits in transplanted muscle likely correlate with decreased axonal supply.

Free muscle transfer: dual innervation

Dual innervation of free muscle transfers with both the masseteric nerve and CFNG has been suggested to optimize both strength and spontaneity of movement (patient example in **Fig. 11**, Video 5). Watanabe and colleagues[69] first reported the use of 1-stage free muscle transfer with double innervation for reanimation of long-standing FP; their study demonstrated improvement in latissimus dorsi muscle contraction by positioning the hilum of the flap in contact with a part of the denuded masseter on the paralyzed side. Several

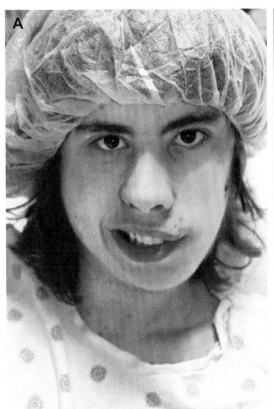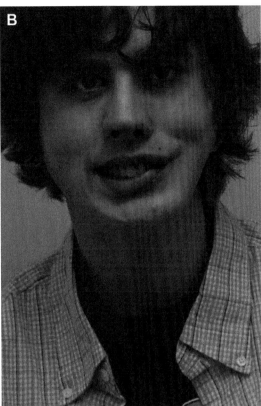

Fig. 11. A 16-year-old boy with complete, irreversible left facial paralysis secondary to Möbius syndrome underwent 2-stage free muscle transfer with dual CFNG and masseteric innervation. Preoperative (*A*) and 1-year postoperative (*B*) results.

recent studies using dual innervation have shown good to excellent outcomes in symmetry at rest as well as volitional/spontaneous movement.[70–72]

Similar questions arise: Is 1-stage versus 2-stage more preferable? What is the ideal coaptation pattern? Biglioli and colleagues[70] and Sforza and colleagues[71] describe a similar *1-stage* procedure whereby the ipsilateral masseteric nerve is coapted by *end-to-end* neurorrhaphy to the obturator nerve and the contralateral, intact facial nerve is coapted *end-to-end* with a CFNG on the healthy side, which is coapted *end-to-side* on the obturator nerve, distal to the masseteric-obturator anastomosis. In the Sforza study,[71] a 3-dimensional optoelectronic motion analyzer was used to find that following dual innervation gracilis surgery, 75% of the normal spontaneous smile was achieved on the paretic side, which increased to 91% when teeth clenching was added, with less than 20% asymmetry.

In contrast, Cardenas-Mejia and colleagues[72] report a *2-stage* gracilis free muscle transfer with dual innervation. In the first stage, a cross-facial nerve graft is harvested. In the second stage, the free gracilis muscle is transferred and the obturator nerve is coapted *end-to-end* to the CFNG and the masseteric nerve is coapted *end-to-side* to the obturator nerve, distal to the obturator-CFNG anastomosis. They think that performing the CFNG-obturator nerve anastomosis in an end-to-end fashion gives the best chance for the contralateral facial nerve to recruit major motor units in the gracilis muscle. Interestingly, the study investigators started performing dual innervation based on their positive experience after adding masseteric nerve transfer in patients with poor response following classic 2-stage (CFNG) muscle transfer.

The optimal method for coaptation in cases of dual innervation is not yet clear, although the intentions are the same: to provide both strength and spontaneity to the gracilis muscle. It is important to recognize that the masseteric nerve has greater axonal density compared with the CFNG and, if given an equal chance, will likely overwhelm the recruitment of motor units. In the authors' anecdotal experience, splitting the obturator nerve for divided coaptation to the CFNG and masseteric nerve has also produced good results.

Dynamic Reinnervation in Incomplete Facial Palsy

In patients with nonflaccid FP, the mainstay treatments tend to be nonsurgical in nature: physical therapy, chemodenervation procedures to improve symmetry and ameliorate synkinesis, and volumizing fillers to improve facial balance, particularly in the midface. Some patients recover with facial tone at rest but diminished or absent excursion with movement and present for dynamic reanimation. The presence of some degree of nerve function makes the decision to intervene and how more complicated because attempts to improve tone and/or movement can put the residual or recovered facial function at risk. The optimal approach in these patients is to functionally upgrade tone and movement without sacrificing any existing function. This approach can be achieved with neural signal upgrading through neurotization procedures, functional muscle upgrading through muscle transfer, and/or static procedures.[22]

Neurotization procedures may be an ideal option for patients in which additional innervation (neural supercharge) is thought to result in more muscle fiber recruitment.[73] Clinically, these patients may have reduced but some present excursion on attempted facial animation with minimal synkinesis. The same decisions regarding the optimal selection of donor nerve apply. For fear of downgrading function, the concept of end-to-side coaptation[74] of the donor nerve to facial nerve branches on the incompletely paralyzed side has been suggested to improve recovery without disrupting native nerve fibers.[75] An alternative option described is direct neurotization, whereby a donor nerve is implanted directly or through an interposition nerve graft into a denervated muscle so as not to sacrifice its native innervation.[9]

If additional innervation is not expected to recruit more facial mimetic motion, functional muscle transfer is a better option. Clinically, these patients are those who have recovered with varying degrees of hyperactivity and synkinesis. Nerve transfer techniques to native facial musculature in these patients are typically less successful than free muscle transfer, possibly because of residual synkinetic input to the muscle, disorganization of muscle units, and focally denervated, adynamic segments within the synkinetic muscles that are not amenable to reinnervation.[5] The authors have used free gracilis muscle transfers for several of these cases, using either the masseteric nerve and/or contralateral facial nerve as the donor, depending on the patients' goals and preferences. In these cases, meticulous care must be taken to identify the correct vector of smile and thin the gracilis muscle based on its fascicular distribution[76] to minimize problems related to excessive bulk.

SUMMARY

Although the complexity of facial expression and intricate synergy of facial mimetic muscles is difficult to fully restore, the ultimate goal of FP treatment is to reestablish facial symmetry and movement. Tremendous progress in dynamic facial reanimation options and outcomes has been made over the past couple of decades, but contemporary management remains fraught with debate. Advances in surgical techniques as well as the consistent use of outcome reporting measures across FP specialists will guide the evolving evidence-based approach to facial reanimation. The future holds additional promise with developing advances in tissue engineering and neural regeneration as well as emerging technologies in bioelectrical interfaces.[77]

SUPPLEMENTARY DATA

Supplementary data related to this article can be found at http://dx.doi.org/10.1016/j.fsc.2016.03.016.

REFERENCES

1. Ishii LE, Godoy A, Encarnacion CO, et al. What faces reveal: impaired affect display in facial paralysis. Laryngoscope 2011;121:1138–43.
2. Lindsay RW, Bhama P, Hadlock TA. Quality-of-life improvement after free gracilis muscle transfer for smile restoration in patients with facial paralysis. JAMA Facial Plast Surg 2014;16:419–24.
3. Hohman MH, Hadlock TA. Etiology, diagnosis, and management of facial palsy: 2000 patients at a facial nerve center. Laryngoscope 2014;124:E283–93.
4. Boahene K, Byrne P, Schaitkin BM. Facial reanimation: discussion and debate. Facial Plast Surg Clin North Am 2012;20:383–402.
5. Jowett N, Hadlock TA. A contemporary approach to facial reanimation. JAMA Facial Plast Surg 2015;17:293–300.
6. Ylikoski J, Hitselberger WE, House WF, et al. Degenerative changes in the distal stump of the severed human facial nerve. Acta Otolaryngol 1981;92:239–48.
7. Boahene K. Reanimating the paralyzed face. F1000Prime Rep 2013;5:49.
8. Malik TH, Kelly G, Ahmed A, et al. A comparison of surgical techniques used in dynamic reanimation of the paralyzed face. Otol Neurotol 2005;26:284–91.

9. Terzis JK, Konofaos P. Nerve transfers in facial palsy. Facial Plast Surg 2008;24:177–93.

10. Guntinas-Lichius O, Streppel M, Stennert E. Postoperative functional evaluation of different reanimation techniques for facial nerve repair. Am J Surg 2006;191:61–7.

11. Verdú E, Ceballos D, Vilches JJ, et al. Influence of aging on peripheral nerve function and regeneration. J Peripher Nerv Syst 2000;5:191–208.

12. Chan JYK, Byrne PJ. Management of facial paralysis in the 21st century. Facial Plast Surg 2011;27:346–57.

13. Jowett N, Hadlock TA. An evidence-based approach to facial reanimation. Facial Plast Surg Clin North Am 2015;23:313–34.

14. Fattah AY, Gavilan J, Hadlock TA, et al. Survey of methods of facial palsy documentation in use by members of the Sir Charles Bell Society. Laryngoscope 2014;124:2247–51.

15. Kang TS, Vrabec JT, Giddings N, et al. Facial nerve grading systems (1985-2002): beyond the House-Brackmann scale. Otol Neurotol 2002;23:767–71.

16. House JW, Brackmann DE. Facial nerve grading system. Otolaryngol Head Neck Surg 1985;93:146–7.

17. Ross BG, Fradet G, Nedzelski JM. Development of a sensitive clinical facial grading system. Otolaryngol Head Neck Surg 1996;114:380–6.

18. Vrabec JT, Backous DD, Djalilian HR, et al. Facial nerve grading system 2.0. Otolaryngol Head Neck Surg 2009;140:445–50.

19. Banks CA, Bhama PK, Park J, et al. Clinician-graded electronic facial paralysis assessment: the eFACE. Plast Reconstr Surg 2015;136:223e–30e.

20. VanSwearingen JM, Brach JS. The facial disability index: reliability and validity of a disability assessment instrument for disorders of the facial neuromuscular system. Phys Ther 1996;76:1288–98.

21. Kahn JB, Gliklich RE, Boyev KP, et al. Validation of a patient-graded instrument for facial nerve paralysis: the FaCE scale. Laryngoscope 2001;111:387–98.

22. Boahene K. Facial reanimation after acoustic neuroma resection: options and timing of intervention. Facial Plast Surg 2015;31:103–9.

23. Rivas A, Boahene KD, Bravo HC, et al. A model for early prediction of facial nerve recovery after vestibular schwannoma surgery. Otol Neurotol 2011;32:826–33.

24. Albathi M, Oyer S, Ishii LE, et al. Early nerve grafting for facial paralysis after cerebellopontine angle tumor resection with preserved facial nerve continuity. JAMA Facial Plast Surg 2016;18(1):54–60.

25. Özmen ÖA, Falcioni M, Lauda L, et al. Outcomes of facial nerve grafting in 155 cases: predictive value of history and preoperative function. Otol Neurotol 2011;32:1341–6.

26. Scaramella LF. Anastomosis between the two facial nerves. Laryngoscope 1975;85:1359–66.

27. Smith JW. A new technique of facial animation. Transactions of the fifth international congress of plastic surgery. Melbourne (Australia): Butterworths; 1971. p. 83–4.

28. Thanos PK, Terzis JK. A histomorphometric analysis of the cross-facial nerve graft in the treatment of facial paralysis. J Reconstr Microsurg 1996;12:375–82.

29. Snyder-Warwick AK, Fattah AY, Zive L, et al. The degree of facial movement following microvascular muscle transfer in pediatric facial reanimation depending on donor motor nerve axonal density. Plast Reconstr Surg 2015;135:370–379e.

30. Terzis JK, Wang W, Zhao Y. Effect of axonal load on the functional and aesthetic outcomes of the cross-facial nerve graft procedure for facial reanimation. Plast Reconstr Surg 2009;124:1499–512.

31. May M. Nerve substitution techniques: XII-VII hook-up, XII-VII jump graft and cross-face graft. In: May M, Schaitkin BM, editors. The facial nerve. 2nd edition. New York: Thieme Medical Publishers; 2000. p. 611–33.

32. Spira M. Anastomosis of the masseteric nerve to lower division of facial nerve for correction of lower facial paralysis. Preliminary report. Plast Reconstr Surg 1978;61:330–4.

33. Klebuc M. Masseter-to-facial nerve transfer: a new technique for facial reanimation. J Reconstr Microsurg 2006;22:A101.

34. Borschel GH, Kawamura DH, Kasukurthi R, et al. The motor nerve to the masseter muscle: an anatomic and histomorphometric study to facilitate its use in facial reanimation. J Plast Reconstr Aesthet Surg 2012;65:363–6.

35. Hwang K, Kim YJ, Chung IH, et al. Course of the masseteric nerve in masseter muscle. J Craniofac Surg 2005;16:197–200.

36. Collar RM, Byrne PJ, Boahene KDO. The subzygomatic triangle: rapid, minimally invasive identification of the masseteric nerve for facial reanimation. Plast Reconstr Surg 2013;132:183–8.

37. Cotrufo S, Hart A, Payne AP, et al. Topographic anatomy of the nerve to masseter: an anatomical and clinical study. J Plast Reconstr Aesthet Surg 2011;64:1424–9.

38. Coombs CJ, Ek EW, Wu T, et al. Masseteric-facial nerve coaptation: an alternative technique for facial nerve reinnervation. J Plast Reconstr Aesthet Surg 2009;62:1580–8.

39. Rubin LR, Rubin JP, Simpson RL, et al. The search for the neurocranial pathways to the fifth nerve nucleus in the reanimation of the paralyzed face. Plast Reconstr Surg 1990;103:1725–8.

40. Lifchez SD, Matloub HS, Gosain AK. Cortical adaptation to restoration of smiling after free muscle

transfer innervated by the nerve to the masseter. Plast Reconstr Surg 2005;115:1472–9.

41. Klebuc MJA. Facial reanimation using masseter-to-facial nerve transfer. Plast Reconstr Surg 2011;127: 1909–15.

42. Schaverien M, Moran G, Stewart K, et al. Activation of the masseter muscle during normal smile production and the implications for dynamic reanimation surgery for facial paralysis. J Plast Reconstr Aesthet Surg 2011;64:1585–8.

43. Manktelow RT, Tomat LR, Zuker RM. Smile reconstruction in adults with free muscle transfer innervated by the masseter motor nerve: effectiveness and cerebral adaptation. Plast Reconstr Surg 2006;118:885–99.

44. Wang W, Yang C, Li Q, et al. Masseter-to-facial nerve transfer: a highly effective technique for facial reanimation after acoustic neuroma resection. Ann Plast Surg 2014;73:S63–9.

45. Conley J, Baker DC. Hypoglossal-facial nerve anastomosis for reinnervation of the paralysed face. Plast Reconstr Surg 1979;63:63–72.

46. Hammerschlag PE. Facial animation with jump interpositional graft hypoglossal facial anastomosis and hypoglossal facial anastomosis: evolution in management of facial paralysis. Laryngoscope 1999; 109:1–23.

47. May M, Sobol SM, Mester SJ. Hypoglossal-facial nerve interpositional-jump graft for facial reanimation without tongue atrophy. Otolaryngol Head Neck Surg 1991;104:818–25.

48. Terzis JK, Tzafetta K. The "babysitter" procedure: minihypoglossal to facial nerve transfer and cross-facial nerve grafting. Plast Reconstr Surg 2009; 123:865–76.

49. Faria JC, Scopel GP, Ferreira MC. Facial reanimation with masseteric nerve. Babysitter or permanent procedure? Preliminary results. Ann Plast Surg 2010;64: 31–4.

50. Bianchi B, Ferri A, Ferrari S, et al. Cross-facial nerve graft and masseteric nerve cooptation for one-stage facial reanimation: principles, indications, and surgical procedure. Head Neck 2014; 36:235–40.

51. Lindsay RW, Edwards C, Smitson C, et al. A systematic algorithm for the management of lower lip asymmetry. Am J Otolaryngol 2011;32:1–7.

52. Gillies H. Experiences with fascia lata grafts in the operative treatment of facial paralysis. Proc R Soc Med 1934;27:1372–82.

53. McLaughlin CR. Surgical support in permanent facial paralysis. Plast Reconstr Surg 1953;11: 302–14.

54. Byrne PJ, Kim M, Boahene K, et al. Temporalis tendon transfer as part of a comprehensive approach to facial reanimation. Arch Facial Plast Surg 2007;9:234–41.

55. Labbé D, Huault M. Lengthening temporalis myoplasty and lip reanimation. Plast Reconstr Surg 2000;105:1289–97.

56. Boahene KD, Farrag TY, Ishii L, et al. Minimally invasive temporalis tendon transposition. Arch Facial Plast Surg 2011;13:8–13.

57. Boahene KD. Principles and biomechanics of muscle tendon unit transfer: application in temporalis muscle tendon transposition for smile improvement in facial paralysis. Laryngoscope 2013;123:350–5.

58. Erni D, Lieger O, Banic A. Comparative objective and subjective analysis of temporalis tendon and microneurovascular transfer for facial reanimation. Br J Plast Surg 1999;52:167–72.

59. Zuker RM, Goldberg CS, Manktelow RT. Facial animation in children with Mobius syndrome after segmental gracilis muscle transplant. Plast Reconstr Surg 2000;106:1–8.

60. Bhama PK, Weinberg JS, Lindsay RW, et al. Objective outcomes analysis following microvascular gracilis transfer for facial reanimation: a review of 10 years' experience. JAMA Facial Plast Surg 2014; 16:85–92.

61. Harii K, Ohmori K, Torii S. Free gracilis muscle transplantation, with micro-neurovascular anastomoses for the treatment of facial paralysis. A preliminary report. Plast Reconstr Surg 1976;57:133–43.

62. Zuker RM, Manktelow RT. A smile for the Mobius syndrome patient. Ann Plast Surg 1989;22:188–94.

63. Kumar PA, Hassan KM. Cross-face nerve graft with free-muscle transfer for reanimation of the paralyzed face: a comparative study of the single-stage and two-stage procedures. Plast Reconstr Surg 2002; 109:451–62.

64. Biglioli F, Frigerio A, Rabbiosi D, et al. Single-stage facial reanimation in the surgical treatment of unilateral established facial paralysis. Plast Reconstr Surg 2009;124:124–33.

65. Urso-Baiarda F, Grobbelaar AO. A comparison of one- versus two-stage surgery in an experimental model of functional muscle transfer with interposed nerve grafting. J Plast Reconstr Aesthet Surg 2009;62:1042–7.

66. Garcia RM, Hadlock TA, Klebuc MJ, et al. Contemporary solutions for the treatment of facial nerve paralysis. Plast Reconstr Surg 2015;135:1025e–46e.

67. Bae YC, Zuker RM, Manktelow RT, et al. A comparison of commissure excursion following gracilis muscle transplantation for facial paralysis using a cross-face nerve graft versus the motor nerve to the masseter nerve. Plast Reconstr Surg 2006;117:2407–13.

68. Hontanilla B, Marre D, Cabello A. Facial reanimation with gracilis muscle neurotized to cross-facial nerve graft versus masseteric nerve: a comparative study using the FACIAL CLIMA evaluating system. Plast Reconstr Surg 2013;131:1241–52.

69. Watanabe Y, Akizuki T, Ozawa T, et al. Dual innervation method using one-stage reconstruction with free latissimus dorsi muscle transfer for reanimation of established facial paralysis: simultaneous reinnervation of the ipsilateral masseter motor nerve and the contralateral facial nerve to improve the quality of smile and emotional facial expressions. J Plast Reconstr Aesthet Surg 2009;62:1343–9.

70. Biglioli F, Colombo V, Tarrabia F, et al. Double innervation in free-flap surgery for long-standing facial paralysis. J Plast Reconstr Aesthet Surg 2012;65:1343–9.

71. Sforza C, Frigerio A, Mapello A, et al. Double-powered free gracilis muscle transfer for smile reanimation: a longitudinal optoelectronic study. J Plast Reconstr Aesthet Surg 2015;68:930–9.

72. Cardenas-Mejia A, Covarrubias-Ramirez JV, Bello-Margolis A, et al. Double innervated free functional muscle transfer for facial reanimation. J Plast Surg Hand Surg 2015;49:183–8.

73. Yamamoto Y, Sekido M, Furukawa H, et al. Surgical rehabilitation of reversible facial palsy: facial-hypoglossal network system based on neural signal augmentation/neural supercharge concept. J Plast Reconstr Aesthet Surg 2007;60:223–31.

74. Viterbo F, Trindaade JC, Hoshino K, et al. Latero-terminal neurorrhaphy without removal of the epineural sheath: experimental study in rats. Rev Paul Med 1992;110:267–75.

75. Frey M, Giovanoli P, Michaelidou M. Functional upgrading of partially recovered facial palsy by cross-face nerve grafting with distal end-to-side neurorrhaphy. Plast Reconstr Surg 2006;117:597–608.

76. Manktelow RT, Zuker RM. Muscle transplantation by fascicular territory. Plast Reconstr Surg 1984;73:751–7.

77. Langhals NB, Urbanchek MG, Ray A, et al. Update in facial nerve paralysis: tissue engineering and new technologies. Curr Opin Otolaryngol Head Neck Surg 2014;22:291–9.

Controversies in the Management of the Trauma Patient

Regina E. Rodman, MD[a],*, Robert M. Kellman, MD[b]

KEYWORDS

- Facial trauma ● Orbital trauma ● Mandibular trauma ● Maxillomandibular fixation ● Condylar fracture
- Endoscopic repair ● Blowout fractures

KEY POINTS

- There is debate about the optimal timing of repair, as well as material chosen to repair orbital floor fractures. There is a trend toward early repair in patients with large, displaced fractures and observation of smaller ones. When choosing a material to repair the fracture, the critical issue is the magnitude of the fracture, with large fractures requiring a stronger, supportive material.
- Intraoperative computed tomographic scan and intraoperative navigation are expensive technologies, but may reduce costs overall by decreasing the number of revision surgeries needed.
- There is still much debate about open versus closed repair of subcondylar fractures. Several studies have shown improvements in facial and ramus heights on the side of the open repair as well as improved occlusion with the open technique. Closed technique carries less risk for facial nerve injury and scar formation.
- Endoscopic-assisted subcondylar repair may be a compromise, allowing the benefits of open repair with lower risks. However, this technique is difficult and has a steep learning curve.
- Maxillomandibular fixation has been used for decades to achieve optimal occlusion during and after mandible repair, but there are new data suggesting this may not always be necessary.

INTRODUCTION

Facial trauma is a significant cause of morbidity in the United States. In one analysis, there were 407,167 Emergency Room (ER) visits for facial fractures with a cost approaching $1 billion.[1] Despite the large volume of trauma surgeries at most academic institutions, there is controversy regarding management of certain traumatic injuries. The literature lacks clear-cut best practices with many fractures. In orbital trauma, there is debate about the optimal timing of repair, preferred biomaterial to be used, and the utility of intraoperative computed tomographic (CT) scans. In mandible fractures, there is debate

regarding open versus closed versus endoscopic repair of the condyle. Maxillomandibular fixation (MMF) has been used for decades to achieve optimal occlusion during and after mandible repair, but there are new data suggesting this may not always be necessary. The purpose of this article is to review the salient points of each side of the debate and cite literature that exists to support each position.

REPAIR OF ORBITAL FRACTURES
Timing

Yadav and colleagues[2] noted that the rate of CT use in the US ERs quadrupled from 1996 to

---

Disclosure: The authors have nothing to disclose.
[a] Facial Plastics and Craniofacial Surgery, SUNY Upstate, 750 East Adams Street, Syracuse, NY 13207, USA;
[b] Department of Otolaryngology, SUNY Upstate, 750 East Adams Street, Syracuse, NY 13207, USA
* Corresponding author.
E-mail address: reginarodman@gmail.com

2007. Patients totaling 4.1 million presented to an ER with, and were treated for, injuries of the eye and face. Of those, 20% (820,252 patients) underwent CT imaging, with 102,999 patients (12.5%) diagnosed with an orbital fracture. Another study reported that although the number of facial traumas has gone up between 1991 and 2007, the number of facial fracture repairs has decreased.[3] Although this may in part be attributed to changing causes of fractures, it is likely that these trends are related to increasing use of CT imaging, resulting in decreasing severity of facial injuries being diagnosed. With an increase in the diagnosis of facial fractures, the question about which fractures should be repaired and which should be observed has grown more complex. For those that are repaired, what is the ideal timing of repair?

The 3 generally accepted categories of repair are immediate (within 24 hours), early (less than 2 weeks), and late (greater than 2 weeks). There is consensus on criteria that necessitate immediate repair. The first is activation of the oculocardiac reflex, with CT evidence of an entrapped muscle or periorbital tissue causing bradycardia, heart block, nausea, vomiting, or syncope. The second is entrapment of the perimuscular tissue with marked limitation of extra ocular movements on upward gaze.[4] There is also a trend toward early repair in patients with large, displaced orbital fracture with increased orbital volume. Several investigators have demonstrated improved postoperative results, with decreased diplopia and enophthalmos by performing early intervention.[5–7] It has been suggested that greater intrinsic damage leads to subsequent fibrosis, which results in poorer motility outcomes despite complete release of soft tissues. There is a suggestion that earlier intervention for such injuries might improve outcomes.[5]

The real question then is, which patients need early orbital reconstruction and which patients are candidates for delayed repair? This uncertainty applies to patients with orbital fractures that have good ocular motility and only slight displacement of the orbital contents. The indication for surgery in solitary medial wall fractures is also controversial. Indications for surgery in these patients who do not have diplopia is usually the development of enophthalmos. However, enophthalmos rarely becomes significant (more than 2 mm) in the first 2 weeks after trauma.[8] Although there is the Jaquiery classification, which describes the extent of the orbital fracture,[9] and Hertel exopthamometry, the literature lacks a 3-dimensional volume-based classification to assist in clinical decision-making. At this time, there is not a clear definition of degree of injury that will or will not necessitate repair. For the patient who does undergo repair, there is some evidence for early repair, but this has not been proven conclusively. A review of the literature by Dubois[4] found 4 studies that indicated some advantageous effects for surgery performed at less than 2 weeks for adults,[10–13] although 5 studies found no significant differences.[14–18] In pediatric patients, one study showed a correlation between earlier repair and diplopia and motility disorders,[19] whereas 5 studies were inconclusive.[20–23] In patients with small fractures, a watchful waiting approach may be appropriate, and surgery may be avoided in some cases.

Materials

The choice of reconstructive material presents another major decision in the care of a patient with an orbital fracture. A perfect biomaterial would be chemically inert, biofriendly, nonallergenic, and noncarcinogenic. It should also be cost-effective to place, readily available and able to be sterilized, and easy to handle, yet have the ability to be stable and retain its shape once manipulated. Preferably, it should be radiopaque to enable radiographic evaluation but without producing artifacts that may mask important features on subsequent radiologic examination.[24] Unfortunately, this ideal graft material does not exist at this time. There are dozens of materials from which to choose.

Materials for repair can be placed into 5 main categories: autogenous, allogenic, alloplastic absorbable, alloplastic nonabsorbable, and xenograft. Autogenous grafts are usually bone, cartilage, or temporalis fascia. Bone grafts may be taken from iliac crest, calvarium, nasal septal bone, rib, maxillary, and mandibular bone. Bone grafts are a popular option because of the strength and rigidity of bone as well as the ability of the body to vascularize and incorporate the tissue with minimal immune reactivity. The major disadvantage of bone is that the rigidity does not allow contouring without fracture. When deciding on a harvest site, the following should be taken into account: iliac crest and rib bone show significant and unpredictable resorption, up to 80%, because of their endochondral origin[25,26]; calvarial bone remains a popular choice because of its accessibility and proximity to the surgical field, various sizes of grafts that can be harvested, and a hidden scar with minimal pain.[27] One study illustrated the use of nasal septal bone, which restored orbital volume and alleviated symptomatic nasal passages.[28]

Cartilage can be harvested from the nasal septum or the concha, with studies showing some preference toward septal cartilage.[29] The advantages of cartilage compared with bone are that cartilage is easier to harvest and is more malleable, and the relative avascularity of this tissue allows for minimal oxygen perfusion and less resorption.[30] The major limitation of this method is the limited size of the tissue harvested. Thus, cartilage is usually preferred for smaller defects. The use of temporalis fascia has been well described. This harvest site also offers minimal morbidity with a well-hidden scar. However, the lack of rigidity makes this material unsuitable for a large defect, and it is best for defects of the orbital floor measuring 2 cm^2 or less.[31]

The use of allografts and xenografts has fallen out of favor because of risk of disease transmission and unpredictable absorption. Xenografts, such as collagen membranes of porcine origin, have a risk of disease transmission and an unpredictable rate of absorption and may not be sufficient for defects larger than 1 cm^2.[32] Allografts that have been historically used are demineralized bone, lyophilized dura, homologous fascia lata, and irradiated rib cartilage. Lyophilized dura was popular because of its strength, absence of donor morbidity, and lack of tissue reaction.[33] Unfortunately, a patient was diagnosed with Creutzfeldt-Jakob prion disease, likely from a dura graft she got 6 years previously.[34] There is also a theoretic risk of other disease transmission such as human immunodeficiency virus and hepatitis C. Furthermore, allografts have a rate of absorption higher than that of autogenous tissue.[35]

Alloplastic materials can be divided into absorbable and nonabsorbable. Popular nonabsorbable materials include titanium, porous polyethylene, silicone, and polytetrafluoroethylene. These implants are popular because they are rigid, can cover a wide defect, and can be molded to fit the defect. Using computer assistance, titanium mesh can be custom designed for patient-specific defects.[36] Absorbable materials include copolymers of polylactic acid and polyglycolic acid, and polydioxanone foil. Absorbable materials also have a high level of customizability and control, providing temporary support, leaving fibrous granulation tissue during their degradation.[37] The risk that goes with all foreign body implantation is infection, foreign body reaction, or extrusion.[6,38–40]

Several reviews have been done to evaluate the data on biomaterials. The results do not show a clear advantage of one material.[8,24,37] Most studies are retrospective, and populations were ill defined, making it difficult to control for the variety of trauma patients in regards to age, mechanism of injury, and comorbidities that may affect healing. In addition, different surgical approaches to the orbit may affect healing, and there is a lack of long-term follow-up. Nonetheless, using the evidence available, investigators were able to produce some guidelines. The critical factor in choosing the right implant material is the magnitude of the defect, determined by the size of the fracture and the orbital volume change.[24] In the case of small defects or linear fractures, the placement of a membrane may be suitable, whereas in larger defects affecting one wall or multiple walls, a stronger, supportive material may be necessary.[8] For small defects, the choice of material is more dependent on biocompatibility. In larger defects, mechanical properties and the contour or form factor needs special consideration as well as biocompatibility.[37]

Intraoperative Computed Tomographic Scans

Even with the ideal reconstructive material, the complex anatomy of the bony orbit makes precise reconstruction of orbital fractures and zygomatico-orbital fractures challenging. Inadequate repair of these injuries often results in excess orbital volume with postoperative diplopia and globe malposition.[41] Intraoperative imaging plays a crucial role in orthopedic surgery during the repair of long bone fractures, giving immediate feedback and allowing for further reduction and corrections to be made while still in the operating room. Given the complexity of the facial skeleton, a transfer of this technology to maxillofacial trauma repair seems logical.

Use of intraoperative CT scanning has been reviewed by several investigators.[41–48] Several investigators suggest using intraoperative CT in all cases of orbital or orbital zygomatic trauma,[42,46–49] whereas others propose reserving the use of intraoperative cone-beam CT to aid in the reduction of complex or secondary zygomaticomaxillary (ZMC) repositioning after a failure of conventional techniques.[45]

Those who argue in opposition of the use of intraoperative CT state cost, exposure to radiation, and additional time spent in the operating room.[45] In regards to radiation exposure, the amount of radiation dosed with new technologies such as cone-beam CT is minimal. Daily background radiation is 8 mSv every 24 hours; cone-beam CT is 40 to 80 mSv, and FAN beam CT is 600 to 800 mSv (a 2-view chest radiograph is 100 mSv for reference). Furthermore, many surgeons will obtain postoperative imaging to evaluate reduction. Intraoperative CT obviates this.

A study by Shaye and colleagues[43] investigated the amount of time used for intraoperative CT scan and found it to be a mean of 14.5 minutes. More importantly, the results of the CT scan led to revisions in 24% of patients, with 8 of 9 of them being classified as "complex" cases. This finding is consistent with the average of 18% revisions, which was calculated based on a meta-analysis.[44] There is no way to determine how many of these cases would have required secondary revision at a later date had they not undergone revision in the operating room. This calculation is difficult to determine, because the threshold to perform revision is much higher once out of the operating room, and discrepancies seen on CT may not have contributed to a postoperative problem that would compel revision surgery. Nevertheless, given the high cost of revision surgery, it would take just a few secondary revisions to justify the cost of intraoperative CT.

A review by van Hout and colleagues[44] set out to assess the value of intraoperative imaging on fracture repair and found that intraoperative imaging does have consequences on the surgical management of ZMC fractures. However, they did not find significant data regarding facial symmetry or fracture reduction. Although it is reasonable to assume that performing intraoperative revisions improves the quality of outcomes, the positive consequences of these revisions are merely implied and yet to be proven.

Use of Navigation Technology

A technique that has been described by several investigators is to "mirror" the normal anatomy of the uninjured orbit to the contralateral injured side and use this as a template for surgical repair.[50] This mirror technique has been used in combination with surgical navigation. Surgical navigation shows promise and is particularly useful when one side of the face is unaffected.[41] A CT scan represents the most appropriate imaging modality for cases of bone abnormality, which is generally the image modality of choice used in the ERs to diagnose these fractures on intake. Relying on symmetry of the face, the patient's CT scan can be imported into the navigation system, and the unaffected side then undergoes an axial flip and is virtually mirrored onto the pathologic side. The navigation probe can be placed along the repair throughout the reconstruction to ensure accurate placement of the implant and/or bony pieces.[41,51,52]

The advantage of this method is that the accuracy of the construct can then be assessed at any stage and again at the end of the process.

Intraoperative CT remains less dynamic than navigation-assisted techniques, consequently delaying surgery and adding radiation exposure.[53] In a facility that already uses a navigation system for neurosurgery or otolaryngology, using the system for maxillofacial trauma may be an easy and affordable addition. However, in a facility that is not familiar with the navigation system, there may be financial and technical difficulties initially. Another disadvantage of this technique is that there is, on average, 1 mm of error in registration in the periorbital area regardless of the method of registration.[54] In addition, it requires a normal contralateral side, which is not often the case in panfacial trauma. A larger clinical series with long-term follow-up will be needed to determine reproducibility and cost-effectiveness.

REPAIR OF MANDIBLE FRACTURES
Open Versus Closed Treatment of Subcondylar Fractures

Mandible fractures are the most common facial fractures after the nasal bone. A large percentage of them require repair.[3] Repair of mandible fractures has evolved significantly throughout the years. Techniques ranging from wire osteosynthesis,[55] lag screw,[56] compression,[57] and noncompression plates[58] have been used. Techniques of repair continue to evolve as new evidence becomes available. However, in some areas, the data show mixed results, and there is controversy among surgeons over best practice.

The anatomic distribution of fractures includes the angle, symphysis, condyle and subcondyle, and body.[59] The area of mandible repair that sparks the most controversy is repair of the condylar fracture. Complications of condylar fracture include pain, restricted mandibular movement, deviation of the mandible, malocclusion, pathologic changes to the temporomandibular joint, osteonecrosis, facial asymmetry, and ankylosis. For many years, closed management and MMF were used to treat these fractures. It should be noted that closed management does not actually reduce these fractures and the term closed reduction is a misnomer. Closed management of these fractures includes stabilizing the fracture and re-establishing occlusion with MMF. This method was preferred treatment for many years. In recent years, open treatment of these fractures has become more common, likely because of advancements in the technology of plate and screw fixation devices and use of the endoscope. There is some evidence that this leads to better outcomes.

Most surgeons agree there are several absolute indications for open treatment. These indications were described in an article by Zide and Kent[60] and include dislocation into the middle cranial fossa or external auditory canal, lateral extracapsular displacement, inability to obtain adequate occlusion, and open joint wound with foreign body or gross contamination. In addition, many investigators agree that other indications for open treatment include bilateral fractures[61,62] and polytrauma, where there are fractures of other areas of the face that compromise occlusion and for which rigid fixation will be used.[63] Similarly, most investigators agree that for mild or moderately displaced condylar fractures, conservative treatment with rigid or elastic MMF is generally adequate. The controversy comes when caring for the patient with a considerably displaced fracture. In 2003, the American Association of Oral and Maxillofacial Surgeons special committee on parameters of care developed indications for open reduction and added the following: physical evidence of a fracture, imaging evidence of a fracture, malocclusion, mandibular dysfunction, abnormal relationship of the jaw, hemotympanum, cerebral spinal fluid otorrhea, effusion, and hemarthrosis.

Several studies have attempted to answer the question of open versus closed reduction and to clarify the variables that help determine which approach may be most appropriate for each patient. Haug and Assael[63] compared 10 patients who underwent open reduction internal fixation (ORIF) to 10 patients who underwent closed treatment with maxillomandibular fixation (CRMMF) and found that ORIF was associated with visible scars and CRMMF was associated with chronic pain. Ellis and Throckmorton[64] compared vertical measure of facial morphology in patients with condyle fractures who had undergone either closed or open repair. They found that the patients treated with closed methods had significantly shorter posterior facial and ramus heights on the side of the injury compared with those treated with open reduction. The same group evaluated occlusal relationships of patients treated with closed or open techniques and found that those treated by closed techniques had a significantly greater percentage of malocclusion.[65]

Villarreal and colleagues[66] reviewed a series of 104 condyle fractures to determine what factors most influenced the clinical variables and postoperative result. They found that the principal factors that determined the treatment decision were the level of the fracture and the degree of displacement. The functional improvement obtained by open methods was greater than that obtained by closed treatment. However, open treatment increased the incidence of postoperative condylar deformities and mandibular asymmetry. Ellis and

colleagues[67] did another study and followed 61 patients who underwent ORIF for unilateral condyle fracture and found that despite being in good reduction after the initial repair, 10% to 20% of condylar processes had postsurgical changes of more than 10°, likely from a loss of fixation. Eckelt and colleagues[68] performed a large randomized, prospective controlled trial of open versus closed treatment in 79 fractures. They examined clinical parameters such as mouth opening and protrusion; radiographic parameters, such as deviation of the fragment, shortening of the ascending ramus; and subjective functional impairment including pain and discomfort. They found that both treatment options for condylar fractures of the mandible yielded acceptable results. However, operative (open) treatment, irrespective of the method of internal fixation used, was superior in all objective and subjective functional parameters. Furthermore, they examined the data for each location of fracture (condylar base, condylar neck, condylar head). They found that although patients had less discomfort overall with ascending level of fracture, for all fracture types, open surgical treatment in connection with anatomically correct reduction and fixation of fragments resulted in significantly better outcomes on a uniformly high level.[69]

Many surgeons recommend closed management because of problems with surgical approach, infection, injury to nerves and blood vessels, and scar formation.[70] Marker and colleagues[71] examined 348 patients who all underwent closed management to see if there were any variables predictive of complications. They found 3% had pain and 2% had malocclusion. Based on this, they determined closed management is safe and reliable in all but a few cases. Santler and colleagues[72] examined 150 patients who were treated with either open or closed management and were examined at 2.5 years follow-up, they found that surgically treated patients showed significantly more weather sensitivity and pain on maximum mouth opening.

A review done by Nussbaum and colleagues[73] was unable to provide definitive answers. They found numerous problems with the information presented in the various articles. These problems included lack of patient randomization, failure to classify the type of condylar fracture, variability within the surgical protocols, and inconsistencies in choice of variables and how they were reported. It is suggested that treatment type should be selected considering patient's age, fracture type, patient's systemic status, other facture, teeth, possibility of occlusal restoration by intermaxillary fixation, and existence of foreign materials. In the final determination of treatment plan, the advantage, disadvantage, risk of each treatment, and risk of complications should be sufficiently discussed with patients.[70]

Endoscopic-Assisted Repair of Subcondylar Fractures

The above arguments illustrate the dilemma faced by the facial plastic surgeon. Many are dissatisfied with the potential complications of open reduction, such as facial scars and injury to the facial nerve, but there is also dissatisfaction with the results of closed management. Endoscopic approach to the subcondylar fracture offers the advantages of both techniques. In several comparison trials, endoscopic reduction has demonstrated equivalent results to open reduction in terms of anterior opening, mandibular deviation, posterior ramal height, and centric occlusion.[74,75] The use of endoscopic assistance allows for minimal if any facial scarring, while also minimizing the risk of facial nerve injury. However, this technique is technically challenging, and there is a steep learning curve. The procedure may be time consuming, especially as the surgeon first attempts it. The senior author reviewed all cases of endoscopic subcondylar fractures and found that of the 48 patients undergoing the procedure, 2 had to be converted to open and 5 were reduced endoscopically but not plated. All of these unsuccessful attempts occurred during the early experience, illustrating the learning curve a surgeon encounters. They also found that this technique is not optimal for high neck, intracapsular issues, or those with medially displaced proximal segments.[76–78] Although it does have some technical challenges, this is a reasonable alternative with lower morbidity compared with the standard extended open reduction.

Use of Maxillomandibular Fixation

The use of MMF has a long tradition. It is described in some version as far back as 1492, when the surgeon would "tie the teeth of the uninjured jaw to the teeth of the injured jaw."[79] However, in recent years, there has been a shift in repair techniques with MMF being used less often. In general, MMF is used to stabilize jaws while the fracture is healing and to establish correct occlusion. It is placed intraoperatively once occlusion is established, before the ORIF of the fracture. It is often left on for a period of weeks after surgery with wires as a way to stabilize the mandible in correct position, to ensure patient compliance with a liquid diet, or in the case of guiding elastics, to correct cases of minor malocclusion. There are recent data indicating that MMF may not be necessary in all cases.[80–84] In several studies, it was demonstrated that MMF offered no advantages.

Postoperative maxillomandibular fixation

Regarding the use of postoperative MMF, in one study, the investigator who previously used MMF and then abandoned the practice compared complications and results in patients with and without postoperative MMF and found no significant difference.[85] In 2 other retrospective studies, both using a matched pairing of identical fractures fixated with identical plating schemes with and without MMF, no significant difference was noted.[80,81] Although it is suggested to use MMF in cases of high subcondylar, condylar, and comminuted fractures, in cases where good reduction is achieved and stabilized with a plate, postoperative MMF may not be needed.

Intraoperative maxillomandibular fixation

In another study, it was suggested that intraoperative MMF may also not be needed. In this review of a decade of trauma experience, it was noted that the use of MMF to achieve occlusion before ORIF had decreased annually, as manual reduction with ORIF became a preferred option. A comparison of the complications between the 2 methods showed no significant differences.[82] Another study compared Erich arch bars, interdental stout wires, and manual reduction and found no significant differences infection, wound dehiscence, or symptomatic hardware requiring removal.[83] These data suggest a shifting trend in mandible fracture management. Although arch bars are still the appropriate treatment for patients with subcondylar fractures, comminuted, significantly displaced, or multiple fractures, as well as midface fractures in addition to mandible fracture, data suggest that a select group of patients may be safely treated without arch bars.

Screw maxillomandibular fixation

Application of arch bars can be tedious, requiring significant time before the fracture repair begins. There is also the risk of blood-borne pathogens transmission via wire stick injuries to the surgeon and operating room staff. The impetus to develop faster and safer techniques to achieve MMF has led to advances in screw MMF. In these cases, the MMF screws are inserted into the bony base of both jaws between the canine and first premolar in all 4 quadrants.[86] The screw heads act as anchor points to fasten wire loops or rubber bands connecting the mandible to the maxilla. In comparison to these tooth-borne appliances, MMF screws shorten the time to achieve intermaxillary fixation considerably and help to reduce the hazards of glove perforation and wire stick injuries.[87] This technique is particularly effective for patients with good dentition and strong intercuspation.

On the downside, MMF screws are attributed with the risk of tooth root damage and a lack of versatility beyond the pure maintenance of occlusion. It is not recommended for use in cases that require stabilizing loose teeth, or fragments of the mandible and alveolar process. The increased distance the intermaxillary fixation wires must travel results in low vector control, which may lead to lingual rotation and poor bone healing.[86] In all cases, there is a risk that the screw may loosen and back out.[87,88] Because the fixation is largely anterior, there may be inadequate posterior stability.

Hybrid maxillomandibular fixation

In an attempt to combine the strength and rigidity of arch bars with the safety and efficiency of MMF screws, a hybrid arch bar has recently been produced. The manufacturer claims that this combination omits the need for interdental wiring, and thereby, reduces the chance of wire stick injuries for health care providers. It also is supposed to save time in application and removal and does not require an additional trip to the operating room for removal. This new technology has not yet undergone controlled trials or studies on the long-term effects, but is a promising new technique in MMF.

SUMMARY

There are still many areas of facial trauma reconstruction that are subject to debate. The lack of guidelines is due to a lack of clinical trials and a high level of evidence, because the most literature is expert opinion and retrospective studies.

REFERENCES

1. Allareddy V, Allareddy V, Nalliah RP. Epidemiology of facial fracture injuries. J Oral Maxillofac Surg 2011; 69(10):2613–8.
2. Yadav K, Cowan E, Wall S, et al. Orbital fracture clinical decision rule development: burden of disease and use of a mandatory electronic survey instrument. Acad Emerg Med 2011;18(3):313–6.
3. VandeGriend ZP, Hashemi A, Shkoukani M. Changing trends in adult facial trauma epidemiology. J Craniofac Surg 2015;26(1):108–12.
4. Dubois L, Steenen SA, Gooris PJJ, et al. Controversies in orbital reconstruction–II. Timing of posttraumatic orbital reconstruction: a systematic review. Int J Oral Maxillofac Surg 2015;44(4):433–40.
5. Harris GJ. Orbital blow-out fractures: surgical timing and technique. Eye (Lond) 2006;20(10):1207–12.
6. Gosau M, Schöneich M, Draenert FG, et al. Retrospective analysis of orbital floor fractures–complications, outcome, and review of literature. Clin Oral Investig 2011;15(3):305–13.
7. Hoşal BM, Beatty RL. Diplopia and enophthalmos after surgical repair of blowout fracture. Orbit 2002;21(1):27–33.
8. Dubois L, Steenen SA, Gooris PJJ, et al. Controversies in orbital reconstruction–I. Defect-driven orbital reconstruction: a systematic review. Int J Oral Maxillofac Surg 2015;44(3):308–15.
9. Jaquiéry C, Aeppli C, Cornelius P, et al. Reconstruction of orbital wall defects: critical review of 72 patients. Int J Oral Maxillofac Surg 2007; 36(3):193–9.
10. Brucoli M, Arcuri F, Cavenaghi R, et al. Analysis of complications after surgical repair of orbital fractures. J Craniofac Surg 2011;22(4):1387–90.
11. Hawes MJ, Dortzbach RK. Surgery on orbital floor fractures. Influence of time of repair and fracture size. Ophthalmology 1983;90(9):1066–70.
12. Harris GJ, Garcia GH, Logani SC, et al. Correlation of preoperative computed tomography and postoperative ocular motility in orbital blowout fractures. Ophthal Plast Reconstr Surg 2000;16(3): 179–87.
13. Shin JW, Lim JS, Yoo G, et al. An analysis of pure blowout fractures and associated ocular symptoms. J Craniofac Surg 2013;24(3):703–7.
14. Matteini C, Renzi G, Becelli R, et al. Surgical timing in orbital fracture treatment: experience with 108 consecutive cases. J Craniofac Surg 2004;15(1): 145–50.
15. Shin KH, Baek SH, Chi M. Comparison of the outcomes of non-trapdoor-type blowout fracture repair according to the time of surgery. J Craniofac Surg 2011;22(4):1426–9.
16. Verhoeff K, Grootendorst RJ, Wijngaarde R, et al. Surgical repair of orbital fractures: how soon after trauma? Strabismus 1998;6(2):77–80.
17. Simon GJB, Syed HM, McCann JD, et al. Early versus late repair of orbital blowout fractures. Ophthalmic Surg Lasers Imaging 2009;40(2):141–8.
18. Dal Canto AJ, Linberg JV. Comparison of orbital fracture repair performed within 14 days versus 15 to 29 days after trauma. Ophthal Plast Reconstr Surg 2008;24(6):437–43.
19. Nowinski D, Di Rocco F, Roujeau T, et al. Complex pediatric orbital fractures combined with traumatic brain injury: treatment and follow-up. J Craniofac Surg 2010;21(4):1054–9.
20. Jordan DR, Allen LH, White J, et al. Intervention within days for some orbital floor fractures: the white-eyed blowout. Ophthal Plast Reconstr Surg 1998;14(6):379–90.

21. Wang N-C, Ma L, Wu S-Y, et al. Orbital blow-out fractures in children: characterization and surgical outcome. Chang Gung Med J 2010;33(3):313–20.

22. Amrith S, Almousa R, Wong WL, et al. Blowout fractures: surgical outcome in relation to age, time of intervention, and other preoperative risk factors. Craniomaxillofac Trauma Reconstr 2010;3(3):131–6.

23. Ethunandan M, Evans BT. Linear trapdoor or 'white-eye' blowout fracture of the orbit: not restricted to children. Br J Oral Maxillofac Surg 2011;49(2):142–7.

24. Gunarajah DR, Samman N. Biomaterials for repair of orbital floor blowout fractures: a systematic review. J Oral Maxillofac Surg 2013;71(3):550–70.

25. Kontio RK, Laine P, Salo A, et al. Reconstruction of internal orbital wall fracture with iliac crest free bone graft: clinical, computed tomography, and magnetic resonance imaging follow-up study. Plast Reconstr Surg 2006;118(6):1365–74.

26. Zins JE, Whitaker LA. Membranous versus endochondral bone: implications for craniofacial reconstruction. Plast Reconstr Surg 1983;72(6):778–85.

27. Ilankovan V, Jackson IT. Experience in the use of calvarial bone grafts in orbital reconstruction. Br J Oral Maxillofac Surg 1992;30(2):92–6.

28. Cavusoglu T, Vargel I, Yazici I, et al. Reconstruction of orbital floor fractures using autologous nasal septal bone graft. Ann Plast Surg 2010; 64(1):41–6.

29. Bayat M, Momen-Heravi F, Khalilzadeh O, et al. Comparison of conchal cartilage graft with nasal septal cartilage graft for reconstruction of orbital floor blowout fractures. Br J Oral Maxillofac Surg 2010;48(8):617–20.

30. Castellani A, Negrini S, Zanetti U. Treatment of orbital floor blowout fractures with conchal auricular cartilage graft: a report on 14 cases. J Oral Maxillofac Surg 2002;60(12):1413–7.

31. Yan Z, Zhou Z, Song X. Nasal endoscopy-assisted reconstruction of orbital floor blowout fractures using temporal fascia grafting. J Oral Maxillofac Surg 2012;70(5):1119–22.

32. Becker ST, Terheyden H, Fabel M, et al. Comparison of collagen membranes and polydioxanone for reconstruction of the orbital floor after fractures. J Craniofac Surg 2010;21(4):1066–8.

33. Luhr HG, Maerker R. Transplantation of homologous dura in reconstruction of the orbital floor. Trans Int Conf Oral Surg 1973;4:340–4.

34. Thadani V, Penar PL, Partington J, et al. Creutzfeldt-Jakob disease probably acquired from a cadaveric dura mater graft. Case report. J Neurosurg 1988; 69(5):766–9.

35. Chowdhury K, Krause GE. Selection of materials for orbital floor reconstruction. Arch Otolaryngol Head Neck Surg 1998;124(12):1398–401.

36. Lieger O, Richards R, Liu M, et al. Computer-assisted design and manufacture of implants in the late

37. Dubois L, Steenen SA, Gooris PJJ, et al. Controversies in orbital reconstruction—III. Biomaterials for orbital reconstruction: a review with clinical recommendations. Int J Oral Maxillofac Surg 2016; 45(1):41–50.

38. Laxenaire A, Lévy J, Blanchard P, et al. Complications of silastic implants used in orbital repair. Rev Stomatol Chir Maxillofac 1997;98(Suppl 1):96–9 [in French].

39. Baumann A, Burggasser G, Gauss N, et al. Orbital floor reconstruction with an alloplastic resorbable polydioxanone sheet. Int J Oral Maxillofac Surg 2002;31(4):367–73.

40. Mauriello JA, Wasserman B, Kraut R. Use of Vicryl (polyglactin-910) mesh implant for repair of orbital floor fracture causing diplopia: a study of 28 patients over 5 years. Ophthal Plast Reconstr Surg 1993; 9(3):191–5.

41. Fuller SC, Strong EB. Computer applications in facial plastic and reconstructive surgery. Curr Opin Otolaryngol Head Neck Surg 2007;15(4):233–7.

42. Wilde F, Lorenz K, Ebner A-K, et al. Intraoperative imaging with a 3D C-arm system after zygomatico-orbital complex fracture reduction. J Oral Maxillofac Surg 2013;71(5):894–910.

43. Shaye DA, Tollefson TT, Strong EB. Use of intraoperative computed tomography for maxillofacial reconstructive surgery. JAMA Facial Plast Surg 2015; 17(2):113–9.

44. van Hout WMMT, Van Cann EM, Muradin MSM, et al. Intraoperative imaging for the repair of zygomaticomaxillary complex fractures: a comprehensive review of the literature. J Craniomaxillofac Surg 2014;42(8):1918–23.

45. Singh M, Ricci JA, Caterson EJ. Use of intraoperative computed tomography for revisional procedures in patients with complex maxillofacial trauma. Plast Reconstr Surg Glob Open 2015;3(7):e463.

46. Heiland M, Schulze D, Blake F, et al. Intraoperative imaging of zygomaticomaxillary complex fractures using a 3D C-arm system. Int J Oral Maxillofac Surg 2005;34(4):369–75.

47. Stanley RB. Use of intraoperative computed tomography during repair of orbitozygomatic fractures. Arch Facial Plast Surg 1999;1(1):19–24.

48. Gülicher D, Krimmel M, Reinert S. The role of intraoperative ultrasonography in zygomatic complex fracture repair. Int J Oral Maxillofac Surg 2006; 35(3):224–30.

49. Cai EZ, Koh YP, Hing ECH, et al. Computer-assisted navigational surgery improves outcomes in orbital reconstructive surgery. J Craniofac Surg 2012; 23(5):1567–73.

50. Gellrich N-C, Schramm A, Hammer B, et al. Computer-assisted secondary reconstruction of unilateral

posttraumatic orbital deformity. Plast Reconstr Surg 2002;110(6):1417–29.

51. Bruneau M, Schoovaerts F, Kamouni R, et al. The mirroring technique: a navigation-based method for reconstructing a symmetrical orbit and cranial vault. Neurosurgery 2013;73(1 Suppl Operative): ons24–8 [discussion: ons28–9].

52. Nyachhyon P, Kim PC. Intraoperative stereotactic navigation for reconstruction in zygomatic-orbital trauma. JNMA J Nepal Med Assoc 2011;51(181): 37–40.

53. Schramm A, Suarez-Cunqueiro MM, Rücker M, et al. Computer-assisted therapy in orbital and mid-facial reconstructions. Int J Med Robot 2009;5(2):111–24.

54. Luebbers H-T, Messmer P, Obwegeser JA, et al. Comparison of different registration methods for surgical navigation in cranio-maxillofacial surgery. J Craniomaxillofac Surg 2008;36(2):109–16.

55. Theriot BA, Van Sickels JE, Triplett RG, et al. Intraosseous wire fixation versus rigid osseous fixation of mandibular fractures: a preliminary report. J Oral Maxillofac Surg 1987;45(7):577–82.

56. Niederdellmann H, Shetty V. Solitary lag screw osteosynthesis in the treatment of fractures of the angle of the mandible: a retrospective study. Plast Reconstr Surg 1987;80(1):68–74.

57. Ellis E, Sinn DP. Treatment of mandibular angle fractures using two 2.4-mm dynamic compression plates. J Oral Maxillofac Surg 1993;51(9):969–73.

58. Ellis E, Walker L. Treatment of mandibular angle fractures using two noncompression miniplates. J Oral Maxillofac Surg 1994;52(10):1032–6 [discussion: 1036–7].

59. Morris C, Bebeau NP, Brockhoff H, et al. Mandibular fractures: an analysis of the epidemiology and patterns of injury in 4,143 fractures. J Oral Maxillofac Surg 2015;73(5):951.e1–12.

60. Zide MF, Kent JN. Indications for open reduction of mandibular condyle fractures. J Oral Maxillofac Surg 1983;41(2):89–98.

61. Banks P. A pragmatic approach to the management of condylar fractures. Int J Oral Maxillofac Surg 1998;27(4):244–6.

62. Tominaga K, Habu M, Khanal A, et al. Biomechanical evaluation of different types of rigid internal fixation techniques for subcondylar fractures. J Oral Maxillofac Surg 2006;64(10):1510–6.

63. Haug RH, Assael LA. Outcomes of open versus closed treatment of mandibular subcondylar fractures. J Oral Maxillofac Surg 2001;59(4):370–5 [discussion: 375–6].

64. Ellis E, Throckmorton G. Facial symmetry after closed and open treatment of fractures of the mandibular condylar process. J Oral Maxillofac Surg 2000;58(7):719–28 [discussion: 729–30].

65. Ellis E, Simon P, Throckmorton GS. Occlusal results after open or closed treatment of fractures of the mandibular condylar process. J Oral Maxillofac Surg 2000;58(3):260–8.

66. Villarreal PM, Monje F, Junquera LM, et al. Mandibular condyle fractures: determinants of treatment and outcome. J Oral Maxillofac Surg 2004;62(2):155–63.

67. Ellis E, Throckmorton GS, Palmieri C. Open treatment of condylar process fractures: assessment of adequacy of repositioning and maintenance of stability. J Oral Maxillofac Surg 2000;58(1):27–34 [discussion: 35].

68. Eckelt U, Schneider M, Erasmus F, et al. Open versus closed treatment of fractures of the mandibular condylar process—a prospective randomized multi-centre study. J Craniomaxillofac Surg 2006; 34(5):306–14.

69. Schneider M, Erasmus F, Gerlach KL, et al. Open reduction and internal fixation versus closed treatment and mandibulomaxillary fixation of fractures of the mandibular condylar process: a randomized, prospective, multicenter study with special evaluation of fracture level. J Oral Maxillofac Surg 2008; 66(12):2537–44.

70. Choi K-Y, Yang J-D, Chung H-Y, et al. Current concepts in the mandibular condyle fracture management part II: open reduction versus closed reduction. Arch Plast Surg 2012;39(4):301–8.

71. Marker P, Nielsen A, Bastian HL. Fractures of the mandibular condyle. Part 2: results of treatment of 348 patients. Br J Oral Maxillofac Surg 2000;38(5): 422–6.

72. Santler G, Kärcher H, Ruda C, et al. Fractures of the condylar process: surgical versus nonsurgical treatment. J Oral Maxillofac Surg 1999;57(4):392–7 [discussion: 397–8].

73. Nussbaum ML, Laskin DM, Best AM. Closed versus open reduction of mandibular condylar fractures in adults: a meta-analysis. J Oral Maxillofac Surg 2008;66(6):1087–92.

74. Khiabani KS, Raisian S, Khanian Mehmandoost M. Comparison between two techniques for the treatment of mandibular subcondylar fractures: closed treatment technique and transoral endoscopic-assisted open reduction. J Maxillofac Oral Surg 2015;14(2):363–9.

75. Nam SM, Kim YB, Cha HG, et al. Transoral open reduction for subcondylar fractures of the mandible using an angulated screwdriver system. Ann Plast Surg 2015;75(3):295–301.

76. Kellman RM, Cienfuegos R. Endoscopic approaches to subcondylar fractures of the mandible. Facial Plast Surg 2009;25(1):23–8.

77. Kellman RM. Endoscopically assisted repair of subcondylar fractures of the mandible: an evolving technique. Arch Facial Plast Surg 2003;5(3):244–50.

78. Kellman RM. Endoscopic approach to subcondylar mandible fractures. Facial Plast Surg 2004;20(3): 239–47.

79. Spina AM, Marciani RD. Maxillofacial surgery: trauma. Philadelphia: WB Saunders; 2000.

80. Valentino J, Marentette LJ. Supplemental maxillomandibular fixation with miniplate osteosynthesis. Otolaryngol Head Neck Surg 1995;112(2):215–20.

81. Kumar I, Singh V, Bhagol A, et al. Supplemental maxillomandibular fixation with miniplate osteosynthesis-required or not? Oral Maxillofac Surg 2011;15(1): 27–30.

82. Kopp RW, Crozier DL, Goyal P, et al. Decade review of mandible fractures and arch bar impact on outcomes of nonsubcondylar fractures. Laryngoscope 2016;126(3):596–601.

83. Bell RB, Wilson DM. Is the use of arch bars or interdental wire fixation necessary for successful outcomes in the open reduction and internal fixation of mandibular angle fractures? J Oral Maxillofac Surg 2008;66(10):2116–22.

84. Gear AJL, Apasova E, Schmitz JP, et al. Treatment modalities for mandibular angle fractures. J Oral Maxillofac Surg 2005;63(5):655–63.

85. Saman M, Kadakia S, Ducic Y. Postoperative maxillomandibular fixation after open reduction of mandible fractures. JAMA Facial Plast Surg 2014; 16(6):410–3.

86. Ansari K, Hamlar D, Ho V, et al. A comparison of anterior vs posterior isolated mandible fractures treated with intermaxillary fixation screws. Arch Facial Plast Surg 2011;13(4):266–70.

87. Cornelius C-P, Ehrenfeld M. The use of MMF screws: surgical technique, indications, contraindications, and common problems in review of the literature. Craniomaxillofac Trauma Reconstr 2010;3(2):055–80.

88. Hashemi HM, Parhiz A. Complications using intermaxillary fixation screws. J Oral Maxillofac Surg 2011;69(5):1411–4.

Postoperative Controversies in the Management of Free Flap Surgery in the Head and Neck

Steven B. Cannady, MD[a],*, Kyle Hatten, MD[b],
Mark K. Wax, MD[c]

KEYWORDS

- Free flap • Head and neck defect • Anticoagulation • Fluid management • Flap monitoring

KEY POINTS

- A variety of postoperative anticoagulation protocols exist in the literature and in practice, yet few data suggest that one is superior to another.
- Anticoagulation protocols to manage underlying hypercoagulable risk or prevent secondary or primary clotting events are becoming standardized with known increases in bleeding complication rates.
- Fluid overload is a known risk factor for flap failure and literature supports conservative fluid use with preference for medication-based blood pressure management if physiologically appropriate.
- Flap monitoring methods vary. With changing training program work hour constraints, frequent monitoring by resident physicians may not afford benefit to flap survival.
- With high success rates in free flap surgery becoming standard, detecting significant changes based on subtly different postoperative protocols is increasingly difficult to power.

INTRODUCTION

With centers now reporting excellent free flap success rates that approach the 90% to 99% range, surgeons strive to pursue methods to ensure the survival of free tissue transfers.[1] There is morbidity for the patients undergoing free tissue transfer both at the donor site, and potentially the defect, especially if a free flap fails. Success of secondary transfers after failed first attempts is less than if the initial flap is viable, making the first attempt the best chance for optimal outcome for the patient.[2] Ross and colleagues[2] reported that second free flaps for head and neck defects had 73% success rate after failed first flap compared with 96% for second flap for recurrence or wound complications. Head and neck cancer patients and others undergoing flap surgery have oncologic and medical considerations that may affect success of surgery, or even cancer treatment pathway.[3–5] After preoperative optimization, the survival of free tissue depends on a technically successful surgery, and postoperative management.

Although intraoperative management is paramount for the successful completion of flap surgery, postoperative management is increasingly a focus of surgeons attempting to manage risk of flap failure. That preoperative assessment is important to patient selection is clear, but controversy

[a] Otorhinolaryngology Head and Neck Surgery, University of Pennsylvania, 800 Walnut Street, 18th Floor, Philadelphia, PA 19107, USA; [b] Head and Neck Surgery, Department of Otorhinolaryngology Head and Neck Surgery, University of Pennsylvania, West 34th Street, Philadelphia, PA 19107, USA; [c] Department of Otolaryngology, Oregon Health Sciences University, Portland, OR 97239, USA
* Corresponding author.
E-mail address: Steven.cannady@uphs.upenn.edu

Facial Plast Surg Clin N Am 24 (2016) 309–314
http://dx.doi.org/10.1016/j.fsc.2016.03.007
1064-7406/16/$ – see front matter © 2016 Elsevier Inc. All rights reserved.

exists within the management of the flap and patient in the postoperative timeframe. Substantial literature has been produced regarding anticoagulation, fluid management, and flap monitoring and is of clear importance in success, and ability to salvage flap problems.

As guidelines are increasingly provided to head and neck surgeons regarding the proper perioperative management of anticoagulation for both high-risk and low-risk patients, the effect of these recommendations and how they interface with flap-based anticoagulation protocols remains controversial.[6–8] The risk of hematoma, or bleeding complications, and their impact on flap survival within the guidelines suggested is a topic of recent debate. Bahl and colleagues[8] demonstrated in a large cohort of patients undergoing otolaryngologic surgery that venous thromboembolism (VTE) carries a low likelihood overall, but a subset of patients with high Caprini risk score had a higher rate of VTE. This was offset by the increased risk of bleeding complications in groups on VTE chemoprophylaxis. The study further outlined patients undergoing free tissue reduced their risk of VTE from 7.7% to 2.1% and increased risk of bleeding from 4.5% to 11.9% when treated with chemoprophylaxis.

Furthermore, patients undergoing major head and neck reconstruction are typically devoid of oral intake for substantial periods postoperatively. As such, intravenous or enteral feedings provide sustenance and fluid balance in the postoperative timeframe. The literature supports that intraoperative fluid administration is an important predictor of flap complications and argues that the postoperative course may be affected by choice of fluid volume in the postoperative timeframe.[9] Poor nutrition, cancer pathology, cachexia, and electrolyte imbalance can all be found in the reconstructive candidate and may result in fluid shifts that affect intravascular/extravascular fluid balance. The result can dictate intravascular fluid, oxygen, and nutrient delivery to the newly placed free flap, or create surrounding tissue edema and pressure on the vascular pedicle and microvascular environment. Inherent to flap surgery is disruption of lymphatic drainage, which may compound edema further; fluid shift impacts the local and regional flap environment.

Early flap problem diagnosis is critical to the salvage and survival of free tissue. Some reports suggest that 80% of flaps can be salvaged if diagnosed early in the process of failure. In addition, it is known that the majority of vascular compromise occurs within the first 72 hours after anastamosis.[10] Monitoring methods in the early and late hospitalization periods should be tailored to allow the care team to identify problems early in their course,

and return a patient to the operating room or medical intervention that may save the flap from failing. Multiple monitoring methods exist, and the low likelihood of failure makes the use of potentially costly monitoring controversial.[11]

Within this review, these controversies are explored in more detail with an effort to more clearly delineate the literature, controversies, and future of managing these important, controllable factors in flap survival.

ANTICOAGULATION FOR THE PREVENTION OF VENOUS THROMBOEMBOLISM

Single-center reports and reviews have demonstrated that postoperative anticoagulation protocols after flap surgery vary. The benefit to the patient is largely in the prevention of secondary events during at-risk time periods such as surgery and hospitalization. The Caprini risk score has been applied to head and neck patients and is noted to stratify risk in head and neck surgery patients.[12] Patients with head and neck cancer are at risk for vasculopathology and postoperative clotting events.[8] Newer guidelines suggest that these patients should be maintained on anticoagulation whenever feasible, unless bleeding complications would be catastrophic. In the head and neck, procedures with high bleeding risk or major sequelae of bleeding may warrant cessation of anticoagulation; these are summarized in **Table 1**.[13] These newer guidelines represent a significant paradigm shift from previous common practice to cease the use of anticoagulation before surgery. Coincidently, the cardiac literature suggests that cessation of medications may result in a hypercoagulability increase that would put the patient at risk for secondary clotting events such as myocardial infarction, stroke, deep venous thrombosis, or pulmonary embolus, yet it remains unanswered whether this would also affect flap survival.[6]

Taken in aggregate, the need for adequate prophylaxis and secondary clot prevention with the risk of hematoma or bleeding event create a controversial issue surrounding flap management in the postoperative period. Continuing anticoagulation in the perioperative period results in increased levels of bleeding complications and an inferred decrease in secondary clotting event risk.[8] The risk of secondary clotting event is low in the head and neck population at large, but when examined closely, is substantial in the at-risk patient. In addition, free flap surgery has been identified as an independent risk factor for thromboembolism. It is understood empirically that, if a patient has a major clotting event that is life threatening, that flap preservation is of little

Table 1
A limited list of procedures with major bleeding risk of prophylaxis for venous thromboembolism with potential sequelae

Procedure	Bleeding Risk	Sequelae
Functional endoscopic sinus surgery	Major epistaxis, ingested blood	Vomiting, major blood loss
Transphenoidal	Hematoma at brain	Optic neuropathy, stroke
Thyroidectomy	Airway pressure	Loss of airway
Major head and neck	Hematoma, carotid or jugular vein compression	Cerebral edema, carotid compression
Free flap	Hematoma, flap bleed	Flap pedicle compromise, blood loss

concern. However, the balance between the risks of a secondary clotting event versus flap failure is delineated unclearly (**Table 2**). With hematoma risk of 11.7 and VTE risk of 2.1% in the chemoprophylaxis flap patient, the impact of risk reduction versus increase in bleeding is a substantial concern. As noted in Hsueh and colleagues' review[13] on perioperative management of antithrombotic therapy, the balance between risks should favor the prevention of the most morbid risk. The risk and cost of flap failure is also substantial and associated with increased need for hospitalization and additional surgery. Ahmad and colleagues[14] described a hematoma rate of 4.7% in a large series of free flaps in the head and neck, with 22.7% causing flap compromise. The flap pedicle could be salvaged in 75% of cases in this study. Thus, the projected increase in hematoma and risk of unsalvageable flap pedicle compromise is known: a 7.4% increase in hematomas × 25% that cannot be saved will result in 1.85 flaps per 100 that will fail owing to the increased risk of hematoma. This calculation does not factor in the risk of catastrophic airway bleeding that can result from head and neck surgery, and may be increased from chemoprophylaxis.

Patient selection becomes key to identify that is high risk for VTE. Shuman and colleagues[12] identified 3 groups of risk based on Caprini risk stratification; they noted that patients with score of greater than 9 have a VTE risk of 18.3% when no chemoprophylaxis is given. The low (score of 6) and intermediate (score of 7 or 8) groups had a low VTE risk of 0.5% and 2.4%. Therefore, to further reduce flap risk from hematoma, it is important to stratify those patients at high risk and use chemoprophylaxis despite the hematoma and flap risk. Prior studies demonstrate the risk of fatal pulmonary embolus after general surgery procedure is 0.9%, but after orthopedic procedures (of which many flaps can be considered) the risk was 5% if no prophylaxis is administered. Hsueh and colleagues[13] recommended that, if a patient has a high risk of VTE (defined as >5%) and high risk of bleeding (defined as 1.5%), medications used in secondary prevention may be reasonably held but with bridging therapy. Interestingly, high-risk patients (Caprini score) may also predict for flap failure (Cannady and Wax, personal communication, 2016).

Thus, the risk of VTE may outweigh the slightly increased risk of flap compromise as a

Table 2
Risk of VTE and bleeding with and without prophylaxis stratified by Caprini risk score and flap or no flap

	Overall	<6	6–7	>8	Flap Specific
Caprini score VTE					
Prophylaxis	1.2 (0.88 DVT, 0.55 PE)	0.5	1.9	1.7	2.1
No prophylaxis	1.3 (0.65 DVT, 0.84 PE)	0.5	2.4	18.3[a]	7.7[a]
Caprini score bleeding risk					
Prophylaxis	3.5	—	—	—	11.9
No prophylaxis	1.2[a]	—	—	—	4.5[a]

Abbreviations: DVT, deep venous thrombosis; PE, pulmonary embolism; VTE, venous thromboembolism.
[a] Denotes significant difference.

result; flap surgeons should consider providing chemoprophylaxis for patients at high risk to prevent the morbidity of VTE at the expense of additional hematoma reoperations and flap failures.

FLAP PROPHYLAXIS REGIMEN

There are multiple flap anticoagulation protocols, with no consensus on which is the best to support flap survival. Over the past 15 years, dextran, low-molecular-weight heparin, prostaglandin E1, heparin drip have all been used in various combinations; these regimens were recently reviewed by Brinkman and colleagues in 2013 and are summarized in **Table 3**. Despite the lack of clear evidence, 96% of surgeons report that they use some sort of regimen.[15] In a recent large series reviewing a single-center experience with salvage of clotted flaps revealed that anticoagulation had no impact.[16] The greatest risk of thrombosis seems to be in the first day after anastomosis when the damage to vessel intima is greatest; 80% of pedicle thrombosis occurs in the first 48 hours (the majority representing venous thrombus), but 90% of arterial thrombosis occurring in the first 24 hours.[10] In addition, 95% of explorations occur within the first 72 hours of anastamosis.[11]

Venous thrombi contain higher fibrin deposition than do arterial clots, which are platelet rich; this makes heparin a better venous anticoagulant and aspirin best for arterial clot prevention.[17,18]

Basic science studies indicate that 100 mg of aspirin is sufficient to create the desired effect, but that prior microvascular protocols use doses from 250 to 1500 mg/d.[15] No randomized, controlled studies show that aspirin is superior to other regimens in for flap survival and retrospective studies show it is not superior to other methods.[11,15] In fact, in a multicenter analysis of radial forearm flap survival, on multivariate analysis, no regimen protected from flap loss.[7]

Anticoagulation protocols do have risks associated with their use. Aspirin can lead to gastric bleeds, strokes, and bleeding complications. Dextran can lead to anaphylactic reaction, kidney damage, pulmonary edema, or respiratory distress. Heparin or low-molecular-weight heparin may lead to higher rates of hematoma or other bleeding complications. Despite these factors, the risk of flap loss prompts most surgeons to use some form of anticoagulation prophylaxis with only level IV evidence available. Although some laboratory evidence of effectiveness for some agents does exist, a clear trial in humans remains difficult to conduct. Few surgeons are willing to expose their patients to the potential for higher flap failure risk in a randomized, controlled trial. In addition, with flap failure rates now as low as 5% at major centers, it will be difficult to detect subtle changes without a multicenter design involving large amounts of patients. Therefore, the regimens used will remain as variable as the surgeons performing these cases and remain a source of significant controversy as patients may be subjected to complications of medications for which little evidence of efficacy exists.

POSTOPERATIVE FLUID MANAGEMENT AND VASOPRESSOR USE

Perioperative fluid management is a critical factor in the safe administration of anesthesia, and postoperative course; medical complication, length of hospital stay, return to operating room, and total flap loss were all adversely affected in level 1b or 2b studies.[17] Amount of acceptable fluid administration varies with some studies indicating greater than 130 mL/kg per 24 hours and the recommendation not to exceed 3.5 to 6 mL/kg per hour in the 24-hour perioperative time frame.[19,20]

Similarly, the administration of colloid was shown by Clark and colleagues[20] to increase the duration of hospital stay independent of other factors such as patient age, comorbidities, and smoking. Coincidently, it is desirable to keep the flap well-perfused postoperatively. Flap surgeons have been relatively averse to the use of vasopressors to maintain hemodynamic stability given the

Table 3
Anticoagulation regimens with methods of action and published flap outcomes expressed in percent (%)

Regimen	Method of Action	Flap Failure	Exploration	Thrombosis
ASA	Inhibits COX decrease PG, TXA formation	2.4	NR	3.2
Dextran	Reduce platelet, erythrocyte aggregation	1.0–6.0	3.8–8	NR
Heparin/LMWH	Binds antithrombin Inactivates factor II, IX, X, XI, XII	5–6.6	3.8–15	8.8–14.1

Abbreviations: ASA, aspirin; COX, cyclooxygenase; LMWH, low-molecular-weight heparin; NR, not reported; PG, prostaglandin; TXA, thromboxane.

hypothetical risk of a denervated flap's sensitivity to vasoconstrictive medicines (**Fig. 1**). Multiple basic science studies suggest this is possible; however, Monroe and colleagues[21] demonstrated that vasopressor use was more common then realized by the surgical team and resulted in no difference in flap outcomes in a prospective observational study. In addition, Brinkman and colleagues[17] and Chen and colleagues[22] both showed no increase in flap complication or total flap loss in patients who received pressors. Therefore, 3 studies with level 2b evidence now exist and suggest that vasopressors do not increase the risk of flap related complications.

The current evidence suggests that normovolemic hemodilution may be beneficial to the free flap, but fluid resuscitation should not exceed 6 mL/kg per hour. If a patient is not underloaded, use of vasopressors seems to be safe and desirable over fluid overload based on the complication profiles of both strategies.[17]

POSTOPERATIVE FLAP MONITORING

Detection of early flap problems predicts for the ability to salvage a flap. Therefore, it is generally recommended that flap patients be transferred to a high-volume flap unit with well-trained staff in the immediate postoperative period. For the first 2 to 4 hours, flap checks should be done every 20 to 30 minutes, followed by every 1 to 2 hours for the next 24 hours.[11] Consensus on the early post anesthesia intense monitoring time period is generally accepted, but methods of flap monitoring are highly variable after that.[17] Methods that are available currently include conventional clinical assessment, implantable Doppler, color duplex ultrasonography, near-infrared spectroscopy, microdialysis, and laser Doppler flowometry.

Conventional methods are largely clinical assessment based and may include use of a handheld Doppler unit. From a cost perspective, this requires only the 1-time purchase of a handheld Doppler unit, and a trained clinical team to assess the flap with accuracy. This method is difficult in the case of buried flaps. Therefore, authors have reported use of the Doppler ultrasonography in the buried flap to ensure appropriate monitoring.[23]

In Wax' large study from 2014 of 1142 flap transfers in the head and neck, an implantable Doppler devices were used in all cases.[1] The series detected intraoperative flow problems 11.7% of the time and led to intraoperative revision. Of those that did not require intraoperative revision, a reexploration rate of 6.1% with 61% salvage rate was reported. Ten false-negative results were encountered that required unnecessary reexploration. Overall, the implantable Doppler technique led to 87% sensitivity for flap flow problems. Some authors choose to place a Doppler device on both the artery and vein(s) to ensure real-time feedback on both vessel's flow.

Laser Doppler flowometry has been used frequently as a method to monitor breast flaps that do not suffer from saliva or a moist environment as in the head and neck. It is noninvasive in nature and reveals a trend in flow to the tissue involved. It has not been used frequently in most head and neck practices owing to the frequent placement of flap skin inside the oral cavity or pharynx.

To date, no monitoring system seems to be able to predict for enhanced flap survival, or salvage rates owing to early detection over any other. In

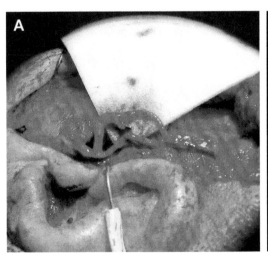
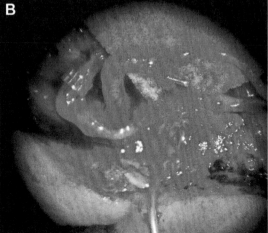

Fig. 1. (*A*) Demonstration of a flap artery in spasm, a hypothetical risk when using pressors in the perioperative period. (*B*) A close up showing the venous coupler with arterial (superior vessel) and venous constriction of vessel.

series in which flap monitoring is not feasible, flap survival suffers overall as a reflection of the inability to save flaps during a take back. With work duty-hour restrictions now affecting resident ability to primarily monitor flap patients, especially in programs with more than 1 hospital to cover, it has become important to train nurses in monitoring. Khariwala and Yueh showed that a protocol to train intensive care unit nurses is effective, and resulted in 100% flap survival. They provided didactics followed by mentorship from a resident instruction session before nurse-led monitoring.

With low rates of flap loss and thrombosis, the ideal monitoring method is that which detects problems earliest within the constraints of the surgeon's practice environment, and with consideration of the available resources (both human capital and instrument availability).

REFERENCES

1. Wax MK. The role of the implantable Doppler probe in free flap surgery. Laryngoscope 2014; 124(Suppl 1):S1–12.
2. Ross G, Yla-Kotola TM, Goldstein D, et al. Second free flaps in head and neck reconstruction. J Plast Reconstr Aesthet Surg 2012;65:1165–8.
3. Simeoni R, Breitenstein K, Esser D, et al. Cardiac comorbidity in head and neck cancer patients and its influence on cancer treatment selection and mortality: a prospective cohort study. Eur Arch Otorhinolaryngol 2015. [Epub ahead of print].
4. Boje CR, Dalton SO, Primdahl H, et al. Evaluation of comorbidity in 9388 head and neck cancer patients: a national cohort study from the DAHANCA database. Radiother Oncol 2014;110:91–7.
5. Boje CR, Dalton SO, Gronborg TK, et al. The impact of comorbidity on outcome in 12 623 Danish head and neck cancer patients: a population based study from the DAHANCA database. Acta Oncol 2013;52: 285–93.
6. Douketis JD, Spyropoulos AC, Spencer FA, et al. Perioperative management of antithrombotic therapy: antithrombotic therapy and prevention of thrombosis, 9th ed: American College of Chest Physicians Evidence-Based Clinical Practice Guidelines. Chest 2012;141:e326S–50S.
7. Swartz JE, Aarts MC, Swart KM, et al. The value of postoperative anticoagulants to improve flap survival in the free radial forearm flap: a systematic review and retrospective multicenter analysis. Clin Otolaryngol 2015;40(6):600–9.
8. Bahl V, Shuman AG, Hu HM, et al. Chemoprophylaxis for venous thromboembolism in otolaryngology. JAMA Otolaryngol Head Neck Surg 2014; 140:999–1005.
9. Macdonald DJ. Anaesthesia for microvascular surgery. A physiological approach. Br J Anaesth 1985;57:904–12.
10. Kroll SS, Schusterman MA, Reece GP, et al. Timing of pedicle thrombosis and flap loss after free-tissue transfer. Plast Reconstr Surg 1996;98:1230–3.
11. Chen KT, Mardini S, Chuang DC, et al. Timing of presentation of the first signs of vascular compromise dictates the salvage outcome of free flap transfers. Plast Reconstr Surg 2007;120:187–95.
12. Shuman AG, Hu HM, Pannucci CJ, et al. Stratifying the risk of venous thromboembolism in otolaryngology. Otolaryngol Head Neck Surg 2012;146: 719–24.
13. Hsueh WD, Hwang PH, Abuzeid WM. Perioperative management of antithrombotic therapy in common otolaryngologic surgical procedures: state of the art review. Otolaryngol Head Neck Surg 2015;153: 493–503.
14. Ahmad FI, Gerecci D, Gonzalez JD, et al. The role of postoperative hematoma on free flap compromise. Laryngoscope 2015;125:1811–5.
15. Prsic A, Kiwanuka E, Caterson SA, et al. Anticoagulants and statins as pharmacological agents in free flap surgery: current rationale. Eplasty 2015;15:e51.
16. Chang EI, Zhang H, Liu J, et al. Analysis of risk factors for flap loss and salvage in free flap head and neck reconstruction. Head Neck 2015 [Epub ahead of print].
17. Brinkman JN, Derks LH, Klimek M, et al. Perioperative fluid management and use of vasoactive and antithrombotic agents in free flap surgery: a literature review and clinical recommendations. J Reconstr Microsurg 2013;29:357–66.
18. Khouri RK, Cooley BC, Kenna DM, et al. Thrombosis of microvascular anastomoses in traumatized vessels: fibrin versus platelets. Plast Reconstr Surg 1990;86:110–7.
19. Zhong T, Neinstein R, Massey C, et al. Intravenous fluid infusion rate in microsurgical breast reconstruction: important lessons learned from 354 free flaps. Plast Reconstr Surg 2011;128:1153–60.
20. Clark JR, McCluskey SA, Hall F, et al. Predictors of morbidity following free flap reconstruction for cancer of the head and neck. Head Neck 2007;29: 1090–101.
21. Monroe MM, Cannady SB, Ghanem TA, et al. Safety of vasopressor use in head and neck microvascular reconstruction: a prospective observational study. Otolaryngol Head Neck Surg 2011;144:877–82.
22. Chen C, Nguyen MD, Bar-Meir E, et al. Effects of vasopressor administration on the outcomes of microsurgical breast reconstruction. Ann Plast Surg 2010;65:28–31.
23. Lindau RH, Detwiller K, Wax MK. Buried free flaps in head and neck surgery: outcome analysis. Head Neck 2013;35:1468–70.

Measuring Nasal Obstruction

Jarrod Keeler, MD, Sam P. Most, MD*

KEYWORDS

- Nasal obstruction • Nasal airway • Rhinomanometry • Nasal resistance • Nasal function

KEY POINTS

- The nose/nasal airway is a complex structure with intricate 3-dimensional anatomy; portions of the structure are composed of skin that has no supporting cartilage or bone.
- The nose functions as a heat and moisture exchanger. The nose also acts as a filter for particles.
- The measurement of nasal obstruction (NAO) can be broken into 3 tools for measurement: patient-derived measurements, physician-observed measurements, and objective measurements.
- The concept of a nasal valve has been key to our understanding of NAO.
- The field of evaluation and surgical treatment for NAO has grown tremendously in the past 4 to 5 decades and will likely continue to grow.

THE NOSE IS A COMPLEX STRUCTURE

The nose and the nasal airway is a highly complex structure with intricate 3-dimensional anatomy resulting in one of the few areas of the body where portions of the structure are composed of skin that has no supporting cartilage or bone. Despite this incomplete substructure, it functions in respiration and filtration in a highly advanced way. This presents difficulty for both patients and clinicians in determining where within the nasal airway perceived obstruction lies.

Nasal obstruction (NAO) is a common complaint in primary care and otolaryngologists' offices. Evaluation of NAO goes back just as far as the published record. The study of obstruction is the study of flow and resistance. The complex intranasal anatomy contains areas of substantial variability in flow (**Fig. 1**). The first published studies on these were using molds of the upper airway and smoke trails in the early 1950s. These studies demonstrated rapid air flow through the areas of the inferior and middle meatus.[1] Further studies in the 1980s, 1990s, and today, using more advanced modeling techniques, demonstrated similar findings.[2,3] However, we are no

closer today to finding the single answer to the cause of NAO than we were decades ago.

FUNCTION AND PHYSIOLOGY

Humans are unique among hominids with increased nasal projection, anterior nasal convexity, expansion of the nasal bone breadth, exaggerated nasal angles, prominence of the anterior nasal spine, and substantial cartilage framework at the nasal tip.[4] These traits began with the *Homo erectus* and continued in our lineage. All of these adaptations are felt to increase the ability of the nose to warm and moisturize the inspired air. These changes afforded the nose the ability to pull increased volumes through a more limited space and increase the contact with mucosa. This evolution is thought to be brought on by migration of early humans to more arid climates.[4] This migration may be the underlying drive towards improving NAO as *Homo erectus* strived to have the air he breathed remain as moist, warm, and pure as it had been in tropical climates.

Studies supporting this hypothesis were hard to generate and were based much on earlier research

Division of Facial Plastic & Reconstructive Surgery, Stanford University School of Medicine, 801 Welch Road, Stanford, CA 94305, USA
* Corresponding author.
E-mail address: smost@ohns.stanford.edu

Facial Plast Surg Clin N Am 24 (2016) 315–322
http://dx.doi.org/10.1016/j.fsc.2016.03.008
1064-7406/16/$ – see front matter Published by Elsevier Inc.

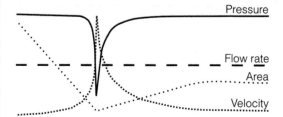

Fig. 1. Bernoulli effect. Pressure varies inversely with velocity for a constant flow rate. Thus, as the area decreases, velocity increases and pressure drops significantly.

of the nasal physiology. Heat and moisture exchange was determined experimentally through evaluation of patients with and without tracheotomies. The nasal physiology is complex, but data from these studies demonstrate air presented to the nostrils at 20°C attains 32°C at the back of the nasopharynx and changes from 45% relative humidity to 98%. The same temperature air only reaches 30°C and 80% humidity if inspired orally.[5] Thus, the ability of the nasal mucosa to moisten air would be key in a more arid climate to prevent dehydration.

Heat and moisture exchanges represents only a small portion of the physiologic purpose for the nose and nasal cavity. The nose also acts as a filter for particles. The earliest studies began in the 1950s and continue currently to evaluate the filtration function of the nose. Through multiple study methods, particles larger than approximately 25 to 30 microns are deposited at near 100% within the nasal cavity.[6–8] This filtration and subsequent chemoreception is sensed in both the olfactory cleft and portions of the anterior nasal cavity.

The loss of thermoreception and chemoreception may represent some of the feelings of NAO when a patient's airway is made overly patent by turbinate surgery. Thermoreceptor TRPM8 function has been implicated in the sensation of NAO with loss of adequate thermal change in the mucosa of the nose resulting in feelings of NAO. The turbinates create nonlaminar flow resulting in the warming of the air by contact with mucosal surfaces. This presents cooling to TRPM8, which is postulated as one of the mechanisms of sensation of nasal patency.[9]

NASAL OBSTRUCTION POORLY CHARACTERIZED

Some of the earliest attempts to measure NAO began with attempts to establish the diagnosis. Early surgeons struggled in patients with persistent symptoms of NAO, but an absence of definitive pathologic findings. The Cottle maneuver

was developed by Heinberg and Kern in the 1970s and named for Dr M.H. Cottle to evaluate patients with NAO.[10] The maneuver is performed by pulling the cheek laterally and is positive when this improves the patient's sensation of nasal airflow.

The Cottle maneuver is a well-known and highly sensitive test with poor specificity. As such, multiple revisions of the technique have been performed to improve specificity with some encouraging results. The use of a small item (ear curette or cotton swab) to support the lateral nasal wall during inspiration was shown to correlate significantly with postoperative results from placement of spreader grafts to improve the nasal airflow.[11]

In our practice, we perform what we call the passive Cottle maneuver. With this maneuver, the examiner's fingers are placed on each side of the nasal sidewall on the skin of the medial maxillary buttress. The examiners fingers are used to simply 'tense' the skin of the lateral nasal wall rather than expand the nasal airway. The patient is then asked to breathe in. If the patient gets relief from this maneuver, it is likely they have dynamic lateral wall insufficiency and would benefit from strengthening the lateral nasal wall.

MEASURING NASAL OBSTRUCTION

The measurement of NAO can be broken into 3 different tools for measurement: patient-derived measurements, physician-observed measurements, and objective measurements. The first is highly important, but a well-known, inexact form of measurement. The second is key in establishing a diagnosis and, although intrarater recognition of findings is fairly consistent, interrater assessment can be variable and is not necessarily correlated with patient symptoms. The third can be very standardized, but also does not necessarily correlate with patient symptoms or patient findings on examination.

PATIENT-DERIVED MEASUREMENTS

Multiple patient reported outcome measures have been used previously for evaluating the symptoms of NAO. Before the current century, no single test was validated, widely accepted, and used. Visual analog scales (VAS) were some of the first to be used. These scales represent patients' overall perception of a problem or group of problems placed on a linear scale from absent to severe. Although this is a useful gauge to determine problem severity, based on its intrarater and interrater variability, its usefulness as a standalone measure is minimal.[12]

In an era where health-related quality-of-life measures are at the forefront of medicine, the most prominent and frequently used in the evaluation of NAO is the Nasal Obstruction Symptom Evaluation (NOSE) score.[13] This quality-of-life scale was created in 2004 out of a need for a reproducible, valid scale to measure a difficult clinical problem. It consists of 5 questions on a scale of 0 to 4 that is multiplied by 5 resulting in a score from 0 to 100 with 100 as the most severe NAO (**Fig. 2**).

Since its inception, the NOSE scale has been validated multiple times for both preoperative and postoperative evaluation of patient symptoms.[13–15] The system has become the gold standard for patient-derived measurements with 64 articles indexed in the English literature featuring this scale at the time of this writing. Unfortunately, the scale correlated poorly with objective measures. In 1 well-performed study of 290 patients with NAO, without sinus disease, were evaluated by acoustic rhinometry (AR), peak nasal flow (PNF), and NOSE score with VAS and no correlations were found of the 16 evaluated.[16] Despite this poor correlation with objective measurement, the NOSE score has an exceedingly useful preoperative and postoperative quality-of-life/patient-reported outcome measure evaluation tool.

Using this system, a severity classification has been created for NAO with cutoff points at 5, 30, 50 and 75 representing patients with mild (5–25), moderate (30–50), severe (55–75), and extreme (>80) obstruction.[15] This classification system was found to have a greater than 90% sensitivity and specificity for evaluating patients with NAO.

Nasal Obstructive Symptoms Evaluation Scale

To the Patient: Please help us to better understand the impact of nasal obstruction on your quality of life by <u>completing the following survey</u>. Thank you!

Over the past <u>ONE</u> month, how much of a <u>problem</u> were the following conditions for you?

Please circle the most correct response

	Not a Problem	Very Mild Problem	Moderate Problem	Fairly Bad Problem	Severe Problem
1. Nasal congestion or stuffiness	0	1	2	3	4
2. Nasal blockage or obstruction	0	1	2	3	4
3. Trouble breathing through my nose	0	1	2	3	4
4. Trouble sleeping	0	1	2	3	4
5. Unable to get enough air through my nose during exercise or exertion	0	1	2	3	4

6. <u>Please mark on this line how troublesome is your difficulty in breathing through your nose:</u>

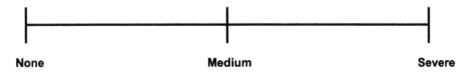

None   Medium   Severe

Fig. 2. Nose questionnaire.

Sinus evaluation has several validated measures, including the Sino-Nasal Outcomes Test. This test was originally designed as a 20-item questionnaire with a score between 0 and 100.[17] In 2009, 2 questions were added to address smell and NAO to create the Sino-Nasal Outcomes Test-22. The scores were validated using other methods such as the NOSE scores and are very useful in patients with chronic sinusitis and concomitant NAO.[17]

PHYSICIAN-DERIVED MEASUREMENTS

Physician-derived measurements for evaluation of NAO began in earnest with Guy de Cehauliac when he referred in his writing to the nasal speculum in the 13th century.[18] The field has changed by leaps and bounds owing to the diligent work of innumerable clinician–scientists; however, we continue to struggle with the physician-derived measurement techniques for NAO.

The concept of a nasal valve has been key to our understanding of NAO. Starting with Bridger in 1970, the nasal valve as a primary site of obstruction was codified. In his work, Bridger illuminated the physics of fluid passing through the nose and the creation of a "flow-limiting segment," which he called the nasal valve at the junction of the caudal edge of the upper lateral cartilage and the nasal septum.[19] Goode continued this work in 1985, describing diagnosis and surgery within this location.[20] Goode went into great detail about the various causes, including septal deviations, iatrogenic causes from cartilage resection or inappropriate osteotomies, weak or recurved cartilage, facial nerve weakness, or vestibular soft tissue insufficiencies.[20]

This structure remains so vitally important in the nasal airway that papers continue to be published on the surgical evaluation and treatment of the nasal valve. In 2010 a clinical consensus statement was released by the American Academy of Otolaryngology—Head and Neck Surgery.[21] This group defined nasal valve compromise as a distinct entity resulting in NAO with a variety of causes. The statement included that history and examination, including anterior rhinoscopy, Cottle maneuver or modified Cottle maneuver, and visualization of the nasal wall during inspiration were sufficient to diagnose nasal valve compromise.

Both Bridger and Goode cited a second area prone to dynamic collapse, which was initially termed alar collapse and later termed external nasal valve collapse. The area is caudal to the internal nasal valve and is composed of the septum, nasal ala, and caudal portion of the lower lateral cartilage. This is a zone defined by the American Academy of Otolaryngology—Head and Neck

Surgery group subject to valve compromise. More recently, this terminology has been modified to be the less ambiguous "lateral wall insufficiency or collapse."[22] The lateral nasal wall and its dynamic collapse or lateral wall insufficiency can be broken into 2 zones, with zone 1 superior to the scroll region of the upper and lower lateral cartilages and zone 2 inferior to that.[22] Zone 2 collapse represents classical alar collapse or external valve collapse. This method of classification allows for previously poorly characterized collapse superior to the region of the external nasal valve, or zone 1, to be evaluated and more adequately treated.[22,23] Most important, a validated, physician-derived grading scale has been developed to quantify the amount of dynamic collapse of the airway in these cases (**Table 1**).[24]

Finally, the inferior turbinates are evaluated frequently in any nasal examination and remain as a substantial portion of the perceived nasal resistance. A recent study looking at turbinate hypertrophy, as well as many other factors in NAO, noted a correlation with severity of turbinate hypertrophy with severity of NOSE scores.[25] There has not been a well-established grading system for turbinate hypertrophy and most fall to subjective categories such as mild, moderate, and severe. To that end, a grading scale was created and validated for the objective evaluation based on a quartile approach to the obstruction of the airway numbered from 1 to 4.[26] This scale is unique in that it rates turbinates on the total nasal airway, independent of septal deviation or spur.

OBJECTIVE MEASURES

Various objective measurement techniques for the evaluation of the nasal flow have been used for the last 5 decades. Pure nasal flow (PNF) was one of the earliest attempted and has the most reproducible results during repeated measurements of 1 subject of all the measurement techniques. The technique initially measured strict nasal breathing, but was fraught with questions of differences in intrathoracic pressure, chest wall movement, and inhalation versus exhalation. Different evaluators

Table 1	
Grading system for lateral wall insufficiency	
Grade	**% Closure Towards Nasal Septum**
0	0 (none)
1	1–33
2	34–66
3	67–100

have reduced some of this bias by creating indices of nasal and oral peak flow.[27,28]

During the same time frame, of the advent of peak flow and in response to many of the criticisms of peak flow, rhinomanometry was created and adapted.[27] Both active and passive methods have been described. Active methods consist of the use of the patient's own respiration for flow. Passive methods involve a pressure placed into the nasal cavity via a mask. Rhinomanometry is also subdivided into anterior and posterior rhinomanometry. The anterior measurement for both types is the pressure at the face mask. In the posterior method, the oropharyngeal pressure is taken as the pressure in the nasopharynx. The resistance is taken as the difference between the two. In anterior rhinomanometry the posterior pressure is measured by sealing off nasal cavity and, in effect, converting the nasal cavity into a tube sampling of the posterior pressure. This technique requires each side to be calculated separately and then parallel resistances are generated by computation.[29] When measured simultaneously in patients, the posterior rhinomanometry gives an average of 16% higher values and more consistent results compared to anterior rhinomanometry.[29,30]

More recently, polyphasic or 4-phase rhinomanometry has been used to evaluate the changes in nasal breathing over time and to obtain what some feel is more consistent results. These results are believed explain differences in the techniques of anterior and posterior—passive and active rhinomanometry.[31,32] The results feature changes in the airway throughout the breathing cycle with an accelerating inspiratory phase, decelerating inspiratory phase, accelerating expiratory phase, and decelerating expiratory phase.[31] Although there is high correlation with classical methods of rhinomanometry, no studies have been performed comparing these systems with patient symptoms.

Owing to some of the limitations of both peak flow and rhinomanometry, a separate method of evaluation known as AR was created using acoustic reflections to evaluate cross-sectional area. Incident waves are released and reflected waves are computationally used to generate a cross-sectional area. AR is based on the assumptions that sound waves propagate as plane waves, viscous losses are negligible, and that the walls behave rigidly.[27] Despite these assumptions results have proven quite reproducible.

Thanks largely to the ease of modern imaging technology and increasing speed and power of computers, a new science of computational fluid dynamics has become increasingly popular in upper airway modeling. High-resolution CT scans are used to generate 3-dimensional models.

Airflow is then simulated with thousands of iterations to generate overall flow loops within the nasal cavity with any parameter altered individually. This may lead to the possibility of virtual surgery, whereby site-specific surgical planning can occur.[33]

CONTROVERSIES IN MEASUREMENT TECHNIQUES

As one would expect with so many ways to evaluate a single symptom, the solution is not simple. Each method has pros and cons. Patient derived measures as explained earlier have been wrought with difficulty. Until very recently, no normative data have existed for patients with NAO or normal controls. A systematic review created normative data for NOSE and VAS scores with mean scores in symptomatic patients of 65 and 6.7 pretreatment and 15 and 2.1 for asymptomatic patients.[13] This correlates well with the senior author's severity classification noted earlier, but still needs large-scale and possibly cross-sectional studies to verify validity.[15]

Although physician-derived measures are useful in indicating those who may have NAO, this is a biased evaluation. Within the group who seek treatment for NAO, we do not surgically treat those without findings that would be improved by surgery; therefore, control groups are impossible. Some of our techniques such as the Cottle maneuver have been evaluated. Those who had a positive Cottle maneuver were show by 1 study to have more correlation with improvement in those patients who had internal nasal valve stenosis compared with those with external valve stenosis, but suffered from a lack of control patients.[11] Similarly, the Cottle maneuver was shown to increase the area of the internal nasal valve by area by an average of 33% when measured by AR.[10] And although these studies are promising, the Cottle maneuver is well-known to be poorly specific.[10,11]

The objective measures are similarly fallible. PNF is a simple, inexpensive, and individually reproducible way of evaluating NAO.[28] It has good correlation with VAS scores in patients with NAO and nasal polyps.[34] Several studies have shown good correlation with symptoms and rhinomanometry, as well.[27,34,35] However, owing to the differences in patient effort, small changes in flow are poorly detected, the results are poorly generalizable, and changes to the nasal airway reach a plateau effect as treatment increases.[35–37]

Rhinomanometry as noted earlier is well-correlated with PNF. The technique is also well-known to demonstrate treatment effect with decongestants.[27] Active rhinomanometry is patient effort dependent. As such, some forms of rhinomanometry are very poorly reproducible.[30,38] Passive rhinomanometry does not respond to changes in dynamic airway form.[30] Unlike PNF, rhinomanometry has a mixed result with correlation with symptoms.[39–41] The equipment for testing is expensive and requires skilled technicians to administer the testing.

AR is very reproducible and not patient dependent. It is known to correlate well with imaging studies and endoscopic findings.[27,42] Similar to rhinomanometry, AR changes in accordance with decongestion and histamine challenges.[27,42,43] However, similar to rhinomanometry, the equipment is expensive and requires an experienced technician to achieve reproducible results.[44] AR is poorly correlated with patient symptoms in some studies.[42,44] In a cross-sectional study, it was unable to distinguish between patients with symptomatic NAO and chronic rhinosinusitis.[45,46] Finally, even though symptom scores improve after septorhinoplasty 1 study found no change in cross-sectional area by AR.[47]

Computational fluid dynamics is a burgeoning science and was well-correlated with results with NOSE and VAS scores, although in a very limited number of patients.[48] The technology is very powerful and has the opportunity to create tailored surgical options for patients, but has the requirements of preoperative and postoperative CT scans to evaluate patients and the validity of the technique with associated risks of radiation exposure.[33,48] The results have not been tested widely and needs far more experimentation to validate this technique.

The field of evaluation and surgical treatment for NAO has grown tremendously in the past 4 to 5 decades and will likely continue to grow. Further frontiers of NAO will push technology ahead. New avenues include further evaluating 4-phase rhinomanometry to examine correlations with patient symptoms, continued research into point of care use of PNF for preoperative and postoperative evaluation to establish treatment effects, use of AR to evaluate dynamic lateral wall changes in patients with lateral wall insufficiency, and finally using computational fluid dynamics analysis to personalize surgery for optimum treatment effect.[27,28,31,33] Recently, we used a randomized control trial study design, along with physician-derived measures and patient-reported outcome measures to study a new method for treatment of NAO. It is our hope that future studies, with proper design and measurement methodology, will help to delineate those treatments with the best efficacy for site-specific problems in NAO.[49]

REFERENCES

1. Proetz AW. Air currents in the upper respiratory tract and their clinical importance. Ann Otol Rhinol Laryngol 1951;60(2):439–67.
2. Elad D, Liebenthal R, Wenig BL, et al. Analysis of air flow patterns in the human nose. Med Biol Eng Comput 1993;31(6):585–92.
3. Zhao K, Jiang J. What is normal nasal airflow? A computational study of 22 healthy adults. Int Forum Allergy Rhinol 2014;4(6):435–46.
4. Franciscus RG, Trinkaus E. Nasal morphology and the emergence of Homo erectus. Am J Phys Anthropol 1988;75(4):517–27.
5. Ingelstedt S. Humidifying capacity of the nose. Ann Otol Rhinol Laryngol 1970;79(3):475–80.
6. Lippmann M. Deposition and clearance of inhaled particles in the human nose. Ann Otol Rhinol Laryngol 1970;79(3):519–28.
7. Smith JR, Birchall A, Etherington G, et al. A revised model for the deposition and clearance of inhaled particles in human extrathoracic airways. Radiat Prot Dosimetry 2014;158(2):135–47.
8. Keeler JA, Patki A, Woodard CR, et al. A computational study of nasal spray deposition pattern in four ethnic groups. J Aerosol Med Pulm Drug Deliv 2016;29(2):153–66.
9. Sozansky J, Houser SM. Pathophysiology of empty nose syndrome. Laryngoscope 2015;125(1):70–4.
10. Tikanto J, Pirila T. Effects of the Cottle's maneuver on the nasal valve as assessed by acoustic rhinometry. Am J Rhinol 2007;21(4):456–9.
11. Fung E, Hong P, Moore C, et al. The effectiveness of modified Cottle maneuver in predicting outcomes in functional rhinoplasty. Plast Surg Int 2014;2014:618313.
12. Andrews PJ, Choudhury N, Takhar A, et al. The need for an objective measure in septorhinoplasty surgery: are we any closer to finding an answer? Clin Otolaryngol 2015;40(6):698–703.
13. Stewart MG, Witsell DL, Smith TL, et al. Development and validation of the Nasal Obstruction Symptom Evaluation (NOSE) scale. Otolaryngol Head Neck Surg 2004;130(2):157–63.
14. Rhee JS, Sullivan CD, Frank DO, et al. A systematic review of patient-reported nasal obstruction scores: defining normative and symptomatic ranges in surgical patients. JAMA Facial Plast Surg 2014;16(3):219–25 [quiz: 232].
15. Lipan MJ, Most SP. Development of a severity classification system for subjective nasal obstruction. JAMA Facial Plast Surg 2013;15(5):358 61.

16. Lam DJ, James KT, Weaver EM. Comparison of anatomic, physiological, and subjective measures of the nasal airway. Am J Rhinol 2006; 20(5):463–70.

17. Hopkins C, Gillett S, Slack R, et al. Psychometric validity of the 22-item sinonasal outcome test. Clin Otolaryngol 2009;34(5):447–54.

18. Tange RA. Some historical aspects of the surgical treatment of the infected maxillary sinus. Rhinology 1991;29(2):155–62.

19. Bridger GP. Physiology of the nasal valve. Arch Otolaryngol 1970;92(6):543–53.

20. Goode RL. Surgery of the incompetent nasal valve. Laryngoscope 1985;95(5):546–55.

21. Rhee JS, Weaver EM, Park SS, et al. Clinical consensus statement: diagnosis and management of nasal valve compromise. Otolaryngol Head Neck Surg 2010;143(1):48–59.

22. Most SP. Trends in functional rhinoplasty. Arch Facial Plast Surg 2008;10(6):410–3.

23. Most SP. Comparing methods for repair of the external valve: one more step toward a unified view of lateral wall insufficiency. JAMA Facial Plast Surg 2015;17(5):345–6.

24. Tsao GJ, Fijalkowski N, Most SP. Validation of a grading system for lateral nasal wall insufficiency. Allergy Rhinol (Providence) 2013;4(2): e66–8.

25. Leitzen KP, Brietzke SE, Lindsay RW. Correlation between nasal anatomy and objective obstructive sleep apnea severity. Otolaryngol Head Neck Surg 2014;150(2):325–31.

26. Camacho M, Zaghi S, Certal V, et al. Inferior turbinate classification system, grades 1 to 4: development and validation study. Laryngoscope 2015; 125(2):296–302.

27. Hilberg O. Objective measurement of nasal airway dimensions using acoustic rhinometry: methodological and clinical aspects. Allergy 2002; 57(Suppl 70):5–39.

28. Holmstrom M, Scadding GK, Lund VJ, et al. Assessment of nasal obstruction. A comparison between rhinomanometry and nasal inspiratory peak flow. Rhinology 1990;28(3):191–6.

29. Jones AS, Lancer JM, Stevens JC, et al. Rhinomanometry: do the anterior and posterior methods give equivalent results? Clin Otolaryngol Allied Sci 1987;12(2):109–14.

30. Dvoracek JE, Hillis A, Rossing RG. Comparison of sequential anterior and posterior rhinomanometry. J Allergy Clin Immunol 1985; 76(4):577–82.

31. Vogt K, Wernecke KD, Behrbohm H, et al. Four-phase rhinomanometry: a multicentric retrospective analysis of 36,563 clinical measurements. Eur Arch Otorhinolaryngol 2016;273(5): 1185–98.

32. Wong EH, Eccles R. Comparison of classic and 4-phase rhinomanometry methods, is there any difference? Rhinology 2014;52(4):360–5.

33. Rhee JS, Pawar SS, Garcia GJ, et al. Toward personalized nasal surgery using computational fluid dynamics. Arch Facial Plast Surg 2011; 13(5):305–10.

34. Hox V, Bobic S, Callebaux I, et al. Nasal obstruction and smell impairment in nasal polyp disease: correlation between objective and subjective parameters. Rhinology 2010;48(4):426–32.

35. Clarke RW, Jones AS. The limitations of peak nasal flow measurement. Clin Otolaryngol Allied Sci 1994;19(6):502–4.

36. Clarke RW, Jones AS, Richardson H. Peak nasal inspiratory flow–the plateau effect. J Laryngol Otol 1995;109(5):399–402.

37. Panagou P, Loukides S, Tsipra S, et al. Evaluation of nasal patency: comparison of patient and clinician assessments with rhinomanometry. Acta Otolaryngol 1998;118(6):847–51.

38. Shelton DM, Pertuze J, Gleeson MJ, et al. Comparison of oscillation with three other methods for measuring nasal airways resistance. Respir Med 1990;84(2):101–6.

39. Cole P. Toronto rhinomanometry: laboratory, field and clinical studies. J Otolaryngol 1988;17(6):331–5.

40. Gleeson MJ, Youlten LJ, Shelton DM, et al. Assessment of nasal airway patency: a comparison of four methods. Clin Otolaryngol Allied Sci 1986; 11(2):99–107.

41. Lund VJ. Objective assessment of nasal obstruction. Otolaryngol Clin North Am 1989; 22(2):279–90.

42. Isaac A, Major M, Witmans M, et al. Correlations between acoustic rhinometry, subjective symptoms, and endoscopic findings in symptomatic children with nasal obstruction. JAMA Otolaryngol Head Neck Surg 2015;141(6):550–5.

43. Hilberg O, Grymer LF, Pedersen OF. Nasal histamine challenge in nonallergic and allergic subjects evaluated by acoustic rhinometry. Allergy 1995;50(2): 166–73.

44. Cannon DE, Rhee JS. Evidence-based practice: functional rhinoplasty. Otolaryngol Clin North Am 2012;45(5):1033–43.

45. Lange B, Thilsing T, Baelum J, et al. Acoustic rhinometry in persons recruited from the general population and diagnosed with chronic rhinosinusitis according to EPOS. Eur Arch Otorhinolaryngol 2014;271(7):1961–6.

46. Proimos EK, Kiagiadaki DE, Chimona TS, et al. Comparison of acoustic rhinometry and nasal inspiratory peak flow as objective tools for nasal obstruction assessment in patients with chronic rhinosinusitis. Rhinology 2015;53(1): 66–74.

47. Edizer DT, Erisir F, Alimoglu Y, et al. Nasal obstruction following septorhinoplasty: how well does acoustic rhinometry work? Eur Arch Otorhinolaryngol 2013;270(2):609–13.

48. Kimbell JS, Garcia GJ, Frank DO, et al. Computed nasal resistance compared with patient-reported symptoms in surgically treated nasal airway passages: a preliminary report. Am J Rhinol Allergy 2012;26(3):e94–8.

49. Weissman J, Most SP. Radiofrequency thermotherapy versus bone anchored suspension for treatment of lateral nasal wall insufficiency: a randomized controlled trial. JAMA Facial Plast Surg 2015;17(2):84–9.

Primary Rhinoplasty

Fred G. Fedok, MD[a,b,*]

KEYWORDS

- Spreader grafts • Autospreader flaps • Open approach • Endonasal approach • Costal cartilage
- Pediatric nasal surgery • Fillers in rhinoplasty • Nonsurgical rhinoplasty

KEY POINTS

- Spreader grafts and other proven methods to manage middle vault deficiencies should be prudently applied in patients at risk of middle vault insufficiency.
- The open and endonasal approaches should both be part of the rhinoplasty surgeon's armamentarium.
- Corrective nasal surgery should be performed even in the very young patient to restore form and function.
- The costal cartilage donor site should be considered when it presents as the optimal donor site in rhinoplasty.
- Fillers can be judiciously used to temporarily correct limited deficiencies in rhinoplasty. Sound principles of application should be followed to limit the risk of complications.

INTRODUCTION

Rhinoplasty is among the most frequently performed cosmetic and elective procedures. This phenomenon is documented in the results of various professional societies' surveys.[1] Along with this frequency, significant advancements have been made in rhinoplasty over the last few decades in the realms of diagnosis, analysis, the development of new surgical technique, and refinements in execution.

Although there are some widely shared and universally recognized aspects of this craft, there are many differences in technique and philosophy regarding rhinoplasty surgery that are reflected in presentations and in print. In this report, several of these current controversies and differences of opinion are examined in an effort to understand and to lend clarity. In many instances, there remains no right or wrong position, and the written opinion expressed on a particular topic is the working opinion of the author based on personal experience and consideration of the viewpoint of other surgeons.

The topics that will be addressed here are the performance of the open approach versus the endonasal rhinoplasty approach, the use of spreader grafts and autospreader flaps in the management of the middle vault in rhinoplasty, corrective rhinoplasty in the younger patient, the use of the rib and other cartilage donor sites for grafting in rhinoplasty, and the use of filler materials in rhinoplasty.

THE OPEN APPROACH AND THE ENDONASAL APPROACH IN RHINOPLASTY

In considering this topic, several questions might be entertained, for instance:

1. Is the endonasal approach "outdated?"
2. Is the open approach "better?"
3. When should one consider doing an endonasal approach? When should one consider doing an open approach?

No pertinent disclosures.
[a] Department of Surgery, The University of South Alabama, 2451 Fillingim Street, Mobile, AL 36617, USA;
[b] Facial Plastic and Reconstructive Surgery, Otolaryngology/Head & Neck Surgery, The Hershey Medical Center, The Pennsylvania State University, 500 University Drive, Hershey, PA 17033, USA
* The McCollough Plastic Surgery Clinic, 350 Cypress Bend Drive, Gulf Shores, AL 36542.
E-mail address: drfredfedok@me.com

Facial Plast Surg Clin N Am 24 (2016) 323–335
http://dx.doi.org/10.1016/j.fsc.2016.03.009
1064-7406/16/$ – see front matter © 2016 Elsevier Inc. All rights reserved.

4. Is the endonasal approach still being taught at an adequate level?

The open rhinoplasty technique has become exceedingly popular. Advantages to this technique include the direct visualization and direct access to structures when executing rhinoplasty maneuvers.[2] Alternatively, others note the disadvantages of the open approach to include the resultant increased swelling of the nose, the transcolumellar scar, possible vascular compromise of the skin, and the unnecessary dissection of much of the nasal anatomy.[3–5]

Passionate discussions between individuals who use the open approach versus those who prefer the endonasal approach are long past in most professional circles; the validity of each approach has been shown.[6] Surgeons commonly practice in a manner consistent with their early training as modified by their additive experience. As in many similar surgical matters, the surgical approach used by an experienced surgeon is the result of these factors in addition to the influence of the tasks at hand and the complexity of a particular operation.

For instance, when the rhinoplasty situation is simple, as when minimal changes are desired, an endonasal approach may be most efficient and appropriate (**Fig. 1**). In another example in which several challenges exist, but the nose is generally symmetric and straight, an endonasal approach again would be appropriate (**Fig. 2**). When the task at hand is more complex because the patient's nose was previously traumatized, is markedly asymmetric, is crooked, or has a congenital deformity, an open approach may be the most appropriate choice (**Fig. 3**). Through the open approach, the surgeon can usually exert more control over the anatomy as it is altered in rhinoplasty. These observations above are reflected in numerous presentations and articles.[7–9]

The most pertinent factor in the endonasal versus the open approach dynamic may be the potential negative impact any bias might have on teaching. Optimal teaching may be adversely influenced if the mentor is an ardent advocate for only one of the approaches. Ideally, facial plastic surgeons should be taught both approaches. The student will then have the requisite surgical acumen to decide on whether an open or endonasal approach is to be used by the consideration of the goals and challenges of each particular case, rather than a limiting prejudice of a teacher.[10]

THE USE OF SPREADER GRAFTS AND THE MANAGEMENT OF THE MIDDLE VAULT

The nasal sidewall must maintain adequate dimensions to support the airway and the anatomic contour of the nose. This integrity of the middle vault depends on several factors, including the actual dimensions and relationships of the lateral nasal wall anatomic structures, the intrinsic resilience and strength of the structures, and the stabilization of the structures afforded by the overlying nasal musculature. The anatomy and physiology of the nasal valve portion of the middle vault have been recognized for several decades. The negative consequences resulting from the disruption of the relationships between the septum and the upper lateral cartilages are recognized and caution is expressed.[11,12]

Middle vault collapse manifests itself as airway obstruction, an aesthetic deficiency in which there is a noticeable disruption in a pleasant contour of the patient's nasal sidewall or both. Patients may present with an inverted V-like deformity that is similar to that seen in saddle nose deformity.

It has been noted in rhinoplasty that there are benefits to recognizing middle vault insufficiency preoperatively and to preventing the iatrogenic creation of a middle vault problem during surgery. Several clinical situations exist in which middle vault insufficiency is commonly seen. The first case is a developmental insufficiency in which a patient has a nasal middle vault that is overly too narrow or has cartilages that are intrinsically too thin or weak to maintain an adequate shape of the middle vault at rest and during inspiration. Another instance is insufficient support of the middle vault after trauma when there has been an avulsion or scarring of the upper lateral cartilage and an iatrogenic collapse of the cartilaginous nasal sidewall. Finally, nasal vault insufficiency may result after nasal surgery in which there has been a disruption of the cartilaginous support of the nasal sidewall or a failure to adequately preserve support in a nose that has anatomic features that might contribute to a tendency to develop middle vault insufficiency.[13]

There is a recognized benefit to stabilizing the middle vault by one of several methods. The management of the middle vault is recommended when there will be a significant surgical manipulation of the nasal dorsum or lateral nasal walls such as with osteotomies or hump reduction. Spreader grafts are found to be a reliable method of addressing both the aesthetic and the functional sequelae of middle vault collapse.[14] Since their introduction, the use of spreader grafts has become exceedingly popular in both aesthetic and functional surgery of the nose. Opinions differ, however, about whether the placement of spreader grafts serve primarily an aesthetic or functional role.[13–15]

Several points of significant controversy surround the use of spreader grafts. These are

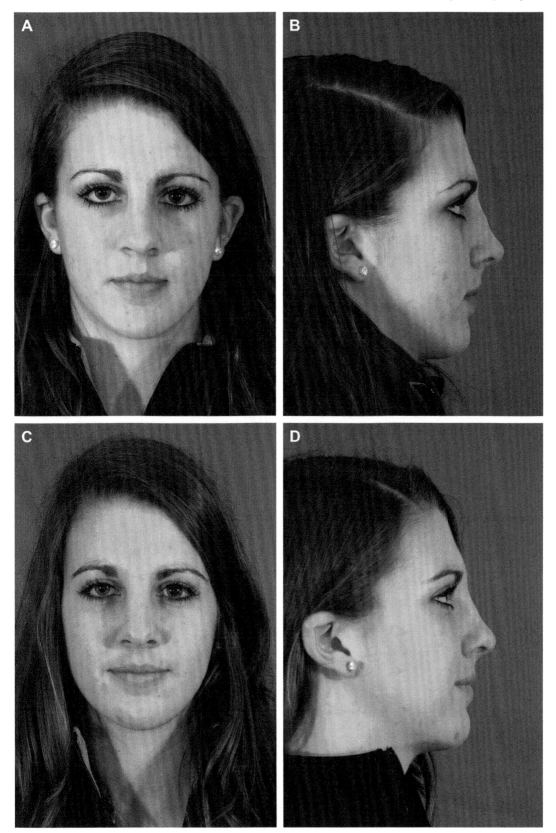

Fig. 1. Clinical images of patient who underwent endonasal rhinoplasty to improve her dorsal profile and minimally narrow her tip with minimal hump reduction, lateral osteotomies, and complete strip. (*A*, *B*) Preoperative images. (*C*, *D*) Postoperative images.

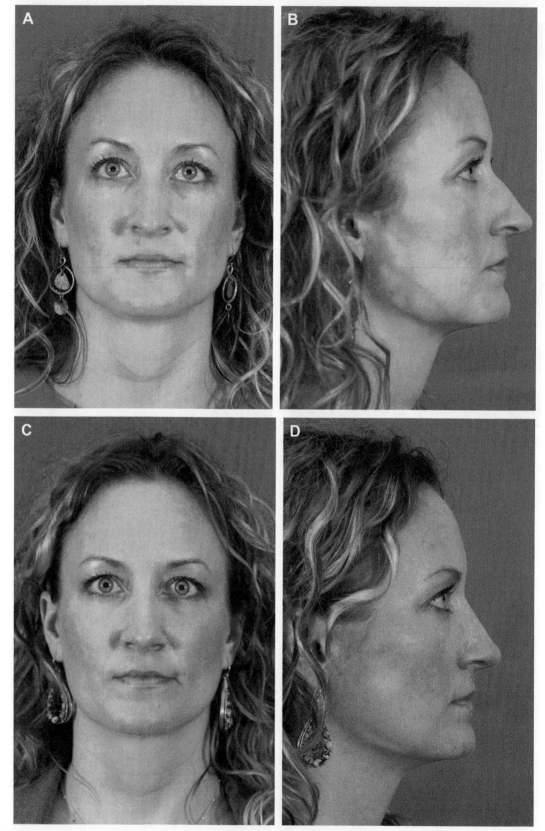

Fig. 2. Clinical images of patient who underwent endonasal rhinoplasty to improve her nasal airway and nasal appearance. The procedure included septoplasty with minimal hump reduction, lateral osteotomies, autospreader flaps, lateral crural overlay, and tongue-in-groove maneuver. (*A, B*) Preoperative images. (*C, D*) Postoperative images.

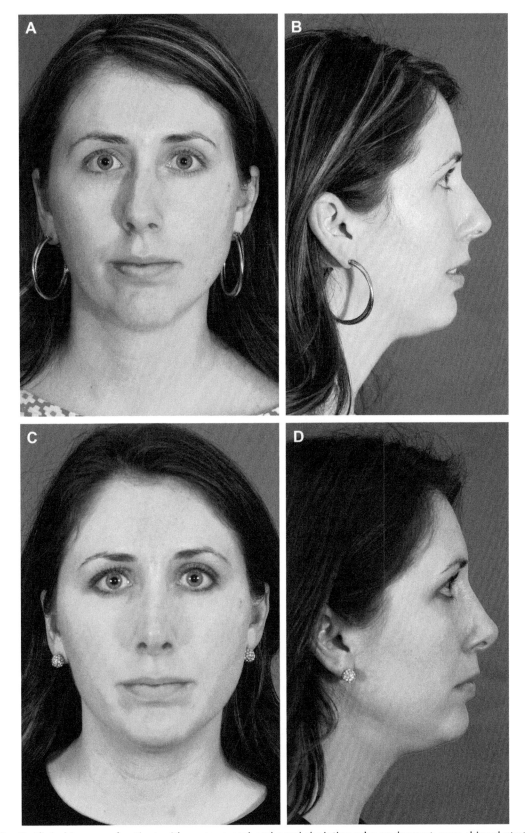

Fig. 3. Clinical images of patient with severe septal and nasal deviation who underwent open rhinoplasty to straighten her nose and improve her nasal airway. The procedure included septoplasty, hump reduction, lateral osteotomies, a transverse osteotomy, autospreader flaps, left lateral crural overlay, and a tip graft. (*A, B*) Preoperative images. (*C, D*) Postoperative images.

unresolved in the literature and are instead more of a topic of individual discussion among surgeons.

Question that remain are:

1. When should spreader grafts be used in primary rhinoplasty?
2. When may it be unnecessary to use spreader grafts in primary rhinoplasty?
3. Does the use of spreader grafts necessitate an open approach?
4. What are reasonable and equivalent alternatives to the use of spreader grafts?

When should spreader grafts be used in primary rhinoplasty? There is a diversity of opinion on this matter. Some experienced surgeons essentially never use them, whereas other experienced surgeons use them in almost every case.

The management of the middle vault of the nose should be considered whenever there is a preexisting deficiency in the integrity of the lateral nasal wall or when it is anticipated that the integrity of the lateral base will be compromised by a surgical maneuver. When a deficiency is detected preoperatively in primary rhinoplasty, spreader grafts are used to correct the deficiency in nasal contour or in the nasal airway (**Fig. 4**). When it is anticipated that the integrity of the lateral nasal wall will be compromised through the rhinoplasty operation, some management technique should probably be entertained. Typical surgical maneuvers that compromise the integrity of the middle vault include the taking down of a dorsal convexity or the separation of the upper lateral cartridges from the septum as might be performed to straighten a crooked nose. When one takes down a dorsal convexity, there is not only a disruption of the attachments between the central cartilaginous septum and the upper level cartilages but also a reduction in the height of the upper lateral cartridges that form the nasal sidewall (**Fig. 5**).

The question about when to use or not to use spreader grafts revolves around 2 different axes. The first axis is diagnostic in which one needs

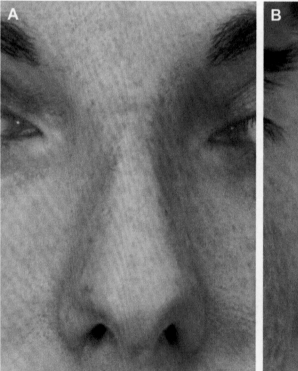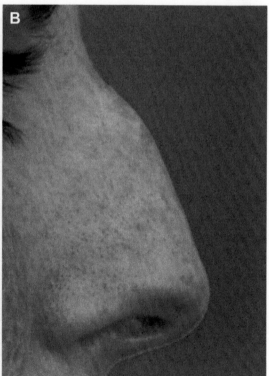

Fig. 4. (*A, B*) Clinical images of a patient's nose that displays characteristics that warrant consideration of the use of spreader grafts or other middle vault stabilizing technique if hump reduction is contemplated during rhinoplasty. These characteristics include short nasal bones noted by the location of the rhinion, an anticipated long nasal sideway predominately supported by the relatively long bilateral upper lateral cartilages, and a nasal profile that might be considered to undergo more than 5 mm of hump reduction. Such a degree of hump reduction without the placement of spreader grafts or other middle vault stabilizing technique would most likely result in middle vault insufficiency and collapse.

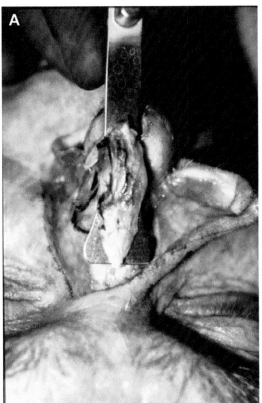
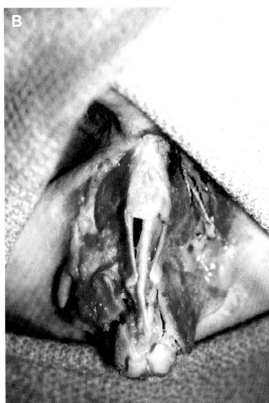

Fig. 5. Laboratory images of cadaver specimen. The skin has been dissected to show the native cartilaginous and bony skeleton. (*A*) Traditional hump reduction is mimicked with both cartilaginous and bony hump reduction. The upper lateral cartilages having been cut, and the line of incision is continued into the nasal bones with a Rubin osteotome. The cartilaginous and bony hump are removed en bloc. (*B*) View of middle vault after hump reduction shows middle vault collapse. Note the instability of the middle vault is present even before lateral osteotomies and infracture of the nasal bones is carried out.

the clinical acumen to judge when the middle vault is stable and will remain stable. Clinically, the concept of short nasal bones has been repeatedly mentioned in presentations and in the literature as a characteristic of a patient that the rhinoplasty surgeon should recognize to be at increased risk for middle vault collapse. Alternatively, patients who are judged to have longer nasal bones will hypothetically have more lateral wall support and be less prone to acquire middle vault collapse. These patients, therefore, may not need spreader grafts to stabilize the middle vault. The concept of short versus long nasal bones has been an arbitrary clinical indicator without an established benchmark of what the normal length of the adult nasal bones are. The study by Setabutr and colleagues,[16] resulted in normative data about the length of normal adult nasal bones in cadavers. There remains, however, little objective evidence to further guide the judgment of the surgeon during surgery.

The other axis that this question revolves around is a surgical/anatomic axis. If there are no dorsolateral nasal wall or osteotomy maneuvers performed, the likelihood of needing some form of middle vault management is lessened. If the relationship between the upper lateral cartilages and the septum is not disrupted, then the middle vault should remain stable, and spreader grafts may not be necessary. Thus, the patient who only has tip maneuvers performed during rhinoplasty may not need spreader grafts or other middle vault maneuvers performed. This statement is made with the caveat that there cannot be a preexisting deficiency, and none of the surgical maneuvers will disrupt the natural relationship between the lateral nasal sidewall and the septum. Primary rhinoplasty in which possibly only a minimal amount of tip procedures are to be performed is an example.

Does the use of spreader grafts necessitate an open approach? It is technically easier to place spreader grafts via an open approach. Alternatively, several investigators found that spreader grafts can be predictably performed through an endonasal approach.[13,17–19]

What are reasonable alternatives to the use of spreader grafts? Spreader grafts are generally described as being paired cartilage grafts that are approximately 4 mm wide by ≥15 mm long. These grafts are sutured on either side of the dorsal midline septum, and in turn, the bilateral upper lateral cartilages are sutured against the spreader grafts. The entire complex can be sutured together with one pair of horizontal mattress sutures. An alternative method is to first suture the spreader grafts to the upper border of the central septum and then secondarily suture the upper lateral cartilages to the spreader grafts. A reasonable alternative method to the use of spreader grafts seems to be the use of autospreader flaps. The creation and utilization of autospreader flaps requires that there is an excess of upper lateral cartilage to contour and suture to the dorsal central septum.[20,21] These flaps seem to serve similar purposes as the use of spreader grafts. The major difference, however, is that in the case of the use of autospreader flaps, the middle vault is stabilized by an excess of bilateral upper lateral cartilage that is recontoured and sutured to the septum. The use of autospreader flaps, by definition, requires that there be an excess of upper lateral cartilage remaining, such as after the reduction of a dorsal hump (**Fig. 6**).

Other surgeons seem to prefer butterfly grafts. These grafts do have utility to improve the nasal airway but are not as suitable when used to change the lateral nasal sidewall contour.[22]

The need to stabilize the middle vault has been fairly well demonstrated. This stabilization can be accomplished using several methods. Every rhinoplasty does not need to involve the placement of spreader grafts. The results of these operations will continue to improve as surgeons recognize and respond to the need in individual cases.

CORRECTIVE NASAL SURGERY AND THE YOUNGER PATIENT

1. Will nasal surgery affect nasal growth?
2. When can one safely do corrective nasal surgery on a child?
3. Can septal surgery be safely performed on the younger child?
4. At what ages is it acceptable to perform cosmetic nasal surgery on a teenager?

Traditional teaching is that nasal surgery should generally be avoided until adolescence to avoid nasal growth disturbances. In practical terms, this meant that many times nasal surgery, even of a corrective nature, was frequently delayed until the teenage years. The development of this

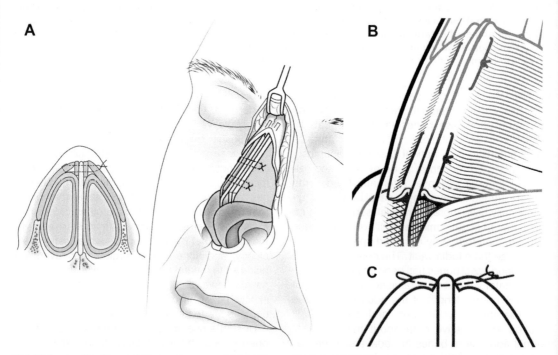

A

B

C

Fig. 6. Two methods to stabilize and improve the integrity of the middle vault in primary rhinoplasty. (*A*) Spreader grafts. (*B, C*), Autospreader flaps. (*From* [*A*] Fedok FG. Managing the overresected dorsum. In: Becker DG, Park SS, editors. Revision rhinoplasty. New York: Thieme Medical Publishers; 2008. p. 102; and [*B, C*] Fedok FG, Garritano F. Management of the middle vault in endonasal rhinoplasty. Facial Plast Surg 2014;30(2):211; with permission.)

principle was the result of several studies that found a decrease of nasal growth in animal groups after surgical intervention of nasal structures. The studies suggested that the septum was a critical growth center in the nose and concluded that surgery of the septum should be especially avoided. In actuality, the findings of many animal studies were somewhat contradictory, with some showing a growth disturbance and others not.

Since the 1950s, several experiments have been performed using animal models to determine the impact of nasal surgery on midface growth. Significant retardation of maxillary and midface growth was noted when resections of septal cartilage were performed in rabbits without preservation of the mucoperichondrium.[23] Impairment in maxillary growth was also found when similar resections of nasal septal cartilage were performed in canines[24]; the canine snout was studied after vomer resection for its impact on the anterior-posterior growth of the maxilla. When compared with controls, the canines with vomer resection were found to have retardation of the anterior-posterior maxillary dimension. Additionally, histologic examination found fibroblast and elastin fiber proliferation in the resected group, suggesting that this proliferation led to a difference in growth patterns.[25] In each of these studies, extensive resections of the nasal septal cartilage were performed.

In contrast, removal of septal cartilage from guinea pigs did not show significant changes to midface growth unless an extensive resection was performed.[26] Bernstein[27] subsequently removed nasal septal cartilage from 4- to 6-week-old canines, preserving the mucoperichondrium. In these canines, no appreciable change in growth was established, and cartilaginous autografts that were performed were found to be viable.[27] Despite these varied opinions and results, conservative recommendations regarding nasal surgery in children were advanced, and it was recommended that elective surgery be delayed until the teenage years after the completion of nasal growth.

Controversy has endured on the topic of the timing of nasal surgery in pediatric patients. One side maintains that nasal surgery should be avoided in this population given its potential impact on nasal and midface growth; the other side points to evidence suggesting that delaying surgery can have negative functional, cosmetic, and social developmental consequences. Since these early studies were reported, considerable experience has been accumulated in the observation of children after trauma and tumor surgery. Clinically, surgery in which aggressive septal surgery is avoided typically fails to demonstrate a significant impact on nasal growth.

The clinical situation will frequently compel a surgical solution. Obstructive nasal septal deformity can lead to chronic mouth breathing, which has is found to affect craniofacial development because it requires an open mouth and lips and a lowered or anterior tongue. It also results in decreased maxillofacial muscle tone. This lack of normal developmental forces causes narrowing of the maxilla, micrognathia, and retrognathia and protrusion of the maxillary incisors. Overall, anterior lower vertical face height is increased in these patients, and posterior facial height is decreased.[28] Additionally, it was found that uncorrected septal deformities will continue to worsen and can impact the frequency of sinusitis and otitis media.[29]

The study by Adil and colleagues[30] supports corrective surgery in the younger patient presenting with significant nasal deformity and obstruction. In general, corrective surgery in the pediatric population is to be considered appropriate and managed in the manner suggested for the management of facial fractures in the pediatric population. There should be an attempt to restore, reposition, and preserve structure. Aggressive surgery of the posterior septum should be avoided. On the other hand, an obvious deformity that is far beyond the normal appearance should be improved. A traumatic deformity should be attended to promptly. A congenital or developmental deformity should be corrected as early as possible. On a practical level, pediatric patients with severe nasal obstruction from a severe septal deviation should have the nasal obstruction corrected. Pediatric patients who suffered deformity secondary to tumor surgery or trauma should undergo corrective surgery to restore their nasal appearance and function to a more normal sphere.

Nasal surgery can be performed safely in selected younger pediatric patients. Goals of surgery should be conservative and aim to maintain the preexisting structural framework, to restore form and function and to maintain or reconstruct the projection of the nose, including the dorsal height and the tip projection and position (**Fig. 7**). Cartilage grafts, obtained from the ear or rib, can be used to strengthen the framework through spreader grafts. With more significant trauma or congenital defects, staged reconstructions may be necessary.

Procedures of a more refined "cosmetic" nature should be delayed until at least 14 years of age in girls and approximately 16 years of age in boys. As with all aspects of surgery, the application of these principles should be individualized and applied with sound judgment.

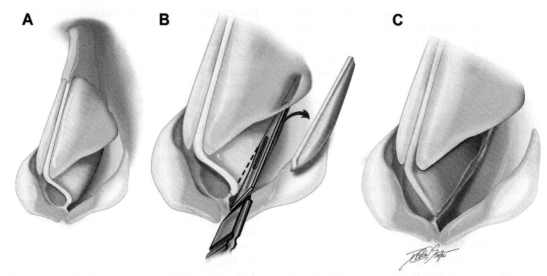

Fig. 7. Conservative septoplasty maneuver in which only the smallest amount of cartilage is removed from the septum to allow repositioning of the septum into the midline. (*A*) Septal spur or buckling of the septum adjacent to the maxillary crest. (*B*) A #15 scalpel is used to excise the narrow strip of redundant or buckled cartilage parallel to and adjacent to the maxillary crest. (*C*) The septum is then repositioned over the maxillary crest. If necessary, the deviated maxillary crest bone may be carefully osteotomized to allow it to be fractured back into a vertical midline position without removal of bone. (*From* Adil E, Goyal N, Fedok FG. Corrective nasal surgery in the younger patient. JAMA Facial Plast Surg 2014;16(3):181; with permission; and *Courtesy of* Devon Medical Art, LLC., Hershey, PA.)

THE USE OF RIB CARTILAGE GRAFTS IN RHINOPLASTY

1. When is the use of rib grafting indicated in primary rhinoplasty?
2. What are the advantages of using rib grafts in rhinoplasty?
3. What are the potential donor site complications?
4. What are the potential recipient site complications?
5. What are the limitations of other cartilage donor sites?

The rib is frequently used as a graft donor site for aesthetic and corrective rhinoplasty.[31] Even in the situation of a primary rhinoplasty, there may be inadequate septal cartilage available to do the necessary grafting. Patients of Asian and African descent possess noses with less adequate septal cartilage.[32,33] In the case of revision rhinoplasty, the paucity of available septal cartilage may be even further compounded.[34] The decision on whether costal cartilage is to be used depends on several factors including the availability of alternative donor sites and other patient factors and an assessment of the relative morbidity.

The preoperative planning for the use of cartilage grafts in rhinoplasty is centered on the goals of the rhinoplasty. If cartilaginous grafting materials are needed, then a donor site must be considered. The reasonably available donor sites are the nasal septum, the ear, and the ribs. Auricular cartilage is available in most patients but has limitations regarding elasticity and curvature. The edges of auricular cartilage grafts are also more likely to show dorsal irregularities through an overlying thin skin envelope compared with septal cartilage and rib cartilage grafts. The amount of auricular cartilage available to be harvested without causing distortion of the ear is also limited compared with what might be harvested from the rib cage; although some surgeons use cadaver rib cartilage, many will not.[35–38]

The limitations of available septal and auricular cartilage may compromise the results of a rhinoplasty procedure when restricted to the use of those two donor sites. The rib cage provides an enormous reserve of costal cartilage that can be carved into a variety of grafts necessary for the successful execution of several rhinoplasty techniques, making it an attractive option in patients with a deficient amount of septal or auricular cartilage. In many circumstances, the available volume and characteristics of costal cartilage is optimal for a successful rhinoplasty operation. If it is decided to use a costal donor site, several considerations must be made including the amount of cartilage that will be needed. The general morbidity of the use of costal cartilage in rhinoplasty has been studied and reported.[39–41] Potential donor site complications include infection, pneumothorax, bleeding, hematoma, and pain. There are also recipient site risks associated with the use of costal cartilage in rhinoplasty. Problems encountered have included inadequate dorsal graft fixation resulting in mobility, asymmetries secondary to prior severe scarring of the soft tissue envelope, dorsal convexities, and prolonged swelling.

Through planning and the successful adherence to recommended techniques, these risks can be minimized. The use of costal cartilage for appropriate candidates is a valuable addition to the toolbox of the rhinoplasty surgeon.

THE USE OF FILLERS IN RHINOPLASTY OR THE NONSURGICAL RHINOPLASTY

Fillers are a new addition to the toolbox for the surgeon performing rhinoplasty. Questions that are still being answered include:

1. What filler materials are used in the primary rhinoplasty situation?
2. What kind of problems can be effectively remedied with injectable filler materials?
3. What is the optimal technique for injection?
4. What are the potential complications?

It is common for patients to present for primary rhinoplasty with various nasal asymmetries and depressions. Essentially, any combination of problems that interfere with the symmetry, balance, and proportion of the nose has presented to a surgeon at some point. The remedy of the problem may be complex or simple depending on the extent of the issue. When the problem does not involve a severe functional issue or a major problem with the nasal structure, lesser remedies have always been preferred.

For problems characterized by a void or volume deficiency, many different filler or grafting materials have been used. At times, the treatment of a small depression warrants the use of cartilage grafting performed as a minimalistic procedure via precision pocket grafting. For even smaller deficiencies, some form of injectable material has frequently been used. In the past, silicone may have been considered to be the filler of choice and ranked as such over several decades. Materials used here include cartilage grafts, fascia grafts, fat grafts, silicone, and others.

As new fillers have been developed, many practitioners have been using the off-the-shelf fillers such as those of a hyaluronic acid and hydroxyapatite derivation. There is considerable literature on the use of the newer fillers in both primary and revision rhinoplasty situations.[42–45] The use of these newer fillers has been more accepted than silicone, although technically, they may have not been scientifically proven to be safer. Fillers have been used as part of a primary approach to rhinoplasty and have been used to lessen the nasal frontal angle, to improve saddle deformity of the dorsum and to change the nasolabial angle.

In spite of the pervasiveness of this use of fillers in the nose, the practice cannot be considered universally accepted, and there are some hazards.[46–49] There have been a significant number of cases reported in which filler injection in the nose has been associated with skin loss, granuloma formation, and deformity. Several recommendations have been made in the literature to avoid complications and include injecting only small amounts, injecting deeply over the cartilaginous skeleton, and avoiding a forceful injection into the nasal tip.[46,50]

These are new practices, and time will tell whether they are enduring or will fall by the wayside. In the meantime, it is this author's recommendation that the use of fillers in the nose be carried out cautiously and with good surgical judgment.

SUMMARY

This report reviews some of the debated issues in rhinoplasty, including the use of spreader grafts and autospreader flaps in the management of the middle vault in rhinoplasty, the performance of the open approach versus the endonasal rhinoplasty approach, corrective rhinoplasty in the younger patient, the use of the rib and other cartilage donor sites for grafting in rhinoplasty, and the use of filler materials in rhinoplasty.

Other ongoing and evolving issues in primary rhinoplasty include (at least) the rhinoplasty management of the traumatized nose, the use of powered instrumentation, the use of absorbable materials in septoplasty, the use of steroids in the perioperative period, and the role of imaging.

What has been presented is a distillation of information from the literature and personal conversations with respected clinicians, lectures, and clinical experience. The various topic conclusions are not meant to dictate clinical application but are instead meant to present one individual's perspective on these issues. Each surgeon will have to do the same as they engage patients who present with problems within these topics. The surgeon as teacher, lifelong learner, and caretaker is best when they avail themselves of all credible information and then judge how the information is best applied to their patients.

REFERENCES

1. AAFPRS. 2013 AAFPRS Membership Study. Philadelphia: International Communications Research; 2013. p. 1–49.

2. Adamson PA. Open rhinoplasty. Otolaryngol Clin North Am 1987;20(4):837–52.

3. Adamson PA, Smith O, Tropper GJ. Incision and scar analysis in open (external) rhinoplasty. Arch Otolaryngol Head Neck Surg 1990;116(6):671–5.

4. Gurlek A, Fariz A, Aydogan H, et al. Effects of different corticosteroids on edema and ecchymosis in open rhinoplasty. Aesthetic Plast Surg 2006;30(2):150–4.

5. Inanli S, Sari M, Yanik M. A new consideration of scar formation in open rhinoplasty. J Craniofac Surg 2009;20(4):1228–30.

6. Perkins SW. The evolution of the combined use of endonasal and external columellar approaches to rhinoplasty. Facial Plast Surg Clin North Am 2004; 12(1):35–50.

7. Gunter JP. The merits of the open approach in rhinoplasty. Plast Reconstr Surg 1997;99(3):863–7.

8. Smith O, Goodman W. Open rhinoplasty: its past and future. J Otolaryngol 1993;22(1):21–5.

9. Zijlker TD, Adamson PA. Open structure rhinoplasty. Clin Otolaryngol Allied Sci 1993;18(2):125–34.

10. Dayan S, Kanodia R. Has the pendulum swung too far?: trends in the teaching of endonasal rhinoplasty. Arch Facial Plast Surg 2009;11(6):414–6.

11. Cottle MH. The structure and function of the nasal vestibule. AMA Arch Otolaryng 1955;62(2):173–81.

12. Haight JS, Cole P. The site and function of the nasal valve. Laryngoscope 1983;93(1):49–55.

13. Fedok FG, Garritano F. Management of the middle vault in endonasal rhinoplasty. Facial Plast Surg 2014;30(2):205–13.

14. Sheen JH. Spreader graft: a method of reconstructing the roof of the middle nasal vault following rhinoplasty. Plast Reconstr Surg 1984;73(2):230–9.

15. Kern EB. Surgical approaches to abnormalities of the nasal valve. Rhinology 1978;16(3):165–89.

16. Setabutr D, Sohrabi S, Kalaria S, et al. The relationship of external and internal sidewall dimensions in the adult Caucasian nose. Laryngoscope 2013; 123(4):875–8.

17. Manavbasi I, Agaoglu G. Endonasal placement of spreader grafts. Plast Reconstr Surg 2007;119(6):1961–2.

18. Pontius AT, Williams EF 3rd. Endonasal placement of spreader grafts in rhinoplasty. Ear Nose Throat J 2005;84(3):135–6.

19. Yoo DB, Jen A. Endonasal placement of spreader grafts: experience in 41 consecutive patients. Arch Facial Plast Surg 2012;14(5):318–22.

20. Byrd HS, Meade RA, Gonyon DL Jr. Using the autospreader flap in primary rhinoplasty. Plast Reconstr Surg 2007;119(6):1897–902.

21. Tellioglu AT. Autospreader flap. Plast Reconstr Surg 2008;122(1):313.

22. Stacey DH, Cook TA, Marcus BC. Correction of internal nasal valve stenosis: a single surgeon comparison of butterfly versus traditional spreader grafts. Ann Plast Surg 2009;63(3):280–4.

23. Sarnat BG, Wexler MR. Growth of the face and jaws after resection of the septal cartilage in the rabbit. Am J Anat 1966;118(3):755–67.

24. Hartshorn D. Facial growth effects of nasal septal cartilage resection in beagle pups. University of Iowa; 1970.

25. Squier CA, Wada T, Ghoneim S, et al. A histological and ultrastructural study of wound healing after vomer resection in the beagle dog. Arch Oral Biol 1985;30(11–12):833–41.

26. Stenström SJ, Thilander BL. Effects of nasal septal cartilage resections on young guinea pigs. Plast Reconstr Surg 1970;45(2):160–70.

27. Bernstein L. Early submucous resection of nasal septal cartilage. A pilot study in canine pups. Arch Otolaryngol Head Neck Surg 1973;97(3):273–8.

28. Harari D, Redlich M, Miri S, et al. The effect of mouth breathing versus nasal breathing on dentofacial and craniofacial development in orthodontic patien. Laryngoscope 2010;120(10):2089–93.

29. Gray L. The development and significance of septal and dental deformity from birth to eight years. Int J Pediatr Otorhinolaryngol 1983;6(3):265–77.

30. Adil E, Goyal N, Fedok FG. Corrective nasal surgery in the younger patient. JAMA Facial Plast Surg 2014; 16(3):176–82.

31. Fedok F. Costal cartilage grafts in rhinoplasty. Clin Plast Surg 2016;43(1):201–12.

32. Nolst Trenite GJ. Considerations in ethnic rhinoplasty. Facial Plast Surg 2003;19(3):239–45.

33. Rohrich RJ, Bolden K. Ethnic rhinoplasty. Clin Plast Surg 2010;37(2):353–70.

34. Fedok FG, Rihani J. Essential Grafting in the Traumatized Nose. Facial Plast Surg 2015;31(3):238–51.

35. Burke AJ, Wang TD, Cook TA. Irradiated homograft rib cartilage in facial reconstruction. Arch Facial Plast Surg 2004;6(5):334–41.

36. Lefkovits G. Irradiated homologous costal cartilage for augmentation rhinoplasty. Ann Plast Surg 1990; 25(4):317–27.

37. Demirkan F, Arslan E, Unal S, et al. Irradiated homologous costal cartilage: versatile grafting material for rhinoplasty. Aesthetic Plast Surg 2003;27(3):213–20.

38. Kridel RW, Ashoori F, Liu ES, et al. Long-term use and follow-up of irradiated homologous costal cartilage grafts in the nose. Arch Facial Plast Surg 2009; 11(6):378–94.

39. Moon BJ, Lee HJ, Jang YJ. Outcomes following rhinoplasty using autologous costal cartilage. Arch Facial Plast Surg 2012;14(3):175–80.

40. Wee JH, Park MH, Jin HR. Post-rib harvesting pain should be considered as a potential significant morbidity in reconstructive rhinoplasty-reply. JAMA Facial Plast Surg 2015;17(3):226.

41. Wee JH, Park MH, Oh S, et al. Complications associated with autologous rib cartilage use in rhinoplasty: a meta-analysis. JAMA Facial Plast Surg 2015;17(1): 49–55.

42. Kurkjian TJ, Ahmad J, Rohrich RJ. Soft-tissue fillers in rhinoplasty. Plast Reconstr Surg 2014;133(2):121e–6e.

43. Jasin ME. Nonsurgical rhinoplasty using dermal fillers. Facial Plast Surg Clin North Am 2013;21(2): 241–52.

44. Cassuto D. The use of Dermicol-P35 dermal filler for nonsurgical rhinoplasty. Aesthet Surg J 2009;29(3 Suppl):S22–4.

45. de Lacerda DA, Zancanaro P. Filler rhinoplasty. Dermatol Surg 2007;33(Suppl 2):S207–12 [discussion: S212].

46. Woodward J, Khan T, Martin J. Facial Filler Complications. Facial Plast Surg Clin North Am 2015; 23(4):447–58.

47. El-Khalawany M, Fawzy S, Saied A, et al. Dermal filler complications: a clinicopathologic study with a spectrum of histologic reaction patterns. Ann Diagn Pathol 2015;19(1):10–5.

48. Park TH, Seo SW, Kim JK, et al. Clinical experience with hyaluronic acid-filler complications. J Plast Reconstr Aesthet Surg 2011;64(7):892–6.

49. Winslow CP. The management of dermal filler complications. Facial Plast Surg 2009;25(2):124–8.

50. Bass LS. Injectable filler techniques for facial rejuvenation, volumization, and augmentation. Facial Plast Surg Clin North Am 2015;23(4):479–88.

Controversies in Revision Rhinoplasty

Eric S. Rosenberger, MD*, Dean M. Toriumi, MD

KEYWORDS

- Revision rhinoplasty • Nasal filler • Cartilage grafting • Dorsal augmentation

KEY POINTS

- Revision rhinoplasty must improve nasal esthetic appearance and airway patency for complete patient satisfaction.
- Key grafts for improving the nasal airway include spreader graft, lateral crural strut graft, and alar batten graft.
- Infection prevention in rhinoplasty should include topical, systemic, or combination therapy, with or without drain management during revision surgery.
- Pros and cons exist regarding potential pitfalls of diced cartilage versus solid cartilage grafting.
- Alloplastic versus autogenous grafting during revision rhinoplasty includes Augmentation of the nasal dorsum.

INTRODUCTION

Surgical rhinoplasty requires manipulation of the structural framework of the nose to elicit desired changes in contour. This procedure is exceedingly complex, especially for the revision rhinoplasty surgeon, because the esthetic outcome desired by the patient may reduce the nasal airway, leading to obstructive symptoms.[1] Multiple variables affect the ultimate outcome, including nasal bone length, strength and resiliency of the upper and lower lateral cartilages, position and shape of the nasal septum, inferior turbinate hypertrophy, and the thickness of the overlying soft tissue envelope.

Over the past 60 years, the approach to revision rhinoplasty has expanded from a primarily reductive procedure, focusing purely on cosmetic outcome, to one that augments the structural components of the nasal skeleton. This evolving method has the ultimate goal of providing improvement in both the nasal airway and the nasal esthetics. Rhinoplasty surgeons seek to refine the techniques and methods that provide the most consistent and long-lasting outcomes. As the structural approach to rhinoplasty evolves, controversies emerge as continuing research applies the scientific method to new technology, surgical maneuvers, and long-term follow-up of surgical outcomes.[2]

CONTROVERSIES IN RHINOPLASTY
Alloplastic Material versus Autologous Grafts in Dorsal Augmentation

Revision rhinoplasty frequently involves correction of iatrogenic nasal deformities, often the result of overresection of the existing nasal cartilaginous skeleton. Surgical correction requires augmentation with material similar to the natural nasal cartilage. The ideal graft material should be sufficient in quantity, strength, resiliency, and ability to be carved. It should be easily removed and unlikely to warp, migrate, become immunogenic, cause infection, or resorb. The source of this ideal graft remains elusive.

Disclosure Statement: The authors have nothing to disclose.
Facial Plastic and Reconstructive Surgery, Department of Otolaryngology, University of Illinois Chicago, 1855 West Taylor Street, Suite 387, Chicago, IL 60612, USA
* Corresponding author.
E-mail address: erosenb3@uic.edu

Facial Plast Surg Clin N Am 24 (2016) 337–345
http://dx.doi.org/10.1016/j.fsc.2016.03.010
1064-7406/16/$ – see front matter © 2016 Elsevier Inc. All rights reserved.

Alloplastic implants are an alternative to autologous grafting. The most popular products currently in use include silicone, porous polyethylene (Medpor, Stryker Inc., Kalamazoo, MI), polytetrafluoroethylene (Proplast, Vitek Inc., Houston, TX), and expanded polytetrafluoroethylene (Gore-Tex, W. L. Gore & Associates Inc, Flagstaff, AZ). The goal of such implants is primarily to address autologous grafting drawbacks related to increased operative time and donor site morbidity. However, alloplastic implants are associated with a unique set of potentially devastating consequences, including infection, rejection, and extrusion.

Silicone and polytetrafluorethylene (Proplast) implants are currently banned by the US Food and Drug Administration (FDA) but continue to be used almost exclusively in Asian augmentation rhinoplasty. Silicone may be produced to almost any consistency (soft to firm), has excellent elastic properties, can be carved, is easily placed, and is also easily removed due to capsule formation in vivo. Significant drawbacks include a reported extrusion/rejection rate of 8% at 160 days.[3] Long-term studies suggest that rates of extrusion also increase with time and are a lifelong risk.[4] The results of extrusion can be severe, including soft tissue loss and scarring of the nasal tip, which make correction to a preoperative state extremely difficult.

Expanded polytetrafluoroethylene (Gore-Tex) is composed of small pores approximately one/tenth the size of porous polyethylene and permits vascular ingrowth. A 3-year large case series (n = 1054) in Southeastern Asian primary rhinoplasty patients reported implant deviation in 1%, visible implant in 0.5%, and infection in 0.4%.[5] However, long-term follow-up is lacking, and recent meta-analysis suggests a 10.6% infection rate with preceding fistula development.[6]

Porous polyethylene (Medpor) has been used for reconstruction of many areas of the head and neck, including orbital fractures, chin and malar bone augmentation, as well as soft tissue augmentation during rhinoplasty and microtia repair. Characteristics include a flexible framework at body temperature, a pore size that permits rapid ingrowth of vascularized tissue, and thermoplastic properties when heated to greater than $85°C$.[7] Long-term follow-up has generally been lacking, but recent meta-analysis suggests that the use of Medpor and Gore-Tex implants has a 3.1% removal rate when used for nasal reconstruction, approximately half that of silicone (6.5%).[8] Further reports have contended that Medpor is a suitable material for nasal spreader grafts.[9]

Drawbacks include difficulty in removal secondary to vascular ingrowth and infection. When Medpor was compared with auricular cartilage spreader grafts in a small case series, of 10 and 8 patients, respectively, 1 case of unilateral infection occurred in the Medpor group (10%).[10] In another study comparing alloplastic to autogenous grafts, the highest infection rate was 23.4% when Medpor was used as a columellar strut graft. The overall autologous versus alloplastic infection rate in recent analysis was 0% versus 12.6%.[11] Use of Medpor in the moveable portions of the nose (lower two-thirds) is fraught with higher infection and extrusion rates because the implant can erode through mucosa or skin. In addition, the Medpor dorsal shell implant is large and very difficult to remove (**Fig. 1**). Once implanted, the skin on the nose is permanently altered and scarred.

Techniques are in development to minimize the risk of infection with alloplastic materials. There is short-term evidence demonstrating increased biocompatibility of synthetic implants is possible with platelet concentrate.[12] The long-term effects of this therapy are unknown.

The current gold standard as well as the majority opinion of many top revision rhinoplasty surgeons favors the use of autologous grafts from the septum, auricle, or costal cartilage for dorsal augmentation. The often cited drawbacks to these sources include increased operative time, donor site morbidity, and inability to predict postoperative graft resorption and warping. However, with experience, graft harvest operative time decreases, nontraumatic technique minimizes donor site morbidity, and experience with carving the cartilage and selecting grafts helps minimize the chances of warping.[13] Most surgeons agree that although alloplastic implants have a role in rhinoplasty, the risk of infection and extrusion must be equal to autologous tissue, with known long-term results, before they are implemented as a true replacement for autologous cartilage grafting.

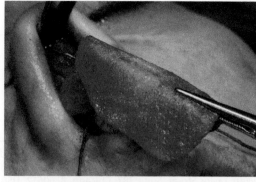

Fig. 1. Medpor shell implant removed from the nasal dorsum. Removal is difficult because the implant covers the entire nasal dorsum and extends onto the ascending process of the maxilla.

Autologous Rib Versus Irradiated Rib for Nasal Reconstruction

The use of irradiated rib has been advocated as an alternative to alloplastic implants and homologous cartilage harvest. The benefits include an ample source of ideal material, replacing like tissue with like tissue, and the absence of donor site morbidity. This process is achieved by applying gamma radiation to cadaver rib, making the final product free of immunogenic and infectious potential. Use of irradiated rib for secondary rhinoplasty has been a source of controversy since its introduction, primarily due to physician concerns of graft resorption, the possibility of rejection by the host, and placement of a nonviable implant that does not become "living tissue." Patient acceptance of a cadaveric donor tissue requires comprehensive consent and education. In addition, universal availability of the graft material may be limited by location and local regulation of donor tissues.

One 15-year retrospective study, published in 1998, concluded that irradiated rib had a high rate of resorption and should be anticipated by those using the material.[14] This report has been contradicted by more recent studies with similar long-term follow-up. Adverse events in this study, from irradiated rib, were reported to be no greater than rhinoplasty complication rates when autologous costal grafts are used. The investigators ultimately concluded that the safety, reliability, and convenience of irradiated grafts are ideal for both primary and revision rhinoplasty.[15]

Proponents of autologous costal cartilage grafts minimize the morbidity of graft harvest and report low risk of infection, extrusion, resorption, and warping. Autologous cartilage also becomes revascularized and can resist infection and resorption to a greater degree than irradiated grafts. Recent meta-analysis found the combined complication rates for autologous costal cartilage grafting were 3.08% (95% confidence interval [CI], 0%–10.15%) for warping, 0.22% (95% CI, 0%–1.25%) for resorption, 0.56% (95% CI, 0%–2.61%) for infection, 0.39% (95% CI, 0%–1.97%) for displacement, 5.45% (95% CI, 0.68%–13.24%) for hypertrophic chest scarring, 0% (95% CI, 0%–0.32%) for pneumothorax, and 14.07% (95% CI, 6.19%–24.20%) for revision surgery.[16] Expert opinion maintains that warping can be controlled through careful selection of cartilage grafts, allowing sufficient time postharvest to witness the tendency of the cartilage to bend, and rigid fixation of the dorsal graft to the bony dorsum. Rigid fixation can be achieved via a perichondrial-bony interface and tight subperiosteal pocket placement (**Fig. 2**).[17]

In a study investigating the effects of carving plane, harvest level, and oppositional suturing techniques on autogenous cartilage warping, the methods used failed to demonstrate statistically significant results for the prevention of warping. However, the study concluded that a balanced approach, with central harvest of the rib, continues to be the most efficacious method for warping prevention because the process was found to continue up to 1 month after implantation and likely continues over time.[18]

The ideal rib for cartilage grafting should have a primarily straight cartilaginous section of ample quantity and quality, be located away from the pleural cavity, and be harvested with minimal donor site morbidity. Based on anatomic study, the seventh rib fits these qualifications and seems to be the most ideal source in most individuals.[19]

Novel application of available endoscopic technology has suggested that hypertrophic scarring of the chest wall associated with rib graft harvest may be eliminated via use of a transumbilical approach to the lower anterior chest wall. Proponents report an associated learning curve and increased operative time for this procedure, averaging 2 to 2.5 hours.[20]

Based on current surgical techniques and available supporting research, autologous costal cartilage seems to be the best available material for complete nasal reconstruction during revision rhinoplasty cases compared with irradiated rib. More studies are required, with long-term

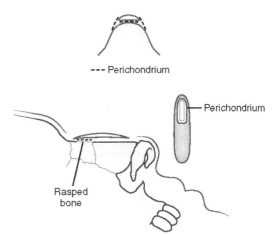

Fig. 2. Dorsal graft fixation. Multiple holes are made in the nasal dorsum using a 2-mm straight osteotome or narrow fine tooth rasp. Then perichondrium is sutured to the undersurface of the dorsal graft and the graft is placed into a tight subperiosteal pocket. Tight adherence of the costal perichondrium against the perforated nasal dorsal bone results in rigid fixation of the graft to the bridge of the nose.

follow-up, before universal acceptance of graft equality. Warping and donor site morbidity, including hypertrophic scarring, are the greatest statistical risks of the autologous harvest procedure and seem to be manageable complications with similar revision rates as those reported for primary rhinoplasty cases.

Diced Cartilage Versus Solid Cartilage Grafting

Diced cartilage dorsal augmentation grafts have been increasingly advocated as an adjunct or alternative to solid cartilage grafting over the past 20 years. The principle is to create a graft that is easy to place and mold, is not prone to warping or resorption, and will not become visible or palpable after tissue edema has subsided, especially in thin-skinned patients. Initially called a "Turkish delight," this graft was composed of Surgicel (oxidized cellulose)-wrapped diced cartilage (0.5–1-mm cubes), sourced from autogenous septum, auricle, or rib. These rolled sleeves were used as dorsal augmentation and dorsal camouflage that were pliable and moldable via finger manipulation. Long-lasting results with few complications, including infection, resorption, or persistent overcorrection, was documented in 2365 patients over 10 years, including revision and primary rhinoplasty patients.[21] Further investigation has failed to demonstrate long-term viability with Surgicel-wrapped grafts compared with grafts wrapped in autologous temporalis fascia, noting that as the Surgicel absorbs, unwanted contour irregularities may form.[22] A rabbit model study replaced Surgicel with Alloderm (acellular dermis) and compared this material versus autologous fascia as a wrap for diced cartilage grafts. The investigators reported equivocal results on histology but cautioned that long-term studies are needed.[23] Autologous tissue glue has also been reported to provide a stable scaffold for diced cartilage grafts with good results in 68 patients at 15 months follow-up.[24]

Diced cartilage wrapped in autologous fascia may prove to be a reliable method of dorsal augmentation, but further long-term follow-up studies are needed to prove graft stability beyond 10 years. At this time, solid cartilage grafting has the advantage of documented long-term stability, structural integrity, and minimal complications with resorption or warping when treated appropriately. Solid cartilage grafting has the additional benefit of in-office needle shaving using local anesthesia if slight dorsal irregularities develop in the postoperative period. An 18-gauge needle provides a simple solution as solid grafts are firm but remain amenable to carving. Diced cartilage

or alloplastic implants do not enjoy the same characteristics and instead must rely on revision surgery or injectable filler to achieve comparable results.

Injectable Cartilage Grafting

Dorsal augmentation with diced cartilage wrapped in fascia or other material requires surgical implantation via an endonasal or open approach with the possibility of postoperative dorsal irregularities due to absorption. Some surgeons think one alternative to diced cartilage is to use available septal, auricular, or costal cartilage to create an injectable cartilage slurry with high chondrocyte viability; this provides the ability to inject cartilage to fill small areas of irregularity while using solid cartilage grafting for structural support. This material should have the fine-tuning characteristics of synthetic injectables but the biocompatibility of autologous cartilage.[25] Tissue engineering is currently lacking the technological advancements necessary to produce this material ex vivo using cell culture. Therefore, alternative methods using autologous cartilage sources have been under investigation.

Results from one study reported an otologic burr as the best instrument for creating uniform (largest dimension 0.44 ± 0.33 mm) cartilage pieces small enough for injection with an 18-gauge needle. Nasal septal cartilage produced the best results with 33% of lacunae containing viable-appearing chondrocytes. Drilled auricular cartilage produced similar size pieces, but only 10% of lacunae were occupied by viable chondrocytes. Other techniques tested (knife, morselizer, and cartilage crusher) did not produce pieces suitable as an injectable cartilage slurry.[26] Additional research has recently been published describing a cartilage shaving technique by hand that produced an injectable cartilage slurry capable of injection through 14- or 18-gauge needles. This material was used to fill all areas of the nose in 128 patients over a 6-year period without a single case of infection, extrusion, displacement, or soft tissue irregularity. However, resorption occurred in almost all patients to some extent, leading to a 5% surgical revision rate.[27]

This area continues to be an area of ongoing research and may have a place in the surgical armamentarium of rhinoplasty surgeons. At this time, long-term follow-up of surgical outcomes is required before wide acceptance as a viable alternative to solid cartilage, diced cartilage, or nasal filler.

Injectables in the Nose

Use of injectable facial fillers, primarily hyaluronic acid and calcium hydroxylapatite (Radiesse), has been used off label to perform "liquid," "nonsurgical," or "injection" rhinoplasty for many years. Although not FDA approved for this location, there are distinct advantages to the use of nonpermanent filler for alleviation of minor cosmetic defects, including minimal pain, avoidance of general anesthesia, short procedure time, quick recovery time, and reversibility with use of hyaluronic acid–based filler. Serious complications are uncommon, but catastrophic vascular compromise can occur via either direct injection of filler into end arterioles or vessel compression, leading to tissue ischemia and skin necrosis.[28]

Short-term prospective studies by rhinoplasty surgeons have reported the use of facial filler, primarily Radiesse, for correction of postoperative deformities with good results and minimal complications that last for at least 1 year.[29] Radiesse has gained increasing favor as the filler of choice for minor nasal augmentation because of its long duration, moldability, high viscosity, elasticity, and low immunogenicity (no allergy testing required).[30] Noted drawbacks with hyaluronic acid intradermal nasal injection include migration and the Tyndall effect, creating a bluish tint in bright light, especially in thin skin.

Liquid silicone was the first off-label permanent filler to be used extensively as an adjunct to rhinoplasty. However, it lost favor in use because of potential long-term issues with chronic inflammation. A recent study using polymethyl methacrylate, used in 19 subjects followed for 1 year, demonstrated good cosmetic results with no serious adverse events other than palpable, but not visible, nodule formation.[31] The product uses bovine collagen as a carrier with a potential risk for allergic reaction or rejection and requires intradermal testing before use. An issue with all permanent injectables includes need for surgical removal, if required, and potential for increased surgical complexity with revision rhinoplasty.

Use of facial filler for primary rhinoplasty or as an adjunct to postoperative irregularity is avoided by the senior author (D.M.T.). Reasons for avoidance are primarily related to the potential for vascular injury to the skin envelope of the nose. Furthermore, most patients present for rhinoplasty with airway complaints and seek improvement in nasal airflow; this requires structural support that injection rhinoplasty cannot provide. Although it is probably a safe practice to inject the nasal dorsum, injection of the nasal tip should be avoided. Nasal tip blood supply is primarily end arterioles, and major reconstruction will be required if intravascular application or local compression leads to tissue necrosis.[32]

Spreader Flap Versus Spreader Grafts

Most reductive rhinoplasty procedures involve the removal of a dorsal hump, consisting of the caudal aspect of the nasal bones as well as the cephalic aspect of the upper lateral cartilages and superior septal cartilage. If a significantly sized hump is removed, generally more than 2 mm, an open roof deformity is created whereby the upper lateral cartilages and septum were resected. Spreader grafts are the traditional solution to addressing the middle vault region but require additional cartilage material that may or may not be available following septoplasty, especially if the procedure is a revision rhinoplasty.[33] The autospreader or spreader flap has been proposed in several case series as a method that makes use of existing upper lateral cartilage during dorsal hump reduction. Proponents advocate this technique as consistently reproducible for preservation of the dorsal esthetic line by keeping the upper lateral intact and scoring the cartilage to allow medial infolding of the upper lateral cartilages onto themselves. The spreader flap is then sutured to the dorsal septum, closing the open roof and simultaneously improving the airway at the internal nasal valve.[34,35]

Controversy with this method exists because of conflicting evidence that the autospreader technique is truly equivalent to traditional spreader grafts carved from septal or costal cartilage. A recent small study demonstrated significant improvement in nasal obstruction symptom evaluation (NOSE) scale and visual analogue scores with the autospreader technique at less than 6 months of follow-up.[36] Another study found no statistical difference in minimal cross-sectional area or by visual analogue scale for esthetic appearance or nasal obstruction at 1-year follow-up when the autospreader technique was used.[37]

A reported drawback of the autospreader technique is inability to address width in the lower third of the nasal dorsum and supratip region. In addition, with smaller dorsal hump reductions, there will be minimal upper lateral cartilage to fold over to create the spreader flap. In another case series, the combination of the autospreader technique was combined with small spreader grafts to increase dorsal width from 5 mm (autospreader only) to 7 mm (combination autospreader/ spreader).[38]

Autospreader or spreader flaps have a role in reduction rhinoplasty, especially with removal of large dorsal humps. At this time, long-term follow-up of this technique is insufficient to recommend their use exclusively over traditional spreader grafting, especially for revision surgery cases. A more prudent approach is combination grafting to achieve a smooth dorsal esthetic line while ensuring that the internal nasal valve remains uncompromised.

Onlay Grafting to Existing Structure Versus Complete Reconstruction

Many surgeons that perform revision rhinoplasty add cartilage to the existing deformed nasal structure to add support and improve contour. This method frequently involves use of alar batten grafts, shield tip grafts, and onlay grafts to the nasal tip. This method can be very effective but does add additional bulk to the structure of the nose and can create extra thickness (**Fig. 3**).

This thickness can add bulk to the nose and also compress internally on the nasal airway resulting in airway obstruction. The senior author (D.M.T.) prefers to rebuild the nasal structure by removing the deformed nasal structures and then rebuild an appropriate nasal supportive framework that provides good nasal contour and maximizes nasal function (**Fig. 4**).

This method of reconstruction is more complex and time consuming and requires more grafting material. In most cases, costal cartilage is used

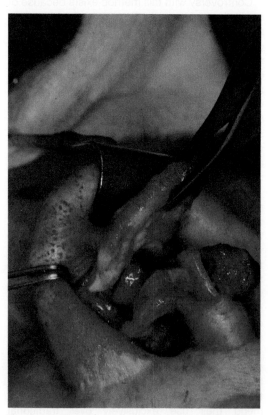

Fig. 3. Layering of cartilage onto the existing structure of nose, resulting in excess thickness of the sidewall of the nose.

for this method of managing the secondary rhinoplasty patient. This method may provide the patient with a more stable, longer-lasting esthetic and functional outcome.

Infection Prevention

Postoperative infection following revision rhinoplasty is a potentially catastrophic event that most surgeons seek to avoid through sterile technique and perioperative antibiotic usage. *Staphylococcus aureus* (SA) can be isolated in 30% of human noses in the asymptomatic general population with a small fraction (0.8%) of those patients harboring methicillin-resistant (MRSA) strains.[39] Perioperative prophylaxis with Mupirocin 2% topical was found and confirmed with subsequent follow-up studies to reduce SA nasal carriage in 97% of patients. However, SA carriage reduction failed to significantly decrease the number of postoperative surgical site infections.[40,41]

There is currently no clear consensus, and controversy exists on the single best regimen for decreasing postoperative infection among revision rhinoplasty patients.

The use of postoperative antibiotics has long been advised following a double-blinded randomized study wherein 100 complicated revision rhinoplasty cases received either placebo or postoperative antibiotics. Results demonstrated statistically significant infection risk in the placebo group with 5 of the 6 serious infections and 9 of 12 local infections identified within this group.[42] Further investigation has suggested that patients at high risk of MRSA colonization should be screened using nasal swab culture and then treated with Mupirocin 2% nasal twice daily during the 5 days before revision rhinoplasty, followed by culture-sensitive antibiotics for 12 days postoperatively.[43] There is some concern that this method may select for MRSA by eliminating the natural flora. A recent follow-up study required 363 patients to use chlorhexidine gluconate to clean the head, neck, and nose, plus topical nasal Mupirocin 5 days before rhinoplasty, followed by nasal swab culture. No additional antibiotics were given if normal flora was isolated. If SA or fecal coliforms were isolated, culture-directed postoperative antibiotics were given. Results of the study found that SA was the most common normal flora organism at 10% and was higher in diabetics. The second most common organisms isolated (7% of cultures) were fecal coliforms, especially from adult acne patients. Postoperative infections were dominated by fecal coliforms (46%) followed by SA (36%), in both primary and revision cases. Notably, MRSA was

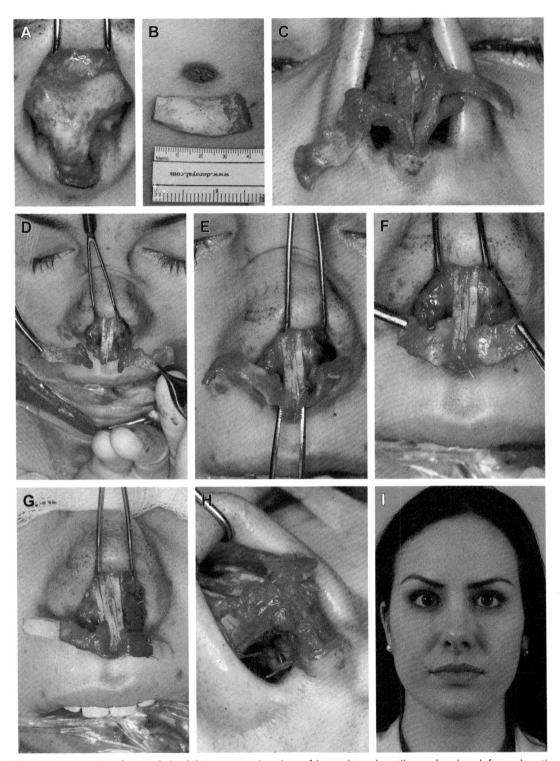

Fig. 4. Restructuring the nasal tip. (*A*) Intraoperative view of lower lateral cartilages showing deformed cartilages. (*B*) Harvesting of costal cartilage from 1.1-cm chest incision. (*C*) Lower lateral cartilages dissected. (*D*) Lateral crura resected. (*E*) Lateral crura in new position. (*F*) Lateral crura resutured to caudal septal extension graft. (*G*) Lateral crural strut grafts sutured in place. (*H*) Lateral crural strut grafts sutured and repositioned. (*I*) Preoperative frontal view. (*J*) Preoperative lateral view. (*K*) Postoperative lateral view. (*L*) Postoperative frontal view.

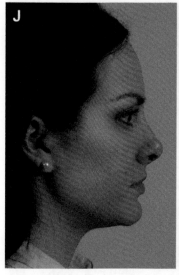
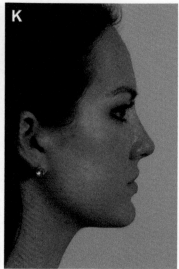
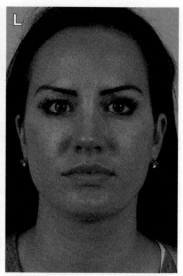

Fig. 4. (*continued*)

only cultured from a single patient. Recommendations suggest that a nasal swab followed by culture-directed antibiotics be performed on all preoperative rhinoplasty patients.[44]

If infection prevention fails, drainage and culture of purulent material are absolutely necessary to prevent cartilage destruction. Most surgeons advocate drain placement and irrigation with an antibiotic solution in addition to culture-directed antibiotics.[45]

SUMMARY

Revision rhinoplasty has undergone considerable changes over the past 40 years. Techniques continue to evolve, but a common trend among experienced rhinoplasty surgeons has shifted from a reductive approach to structural grafting and combination techniques, which simultaneously improve cosmetic and functional outcomes.[46] Continued long-term follow-up is required of the previously discussed techniques and methods currently comprising controversial topics in revision rhinoplasty.

REFERENCES

1. Park SS. Fundamental principles in aesthetic rhinoplasty. Clin Exp Otorhinolaryngol 2011;4(2):55–66.
2. Angelos PC, Been MJ, Toriumi DM. Contemporary review of rhinoplasty. Arch Facial Plast Surg 2012; 14(4):238–47.
3. Tham C, Lai YL, Weng CJ, et al. Silicone augmentation rhinoplasty in an Oriental population. Ann Plast Surg 2005;54:1–7.
4. Loyo M, Ishii LE. Safety of alloplastic materials in rhinoplasty. JAMA Facial Plast Surg 2013;15(3):162–3.
5. Yap EC, Abubakar SS, Olveda MB. Expanded polytetrafluoroethylene as dorsal augmentation material in rhinoplasty on Southeast Asian noses: three-year experience. Arch Facial Plast Surg 2011;13(4):234–8.
6. Berghaus A, Stelter K. Alloplastic materials in rhinoplasty. Curr Opin Otolaryngol Head Neck Surg 2006; 14(4):270–7.
7. Niechajev I. Facial reconstruction using porous high-density polyethylene (Medpor): long-term results. Aesthetic Plast Surg 2012;36(4):917–27.
8. Peled ZM, Warren AG, Johnston P, et al. The use of alloplastic materials in rhinoplasty surgery: a meta-analysis. Plast Reconstr Surg 2008;121(3):85e–92e.
9. Gurlek A, Celik M, Fariz A, et al. The use of high-density porous polyethylene as a custom-made nasal spreader graft. Aesthetic Plast Surg 2006;30:34–41.
10. Reiffel AJ, Cross KJ, Spinelli HM. Nasal spreader grafts: a comparison of Medpor to autologous tissue reconstruction. Ann Plast Surg 2011;66(1):24–8.
11. Winkler AA, Soler ZM, Leong PL, et al. Complications associated with alloplastic implants in rhinoplasty. Arch Facial Plast Surg 2012;14(6):437–41.
12. Sclafani AP, Romo T, Ukrainsky G, et al. Modulation of wound response and soft tissue ingrowth in synthetic and allogeneic implants with platelet concentrate. Arch Facial Plast Surg 2005;7:163–9.
13. Adamson PA, Warner J, Becker D, et al. Revision rhinoplasty: panel discussion, controversies, and techniques. Facial Plast Surg Clin North Am 2014;22(1): 57–96.
14. Welling DB, Maves MD, Schuller DE, et al. Irradiated homologous cartilage grafts: long-term results. Arch Otolaryngol Head Neck Surg 1998;11(6):378–94.

15. Kridel RW, Ashoori F, Liu ES, et al. Long-term use and follow-up of irradiated homologous costal cartilage grafts in the nose. Arch Facial Plast Surg 2009; 11(6):378–94.

16. Wee J, Park M, Oh S, et al. Complications associated with autologous rib cartilage use in rhinoplasty: a meta-analysis. JAMA Facial Plast Surg 2015;17(1): 49–55.

17. Toriumi DM. Autogenous grafts are worth the extra time. Arch Otolaryngol Head Neck Surg 2000;126: 562–4.

18. Farkas JP, Lee MR, Lakianhi C, et al. Effects of carving plane, level of harvest, and oppositional suturing techniques on costal cartilage warping. Plast Reconstr Surg 2013;132(2):319–25.

19. Jung DH, Choi SH, Moon HJ, et al. A cadaveric analysis of the ideal costal cartilage graft for Asian rhinoplasty. Plast Reconstr Surg 2004;114(2):545–50.

20. Ching WC, Hsiao YC. Transumbilical endoscopic costal cartilage harvesting: a new technique. Ann Plast Surg 2014;72(4):423–7.

21. Erol OO. The Turkish delight: a pliable graft for rhinoplasty. Plast Reconstr Surg 2000;105(6):2229–41.

22. Brenner KA, McConnell MP, Evans GR, et al. Survival of diced cartilage grafts: an experimental study. Plast Reconstr Surg 2006;117(1):105–15.

23. Kim HK, Chu LS, Kim JW, et al. The viability of diced cartilage grafts wrapped in autogenous fascia and AlloDerm in a rabbit model. J Plast Reconstr Aesthet Surg 2011;64(8):e193–200.

24. Bullocks JM, Echo A, Guerra G, et al. A novel autologous scaffold for diced-cartilage augmentation rhinoplasty. Aesthetic Plast Surg 2011;35:569–79.

25. Dobratz EJ, Kim SW, Voglewede A, et al. Injectable cartilage using alginate and human chondrocytes. Arch Facial Plast Surg 2009;11(1):40–7.

26. Noordzij JP, Cates JM, Cohen SM, et al. Preparation techniques for the injection of human autologous cartilage: an ex vivo feasibility study. Laryngoscope 2008;118:185–8.

27. Manafi A, Hamedi ZS, Manafi A, et al. Injectable cartilage shaving: an autologous and long lasting filler material for correction of minor contour deformities in rhinoplasty. World J Plast Surg 2015;4(2): 93–100.

28. Manafi A, Barikbin B, Manafi A, et al. Nasal alar necrosis following hyaluronic acid injection into nasolabial folds: a case report. World J Plast Surg 2015; 4(1):74–8.

29. Stupak HD, Moulthrop TH, Wheatley P, et al. Calcium hydroxylapatite gel (Radiesse) injection for the correction of postrhinoplasty contour deficiencies and asymmetries. Arch Facial Plast Surg 2007;9: 130–6.

30. Jasin ME. Nonsurgical rhinoplasty using dermal fillers. Facial Plast Surg Clin North Am 2013;21: 241–52.

31. Rivkin A. A prospective study of non-surgical primary rhinoplasty using a polymethylmethacrylate injectable implant. Dermatol Surg 2014;40(3):305–13.

32. Humphrey CD, Arkins JP, Dayan SH. Soft tissue fillers in the nose. Aesthet Surg J 2009;29:477–84.

33. Sheen JH. Spreader graft: a method of reconstructing the roof of the middle nasal vault following rhinoplasty. Plast Reconstr Surg 1984;73:230.

34. Byrd HS, Meade RA, Gonyon DL. Using the autospreader flap in primary rhinoplasty. Plast Reconstr Surg 2007;119(6):1897–902.

35. Pepper JP, Baker SR. The autospreader flap in reduction rhinoplasty. Arch Facial Plast Surg 2011; 13(3):172.

36. Yoo S, Most SP. Nasal airway preservation using the autospreader technique: analysis of outcomes using a disease-specific quality of life instrument. Arch Facial Plast Surg 2011;13(4):231–3.

37. Saedi B, Amali A, Gharavis V, et al. Spreader flaps do not change early functional outcomes in reduction rhinoplasty: a randomized control trial. Am J Rhinol Allergy 2014;28(1):70–4.

38. Manavbasi YI, Basaran I. The role of upper lateral cartilage in dorsal reconstruction after hump excision: section 1. Spreader flap modification with asymmetric mattress suture and extension of the spreading effect by cartilage graft. Aesthetic Plast Surg 2011;35(4): 487–93.

39. Kuehnert MJ, Kruszon-Moran D, Hill HA, et al. Prevalence of Staphylococcus aureus nasal colonization in the United States, 2001-2002. J Infect Dis 2006; 193:172–9.

40. Perl TM. Prevention of Staphylococcus aureus infections among surgical patients: beyond traditional perioperative prophylaxis. Surgery 2003;134:S10–7.

41. van Rijen M, Bonten M, Wenzel R, et al. Mupirocin ointment for preventing Staphylococcus aureus infection in nasal carriers. Cochrane Database Syst Rev 2008;(4):CD006216.

42. Pirsig W, Schafer J. The importance of antibiotic treatment in functional and aesthetic rhinosurgery. Rhinol Suppl 1988;4:3–11.

43. Angelos PC, Wang TD. Methicillin-resistant Staphylococcus aureus infection in septorhinoplasty. Laryngoscope 2010;120(7):1309–11.

44. Yoo DB, Peng GL, Azizzadeh B, et al. Microbiology and antibiotic prophylaxis in rhinoplasty: a review of 363 consecutive cases. JAMA Facial Plast Surg 2015;17(1):23–7.

45. Walton RL, Wu LC, Beahm EK. Salvage of infected cartilage grafts for nasal reconstruction with a through-and-through irrigation system. Ann Plast Surg 2005;54:445–9.

46. Sepehr A, Chauhan N, Alexander AJ, et al. Evolution in nasal tip contouring techniques: a 10-year evaluation and analysis. Arch Facial Plast Surg 2011; 13(3):217–9.

Antibiotic Use in Facial Plastic Surgery

Javier González-Castro, MD[a],*, Jessyka G. Lighthall, MD[b]

KEYWORDS

- Antibiotics • Facial plastic surgery • Rhinoplasty • Facelift • Blepharoplasty • Implants
- Resurfacing • Trauma

KEY POINTS

- Reported infection rates are low for most procedures, though reporting is confounded by inconsistent antibiotic regimens.
- Survey studies show a significant increase in the use of prophylactic antibiotics in facial plastic and reconstructive surgeries.
- Available literature is generally of low quality and inadequate to make a legitimate argument for or against antibiotic prophylaxis.

INTRODUCTION

The discovery of antibiotics marked one of the greatest milestones in human history. The advances that followed have saved countless millions of lives around the globe. These advances have contributed to the evolution of surgery from a practice that was used only when necessary, carrying great risk of death and morbidity, to what we know today. Cosmetic surgery may never have become as mainstream as it currently is if not for advances in prevention and treatment of infections.

Antibiotic use, however, is not without risk. Allergic reactions, side effects, opportunistic infections, increased health care costs, and most importantly the emergence of drug resistance have led many to question whether we are overusing antibiotics. The National Action Plan for Combating Antibiotic-resistant Bacteria developed in response to Executive Order 13,676 by President Barack Obama highlights the importance of this matter.[1]

In 1999 the Centers for Disease Control and Prevention issued the "Guideline for prevention of surgical site infection."[2] In their report, they advocate for the use of an antimicrobial prophylaxis agent for all operations or classes of operations in which its use has been shown to reduce surgical site infection (SSI) rates based on evidence from clinical trials or for those operations after which an SSI would represent a catastrophe. In the following sections the authors discuss the most commonly performed procedures in facial plastic surgery with one question in mind: Is antimicrobial prophylaxis indicated for these procedures based on the available literature?

Preoperative antibiotic administration is defined as any dose given before surgery; perioperative antibiotics are those given within 1 hour of incision and continuing less than 24 hours after the procedure, and postoperative antibiotics are administered 24 hours or more after surgery.[3]

SEPTOPLASTY/RHINOPLASTY

The nasal cavity comes into contact with everything we breathe and is well known to harbor bacterial pathogens.[2,4–6] Studies have demonstrated a clear correlation between nasal bacterial colonization and SSI in general.[6] But is the same true for nasal

Disclosures: Nothing to disclose.
[a] Department of Otolaryngology-Head and Neck Surgery, University of Puerto Rico, PO Box 16423, San Juan, PR 00908, USA; [b] Division of Otolaryngology-Head and Neck Surgery, Penn State Hershey Medical Center, 500 University Drive H091, Hershey, PA 17033, USA
* Corresponding author.
E-mail address: jgonzalez@facialplasticspr.com

Facial Plast Surg Clin N Am 24 (2016) 347–356
http://dx.doi.org/10.1016/j.fsc.2016.03.011

surgery; is antibiotic prophylaxis indicated for these cases?

The incidence of postseptoplasty/rhinoplasty infection found in current literature fluctuates significantly between 0% and 18%, but in general 2% is considered acceptable.[7,8] Although indications are still a topic of debate, various survey studies have shown that, in practice, prophylactic antibiotic use is favored by most physicians performing rhinoplasty.[9–11] Lyle and colleagues[10] found a 200% increase in antibiotic prophylaxis use between 1985 and 2000. Despite their limitation of survey studies with relatively low response rates, these studies demonstrate that prescribing prophylactic antibiotics is becoming more common in today's rhinoplasty practice.

Table 1 shows studies that evaluated patients who did not receive any antibiotics.[12–15] The complication rate for this group fluctuated between 0% and 0.6%. If one looks at these data in isolation, one could make a compelling argument that risk of infection is so low that there is no need for antibiotics. However, 2 studies had well less than 100 patients, which limits their reliability and reproducibility.[13,14] Cabouli and colleagues[12] had larger numbers but were limited by recall bias; of the 12 patients who developed infections, only 5 were well documented. Interestingly, Yoder and Weimart reported a 0.48% (5 of 1040) infection rate without the use of antibiotics or surgical preparation solution.[15]

Table 2 shows studies that prospectively compared patients who received antibiotics with those who received either placebo or nothing at all.[16–19] All had low sample sizes, which limited their power. Three of the studies show no difference between groups, which would support the argument that antibiotic prophylaxis is not helpful. Conversely, Schäfer and Pirsig found a significant difference between groups, whereby the placebo group had a 27% (14 of 52) infection rate, whereas

Table 1
Rhinoplasty/septoplasty literature whereby no antibiotic prophylaxis was given

Authors	Infection Rate	Design	Results	Conclusions/ Recommendations
Okur et al,[13] 2006	0% 0 of 60	Examined 30 septoplasty and 30 open septorhinoplasty patients free of antibiotic ≥20 d	• Preoperative/ postoperative cultures negative • Intraoperative culture positive in 3 Rhinoplasty and 1 Septoplasty • 0 of 60 Had clinical evidence of infection	• Transient bacteremia develops during rhinoplasty. • Precautions should be taken in patients with high cardiovascular risk.
Yoder & Weimert,[15] 1992	0.48% 5 of 1040	1040 Patients with septoplasty/ septorhinoplasty without antibiotics or topical surgical preparation solution	• Minor nasal infection that resolved with antibiotics in 5 patients	• It is safe and acceptable to use no prophylactic antibiotic or surgical prep solution in Septoplasty/ Septorhinoplasty.
Cabouli et al,[12] 1986	0.6% 12 of 2000	Looked back at their last 2000 cases over 6 y without antibiotics	• 12 Cases of infection • Only 5 of which were well documented and reviewed in detail (limitation)	• The danger of drug toxicity exceeds the incidence of infection.
Slavin et al,[14] 1983	0% 0 of 52	Studied the incidence of bacteremia in patients free of antibiotics ≥2 wk before surgery	• 1 Positive culture • 0 of 52 Infections in 60-d follow-up period	• The value of perioperative antibiotic prophylaxis is questionable.

Table 2
Rhinoplasty/septoplasty literature comparing antibiotic prophylaxis with placebo or no treatment

Authors	Infection Rate	Design	Results	Conclusions/ Recommendations
Caniello et al,[16] 2005	0% 0 of 35	• 35 Patients split in 3 groups: ◦ No antibiotics (n = 16) ◦ 1 g Cefazolin at induction (n = 11) ◦ Cefazolin 1 g IV at induction and cephalexin orally for 7 d (500 mg every 6 h) (n = 8)	• No infections in any group	• Septoplasties do not require prophylactic use of antibiotics because of the low risk of postoperative infection.
Mäkitie et al,[17] 2000	12% 12 of 100	100 Septoplasties, 21 received prophylactic antibiotics	• 12 Infections • 14.3% (3 of 21) Infection rate with antibiotics • 11.4% (9 of 79) Infection rate without antibiotics	• There were higher-than-average infection rates. • There were no significant difference between groups.
Schäfer & Pirsig,[18] 1988	18% 18 of 100	100 Revision rhinoplasties; 48 patients received 3 mega units of oral propicillin for 12 days and 52 patients received placebo	• Infection in 18 patients • 14 of 52 (27%) In placebo group • 4 of 48 (8%) In the antibiotic group	Postoperative propicillin seems to be able to prevent nasal infections.
Weimert & Yoder,[19] 1980	2.3% 4 of 174	75 Randomly assigned prophylactic antibiotics, began 12 h preoperatively and continued for 5 postoperative days; 99 patients had no antibiotics	• Minor infections in 2 from each group • 2.7% Antibiotics group • 2.2% No antibiotic group	The incidence and danger of infection resulting from intranasal surgery is not sufficient to warrant the use of prophylactic antibiotics.

Abbreviation: IV, intravenous.

the antibiotic group had an 8% (4 of 48) infection rate.[18] If evaluated in isolation one could say that this study makes a compelling argument favoring antibiotic prophylaxis. However, it is important to note the high infection rate relative to that published in the literature. The investigators attribute the high infection rate to the fact that all cases were complex revisions, but this could also be an effect of the broad definition of infection used in this study.

Table 3 compared groups whereby all patients received antibiotics of some sort.[8,20,21]

Interestingly, Andrews and colleagues[20] commented that they did not include a placebo arm because they thought it would be "unethical to do so given the high infection rates in published literature." Two of these articles found no added benefit in using postoperative antibiotics in addition to the perioperative therapy, but all investigators think that antibiotic prophylaxis is indicated in rhinoplasty surgery.

Although available literature does not support routine antibiotic prophylaxis, it is not sufficient to make a legitimate argument against their use either.

Table 3
Rhinoplasty/septoplasty literature whereby all patients received antibiotic prophylaxis

Authors	Infection Rate	Design	Results	Conclusions/ Recommendations
Yoo et al,[8] 2015	3% 11 of 363	All patients were washed with chlorhexidine gluconate (Hibiclens) and applied mupirocin daily for 5 d before surgery. All patients received 1 g of cefazolin sodium (Ancef) or 450 mg of clindamycin 30 min before incision. All nasal cavities cultured before surgery, and those with pathologic bacteria received organism-specific antibiotics preoperatively.	Infection rate higher in primary than revision rhinoplasty	Culture-directed treatment
Andrews et al,[20] 2006	9.1% 15 of 164	164 Patients: half received prophylactic antibiotics and half received postop antibiotics.	6 of 82 (7%) Infection in prophylactic arm 9 of 82 (11%) Infection in postop arm infection	Recommend use of prophylactic antibiotics in patients undergoing complex septorhinoplasty Extended postop not needed
Rajan et al,[21] 2005	1.5% 3 of 200	100 Patients got a single preop shot of antibiotics. 100 Patients got a preop shot of antibiotics and a 7-d course of oral antibiotics.	3 of 100 Infection in combined treatment group 0 of 100 Infection in single-shot group	Single-shot antibiotics adequate Statistically significant decrease in price and side effects with single shot

Abbreviations: postop, postoperative; preop, preoperative.

Furthermore, the national tendency to routinely give antibiotics highlights the fact that further data are required in order to draw any significant conclusions.

BLEPHAROPLASTY

The periocular region is considered a clean area. Rich vascularity and ease of preoperative surgical site preparation makes the need for antibiotic prophylaxis questionable. The incidence of infection following blepharoplasty is less than 1%.[22] However, several case reports have described severe postblepharoplasty infections that result in significant morbidity even when treated early.[23–26]

In 2003 Lyle and colleagues[10] found a greater than 200% increase in antibiotic use from 1985 to 2000 in patients undergoing blepharoplasty. In the 1985 survey 11% of respondents admitted to using antibiotic prophylaxis in more than 50.0% of their cases, whereas 46.9% did so in the survey done in 2000. Interestingly this increase came about without any literature to support such an increase. Hauck and Nogan[9] published a similar survey in 2013 whereby they found that 64% of respondents used antibiotics greater than 50% of the time, 51% of respondents always used antibiotic prophylaxis, and 21% never used them. It is important to note that these studies referred to systemic antibiotics not topical. In 2015, Fay and colleagues[27] published their multinational survey directed specifically to members of the oculoplastic societies worldwide. They found that topical antibiotic use was common in all regions (85.2%), whereas perioperative systemic antibiotic was uncommon in all regions (13.5%).

In 2003 Carter and colleagues[22] published a retrospective review of 1627 patients who underwent blepharoplasty. All received topical antibiotics, but only 11 patients received an oral course prophylactically because of prosthetic joints or heart valves. The infection rate was 0.2% (4 of 1627), all of which resolved with a course of antibiotics. They, therefore, concluded that topical postoperative antibiotic prophylaxis alone is sufficient for routine blepharoplasty.

With the evidence available, it is difficult to show that use of antibiotics can decrease an already low complication rate in blepharoplasty. It is the authors' impression that systemic antibiotics are not advantageous in blepharoplasty, but high-quality evidence would be beneficial in order to draw a definitive conclusion and convince physicians to change their practice patterns.

RHYTIDECTOMY

For many years, facial rejuvenation has been a well-sought-after area in facial plastic surgery fueled by patients' interest in maintaining a youthful appearance. Many variations exist between surgeons, including surgical technique, preoperative care, and postoperative care. Scarce published data are available examining the role of antibiotic prophylaxis. With the extensive vascularity of the face, postoperative infection is extremely rare (<1%).[28,29] Nonetheless, an infection can result in wound breakdown, loss of skin, and adverse scarring, which would be considered catastrophic complications for cosmetic patients. With this in mind, it is no surprise that most surgeons elect to use some form of antibiotic prophylaxis.

The most recent study on the subject came in the form of a survey done by Stacey and colleagues[30] in 2010. This survey was a multi-specialty survey distributed to societies in which surgeons perform rhytidectomy. The investigators found that 11% of surgeons give no antibiotics at all, 21% give perioperative antibiotics only, and 68% give some combination of perioperative and postoperative antibiotics for up to 7 days. These findings are similar to those reported by Hauck and Nogan[9] who found that 84% of respondents to their survey use prophylaxis greater than 50% of the time. In this

group 73% used antibiotics in every case, whereas only 9% never used antibiotic prophylaxis.

To the authors' knowledge, there are no clinical trials comparing infection rates in patients who received antibiotic prophylaxis versus those who did not. Although further research is needed to draw definitive conclusions, it is not likely that antibiotic prophylaxis decreases an already low infection rate. It is apparent that most surgeons currently use prophylactic antibiotics in rhytidectomy and additional high-quality research is needed to further elucidate their role.

ALLOPLASTIC IMPLANTATION

The use of synthetic materials for augmentation in aesthetic and reconstructive facial plastic surgery is common. It is generally accepted that sterile technique and proper patient and implant selection decrease the chance of infection and implant exposure. Other maneuvers to decrease the risk of infection include perioperative and postoperative antibiotics, soaking the implant and irrigating the pocket with antibiotic solution, and impregnating the implant with antibiotic solution.[31] The risk of implant infection is a 2-phase process.[32] Phase one involves bacterial adhesion to the implant mostly influenced by sterile operative technique and mechanically removing adhered bacteria by irrigation. The second phase involves firm adherence of bacteria and colonization. Available biomaterials vary significantly in hydrophilicity/hydrophobicity, porosity, surface characteristics, and tissue reactivity, all affecting their risk of infection.

Current literature is of low quality, largely involving case reports and retrospective reviews, many of which do not directly address the antibiotic regimen used.[33–36] Nearly all studies use intraoperative antibiotic treatment techniques and perioperative antibiotics with varying postoperative antibiotic regimens. One meta-analysis reviewed the available literature on implants in rhinoplasty and found infection rates ranging from 0% to 10%.[33] Infection rates are higher in revision cases, cases with coexisting septal perforation or diabetes mellitus, and when a more porous implant is used.[35–37] No good studies were identified comparing patients with versus without prophylaxis. An evidence-based consensus statement did report trends based on survey results and showed increasing postoperative antibiotic prescribing patterns for malar, chin, and nasal implant use.[38] Despite the increasing numbers of providers using antibiotic prophylaxis in these cases, very little research exists to support the increased use.

Implant infection typically results in significant morbidity, including implant removal; thus, most studies and physicians in general use antibiotics of some sort, making a comparison impossible. With the lack of high-quality comparative data, no expert consensus recommendations can be provided. Further research is necessary to elucidate the role antibiotics play in the prevention of implant infection.

RESURFACING

Multiple techniques for facial resurfacing exist, including mechanical dermabrasion, lasers, and chemical peels, which induce an injury to the skin of varying degrees. There is concern with delayed wound healing, prolonged erythema, and increased risk of scarring due to infection[39]; however, very little is available in the literature to help guide antibiotic use in resurfacing procedures. Most of the available literature addresses laser resurfacing. Meticulous sterile technique, skin preparation, and postoperative wound care is critical in the prevention of bacterial infection. Even then, bacterial infection rates after laser skin resurfacing have been reported between 0% and 8.3%.[39–43] Studies typically involve case reports, retrospective reviews, and prospective observational studies with wide variation in topical and systemic antibiotic regimens, decreasing generalizability.

One systematic review of randomized controlled trials in dermatologic procedures compared postoperative topical antibiotics with petroleum ointment and found no difference in infection rates but did note a high incidence of contact dermatitis in the topical antibiotic group.[44] The investigators recommended against topical antibiotic formulations. In regard to oral antibiotic prophylaxis, controversy exists even though these tend to be clean procedures with a low overall infection rate. Some investigators report a decrease in bacterial infection in patients treated with postoperative antibiotics,[40,41,45] whereas others note a significant increase in infection rates in patients treated with systemic therapy, raising the concern for possible induction of antibiotic resistance and superinfection.[46] Despite the low risk of infection and available literature, a 2015 evidence-based consensus statement identified an increase in antibiotic prescribing practices from 17% in 1985 to greater than 49% in 2003 for chemical peels, 74% for laser skin resurfacing, and 60% for dermabrasion.[38]

A literature review of complications after laser resurfacing in 2010 recommended antibiotic prophylaxis only in high-risk patients.[47] The investigators recommend against topical antibiotics and recommend only culture-directed antibiotic therapy for patients with clinical signs and symptoms of postoperative wound infection. Postoperative infections if they occur are typically identified early

and when treated appropriately result in no adverse sequelae.[43,48] Although the available literature is generally of lower quality and controversy exists, the trend in the literature seems to be against routine oral antibiotic prophylaxis except in higher risk patients.

MAXILLOFACIAL TRAUMA

It seems intuitive that patients with facial trauma may experience a higher frequency of wound infections based on the type of injuries, involvement of mucous membranes or sinus cavities, potential for contamination of wounds, and possible delays in treatment. Many articles cite a prospective, randomized clinical trial performed by Chole and Yee[49] in 1987 who evaluated the role antibiotics in 101 patients with facial fractures undergoing open or closed reduction. Patients received either no antibiotics or 2 perioperative doses of cefazolin. The investigators reported a decrease in infection rates from 42.2% to 8.9% when antibiotics were administered. They also note that nearly all of the infections occurred in patients with mandible fractures, particularly those treated with open reduction. As a result, perioperative antibiotic prophylaxis in patients with facial fractures has become standard. Multiple studies have since evaluated the role of antibiotics in facial fractures of varying patterns and have recently been reviewed.[3,50–54]

A recent systematic review evaluating studies published before June 2013 provides evidence-based recommendations based on available literature and compares this with clinical prescribing practices of senior surgeons experienced at treating maxillofacial trauma.[3] Of the studies reviewed, most of them were poor quality, thereby precluding a formal analysis. Despite this, the investigators provide a recommendation supporting the use of preoperative antibiotics for comminuted mandible fractures and perioperative antibiotics in fractures involving all facial thirds. Postoperative antibiotics were not recommended for any fractures.

Since this review, additional studies have been published, including prospective cohort studies, retrospective reviews, and randomized controlled pilot clinical studies evaluating the benefit of postoperative antibiotics (**Table 4**).[50–54] Although these studies are largely underpowered or have significant limitations, they all report no benefit to postoperative antibiotics when perioperative antibiotics are given for facial fractures.

In an expert practice survey of senior surgeons experienced with maxillofacial trauma repair, Mundinger and colleagues[3] found that despite the available literature and recommendations, surgeons reported prescribing preoperative antibiotics 47%

Table 4
Highest-quality studies evaluating antibiotic use for maxillofacial trauma including the systematic review by Mundinger and colleagues and subsequent studies

Authors	Infection Rate (%)	Design	Results	Conclusions/Recommendations
Mundinger et al,[3] 2015	Not Applicable	Systematic review and expert practice survey 44 Included of overall poor quality precluding analysis Survey of antibiotic prescribing practices among senior surgeons	• Penicillin, cephalosporins, clindamycin most commonly prescribed: no superiority could be determined • Grade A recommendations: ○ Periop antibiotics in all facial thirds ○ Preop antibiotics for comminuted mandible fractures ○ Postop antibiotics not recommended for mandible • Grade D recommendation: ○ Inconsistent low level evidence supporting antibiotics in sinusitis	• Use preoperative antibiotics for comminuted mandible fractures only. • Use perioperative antibiotics for all facial fractures. • There is no support for postoperative antibiotics. • Clinical prescribing practices do not adhere to current literature recommendations.
Schaller et al,[53] 2013	20	Prospective randomized, double-blind, placebo-controlled pilot study 59 Patients with mandibular fracture involving the dentoalveolar segment requiring ORIF; all patients received perioperative antibiotics: group 1: only periop, group 2: additional 4 d of postop antibiotics	No difference in infection rate, 19% in the periop group and 20% in the 5-d group	• There is no benefit to postoperative antibiotics. • It is an underpowered study. • Additional research is required.
Baliga et al,[50] 2014	0.3	Prospective study 60 Patients undergoing ORIF of Zygomaticomaxillary complex and mandible fractures Group 1 preop, intraop & postop antibiotics Group 2 preop & intraop but no postop antibiotics Excluded severely comminuted/displaced fractures, infected fractures, immunocompromised	1 Patient each group developed infection	• They recommend against postoperative antibiotics in ORIF of ZMC and mandible fractures.

(continued on next page)

Table 4
(continued)

Authors	Infection Rate (%)	Design	Results	Conclusions/Recommendations
Soong et al,[54] 2014	4.0	Prospective randomized, double-blind, placebo-controlled pilot study 94 Patients with LeFort (35) and zygomatic (59) fractures requiring ORIF; all patients received perioperative antibiotics; group 1: only periop, group 2: additional 4 d of postop antibiotics	No difference in infection rate (4% in the periop group and 4% in the 5-d group)	• There is no benefit to postoperative antibiotic regimen. • It is an underpowered study. • Additional research is required.
Mottini et al,[52] 2014	3.54	Retrospective review of 339 patients receiving 1 vs 5 d of postoperative antibiotics All patients received IV antibiotics on admission through 24 h postop Group 1 received no additional antibiotic; group 2 received an additional 4 d	42% Zygomatic fractures, 34% orbital floor, 23% mandible, 1% Le Fort No difference in infection rate between groups (4% group 1, 3.27% group 2) 92% Occurred in mandible fractures 67% Of infected mandible fractures comminuted	• There is no benefit to postoperative antibiotic regimen.
Campos et al,[51] 2015	9.3	Prospective randomized controlled study evaluating 74 patients undergoing ORIF of facial fractures receiving either a single perioperative dose of antibiotics or 24 h of IV antibiotics	No statistical difference in infection rate between groups for upper or midfacial fractures, but P<.02 for mandible fractures favoring 24 h of antibiotics	• They recommend 24 h of perioperative antibiotics in mandibular fractures and a single perioperative dose for upper and midface fractures. • Larger studies are needed.

Abbreviations: IV, intravenous; ORIF, open reduction and internal fixation; periop, perioperative; postop, postoperative; preop, preoperative.

to 69% of the time, perioperative antibiotics 94% to 100%, and postoperative antibiotics 65% to 71% of the time. They postulated that the inconsistencies with current literature recommendations are a lack of awareness of available literature and the overall lower quality of available studies.

Although the literature in facial trauma is of higher quality than other areas of facial plastic surgery, significant controversy still exists regarding the appropriate indications, duration, and overall efficacy.

SUMMARY

In evaluating the available literature regarding the use of antibiotic prophylaxis within facial plastic surgery, one fact is abundantly clear: There is not sufficient evidence to clearly support the use or abstinence of antimicrobial prophylaxis. Therefore, prophylactic use in this patient population would be indicated if an SSI would represent a catastrophe. But who defines a catastrophe? Most patients and surgeons would likely classify a rhinoplasty infection resulting in saddle nose, loss of facial skin, or disfiguring hypertrophic scarring after a facelift or infection of an alloplast requiring removal as a devastating complication. So in this light one could make the argument that antimicrobial prophylaxis is indicated. Others, however, may argue that these complications are trivial or that overall infection rates are low, thus prophylaxis is not indicated. Further research is needed in order to take a solid stance for or against antimicrobial prophylaxis.

REFERENCES

1. House W. National action plan for combating antibiotic-resistant bacteria. Washington, DC: White House; 2015.
2. Mangram AJ, Horan TC, Pearson ML, et al. Guideline for prevention of surgical site infection, 1999. Centers for Disease Control and Prevention (CDC) Hospital Infection Control Practices Advisory Committee. Am J Infect Control 1999;27(2):97–132 [quiz: 133–4; discussion: 196].
3. Mundinger GS, Borsuk DE, Okhah Z, et al. Antibiotics and facial fractures: evidence-based recommendations compared with experience-based practice. Craniomaxillofac Trauma Reconstr 2015;8(1):64–78.
4. Bode LG, Kluytmans JA, Wertheim HF, et al. Preventing surgical-site infections in nasal carriers of Staphylococcus aureus. N Engl J Med 2010; 362(1):9–17.
5. Gluck U, Gebbers JO. The nose as bacterial reservoir: important differences between the vestibule and cavity. Laryngoscope 2000;110(3 Pt 1):426–8.
6. Weinstein HJ. The relation between the nasal-staphylococcal-carrier state and the incidence of postoperative complications. N Engl J Med 1959; 260(26):1303–8.
7. Bandhauer F, Buhl D, Grossenbacher R. Antibiotic prophylaxis in rhinosurgery. Am J Rhinol 2002; 16(3):135–9.
8. Yoo DB, Peng GL, Azizzadeh B, et al. Microbiology and antibiotic prophylaxis in rhinoplasty: a review of 363 consecutive cases. JAMA Facial Plast Surg 2015;17(1):23–7.
9. Hauck RM, Nogan S. The use of prophylactic antibiotics in plastic surgery: update in 2010. Ann Plast Surg 2013;70(1):91–7.
10. Lyle WG, Outlaw K, Krizek TJ, et al. Prophylactic antibiotics in plastic surgery: trends of use over 25 years of an evolving specialty. Aesthet Surg J 2003;23(3):177–83.
11. Shadfar S, Deal AM, Jarchow AM, et al. Practice patterns in the perioperative treatment of patients undergoing septorhinoplasty: a survey of facial plastic surgeons. JAMA Facial Plast Surg 2014;16(2):113–9.
12. Cabouli JL, Guerrissi JO, Mileto A, et al. Local infection following aesthetic rhinoplasty. Ann Plast Surg 1986;17(4):306–9.
13. Okur E, Yildirim I, Aral M, et al. Bacteremia during open septorhinoplasty. Am J Rhinol 2006;20(1):36–9.
14. Slavin SA, Rees TD, Guy CL, et al. An investigation of bacteremia during rhinoplasty. Plast Reconstr Surg 1983;71(2):196–8.
15. Yoder MG, Weimert TA. Antibiotics and topical surgical preparation solution in septal surgery. Otolaryngol Head Neck Surg 1992;106(3):243–4.
16. Caniello M, Passerotti GH, Goto EY, et al. Antibiotics in septoplasty: is it necessary? Braz J Otorhinolaryngol 2005;71(6):734–8.
17. Makitie A, Aaltonen LM, Hytonen M, et al. Postoperative infection following nasal septoplasty. Acta Otolaryngol Suppl 2000;543:165–6.
18. Schafer J, Pirsig W. Preventive antibiotic administration in complicated rhinosurgical interventions–a double-blind study. Laryngol Rhinol Otol (Stuttg) 1988;67(4):150–5 [in German].
19. Weimert TA, Yoder MG. Antibiotics and nasal surgery. Laryngoscope 1980;90(4):667–72.
20. Andrews PJ, East CA, Jayaraj SM, et al. Prophylactic vs postoperative antibiotic use in complex septorhinoplasty surgery: a prospective, randomized, single-blind trial comparing efficacy. Arch Facial Plast Surg 2006;8(2):84–7.
21. Rajan GP, Fergie N, Fischer U, et al. Antibiotic prophylaxis in septorhinoplasty? A prospective, randomized study. Plast Reconstr Surg 2005;116(7):1995–8.
22. Carter SR, Stewart JM, Khan J, et al. Infection after blepharoplasty with and without carbon dioxide laser resurfacing. Ophthalmology 2003;110(7):1430–2.
23. Goldberg RA, Li TG. Postoperative infection with group A beta-hemolytic Streptococcus after blepharoplasty. Am J Ophthalmol 2002;134(6):908–10.

24. Juthani V, Zoumalan CI, Lisman RD, et al. Successful management of methicillin-resistant Staphylococcus aureus orbital cellulitis after blepharoplasty. Plast Reconstr Surg 2010;126(6):305e–7e.

25. Moorthy RS, Rao NA. Atypical mycobacterial wound infection after blepharoplasty. Br J Ophthalmol 1995; 79(1):93.

26. Suner IJ, Meldrum ML, Johnson TE, et al. Necrotizing fasciitis after cosmetic blepharoplasty. Am J Ophthalmol 1999;128(3):367–8.

27. Fay A, Nallasamy N, Bernardini F, et al. Multinational comparison of prophylactic antibiotic use for eyelid surgery. JAMA Ophthalmol 2015;133(7):778–84.

28. LeRoy JL Jr, Rees TD, Nolan WB 3rd. Infections requiring hospital readmission following face lift surgery: incidence, treatment, and sequelae. Plast Reconstr Surg 1994;93(3):533–6.

29. Sullivan CA, Masin J, Maniglia AJ, et al. Complications of rhytidectomy in an otolaryngology training program. Laryngoscope 1999;109(2 Pt 1):198–203.

30. Stacey DH, Warner JP, Duggal A, et al. International interdisciplinary rhytidectomy survey. Ann Plast Surg 2010;64(4):370–5.

31. Eppley BL. Alloplastic implantation. Plast Reconstr Surg 1999;104(6):1761–83 [quiz: 1784–5].

32. An YH, Friedman RJ. Concise review of mechanisms of bacterial adhesion to biomaterial surfaces. J Biomed Mater Res 1998;43(3):338–48.

33. Peled ZM, Warren AG, Johnston P, et al. The use of alloplastic materials in rhinoplasty surgery: a meta-analysis. Plast Reconstr Surg 2008;121(3):85e–92e.

34. Ridwan-Pramana A, Wolff J, Raziei A, et al. Porous polyethylene implants in facial reconstruction: outcome and complications. J Craniomaxillofac Surg 2015;43(8):1330–4.

35. Wang TD. Gore-Tex nasal augmentation: a 26-year perspective. Arch Facial Plast Surg 2011;13(2): 129–30.

36. Winkler AA, Soler ZM, Leong PL, et al. Complications associated with alloplastic implants in rhinoplasty. Arch Facial Plast Surg 2012;14(6):437–41.

37. Godin MS, Waldman SR, Johnson CM Jr. The use of expanded polytetrafluoroethylene (Gore-Tex) in rhinoplasty. A 6-year experience. Arch Otolaryngol Head Neck Surg 1995;121(10):1131–6.

38. Ariyan S, Martin J, Lal A, et al. Antibiotic prophylaxis for preventing surgical-site infection in plastic surgery: an evidence-based consensus conference statement from the American Association of Plastic Surgeons. Plast Reconstr Surg 2015;135(6):1723–39.

39. Alster TS. Against antibiotic prophylaxis for cutaneous laser resurfacing. Dermatol Surg 2000;26(7): 697–8.

40. Manuskiatti W, Fitzpatrick RE, Goldman MP, et al. Prophylactic antibiotics in patients undergoing laser resurfacing of the skin. J Am Acad Dermatol 1999; 40(1):77–84.

41. Sriprachya-Anunt S, Fitzpatrick RE, Goldman MP, et al. Infections complicating pulsed carbon dioxide laser resurfacing for photoaged facial skin. Dermatol Surg 1997;23(7):527–35 [discussion: 535–6].

42. Bernstein LJ, Kauvar AN, Grossman MC, et al. The short- and long-term side effects of carbon dioxide laser resurfacing. Dermatol Surg 1997;23(7):519–25.

43. Gilbert S, McBurney E. Use of valacyclovir for herpes simplex virus-1 (HSV-1) prophylaxis after facial resurfacing: a randomized clinical trial of dosing regimens. Dermatol Surg 2000;26(1):50–4.

44. Saco M, Howe N, Nathoo R, et al. Topical antibiotic prophylaxis for prevention of surgical wound infections from dermatologic procedures: a systematic review and meta-analysis. J Dermatolog Treat 2015; 26(2):151–8.

45. Ross EV, Amesbury EC, Barile A, et al. Incidence of postoperative infection or positive culture after facial laser resurfacing: a pilot study, a case report, and a proposal for a rational approach to antibiotic prophylaxis. J Am Acad Dermatol 1998;39(6):975–81.

46. Walia S, Alster TS. Cutaneous CO2 laser resurfacing infection rate with and without prophylactic antibiotics. Dermatol Surg 1999;25(11):857–61.

47. Metelitsa AI, Alster TS. Fractionated laser skin resurfacing treatment complications: a review. Dermatol Surg 2010;36(3):299–306.

48. Gaspar Z, Vinciullo C, Elliott T. Antibiotic prophylaxis for full-face laser resurfacing: is it necessary? Arch Dermatol 2001;137(3):313–5.

49. Chole RA, Yee J. Antibiotic prophylaxis for facial fractures. A prospective, randomized clinical trial. Arch Otolaryngol Head Neck Surg 1987;113(10):1055–7.

50. Baliga SD, Bose A, Jain S. The evaluation of efficacy of post-operative antibiotics in the open reduction of the zygomatic and mandibular fracture: a prospective trial. J Maxillofac Oral Surg 2014;13(2):165–75.

51. Campos GB, Lucena EE, da Silva JS, et al. Efficacy assessment of two antibiotic prophylaxis regimens in oral and maxillofacial trauma surgery: preliminary results. Int J Clin Exp Med 2015;8(2):2846–52.

52. Mottini M, Wolf R, Soong PL, et al. The role of postoperative antibiotics in facial fractures: comparing the efficacy of a 1-day versus a prolonged regimen. J Trauma Acute Care Surg 2014;76(3):720–4.

53. Schaller B, Soong PL, Zix J, et al. The role of postoperative prophylactic antibiotics in the treatment of facial fractures: a randomized, double-blind, placebo-controlled pilot clinical study. Part 2: mandibular fractures in 59 patients. Br J Oral Maxillofac Surg 2013;51(8):803–7.

54. Soong PL, Schaller B, Zix J, et al. The role of postoperative prophylactic antibiotics in the treatment of facial fractures: a randomised, double-blind, placebo-controlled pilot clinical study. Part 3: Le Fort and zygomatic fractures in 94 patients. Br J Oral Maxillofac Surg 2014;52(4):329–33.

Facelift Controversies

Dane M. Barrett, MD[a,*], Deniz Gerecci, MD[a], Tom D. Wang, MD[b,*]

KEYWORDS

- Facelift • Rhytidectomy • Facial rejuvenation • Autologous fat grafting • Aging face
- Deep-plane rhytidectomy • Midface augmentation • Controversy

KEY POINTS

- Smoking cessation should be encouraged before surgery, though smoking may not be an absolute contraindication if a deep-plane technique is used.
- Incision placement should be determined by patient factors and degree of skin excision to be performed. Incisions into hair-bearing scalp should be avoided if significant skin or scalp excision is anticipated.
- A variety of techniques are available to the aesthetic surgeon. These are classified in relation to manipulation of the superficial musculoaponeurotic system and extent of dissection.
- No technique has been definitively shown to be superior to others. Selection of surgical technique should be guided by the surgeon's experience and patient factors.
- There are several options available for midface rejuvenation. Autologous fat grafting is a simple and reliable technique used by many aesthetic surgeons with good results.

INTRODUCTION

Numerous variations in techniques of facelift surgery have been described. Elements of the historical procedures have been adopted, molded, or abandoned, culminating in the modern techniques that exist today. A greater understanding of the process of aging, as well as facial anatomy, has advanced both the quality and duration of postoperative results.

Though advancements have been made, there is no consensus on a best facelift technique. This is abundantly evident in the literature and is hotly debated in panel discussions at aesthetic conferences. Most would agree that the ideal facelift would encompass the following: technical ease, minimal operative time, short patient convalescence, minimal risk and complications, durable efficacy, and maximal patient satisfaction. This article reviews the controversies in facelift surgery and relevant literature to provide clarity to this complex subject (**Box 1**).

> **Box 1**
> **Controversies in facelift**
>
> Patient Candidacy
>
> Incisions
>
> Plane of dissection, length of flap, vector of pull
>
> Management of the midface and volume restoration
>
> Management of the neck

HISTORICAL PERSPECTIVE

In contrast to the openness regarding aesthetic surgery in modern times, the beginnings of the rhytidectomy were secretive in nature. Publication of surgical techniques was avoided for years due to fear of ridicule. Eugen Hollander[1] and Erich Lexer,[2] both German surgeons, are most frequently credited with performing the first facelift. Each

---

Disclosures: The authors have no commercial or financial disclosures.

[a] Department of Otolaryngology-Head and Neck Surgery, Oregon Health and Science University, 3181 Southwest Sam Jackson Park Road, SJH01, Portland, OR 97239, USA; [b] Division of Facial Plastic & Reconstructive Surgery, Department of Otolaryngology-Head and Neck Surgery, Oregon Health and Science University, 3181 Southwest Sam Jackson Park Road, SJH01, Portland, OR 97239, USA

* Corresponding authors.

E-mail addresses: Barredan@ohsu.edu; Wangt@ohsu.edu

Facial Plast Surg Clin N Am 24 (2016) 357–366
http://dx.doi.org/10.1016/j.fsc.2016.03.012

claimed to have completed their operations at the turn of the twentieth century, though neither admitted it until decades later.

Facelift surgery saw more prodigious growth in the wake of the First World War. Increases in surgeons, american prosperity, and quality of anesthesia cultivated a more favorable climate for aesthetic surgery. Early techniques involved small local skin excisions near the hairline in natural skin creases without undermining. In 1920, Bettman[3] described a continuous temporal scalp, periauricular, and mastoid incision incorporating undermining of a large random skin flap. This was the predominant technique until the 1960s when surgeons began addressing the deeper tissues to compensate for the limitations of the subcutaneous lift.

In 1960, Aufrict was first to promote suturing deep to the superficial fat.[4] Skoog[5] is credited as the first to pioneer actual dissection of the deeper facial layers. In 1976, Mitz and Peyronie[6] defined the superficial musculoaponeurotic system (SMAS) as a fascial layer continuous with the platysma and temporoparietal fascia, enveloping the facial mimetic musculature. Discovery of this important fascial layer, distinct from the parotidomasseteric fascia, paved the way for modern facelifting techniques. Procedures using plication or imbrication of the SMAS were the dominant techniques for decades and are still in widespread use.

In 1989, Furnas[7] described the midfacial ligaments, which allowed greater progress in facial rejuvenation. Knowledge of the midfacial ligaments improved understanding of the facial tissue support system as it relates to the aging process. Modifications of facelifting ensued with a focus on retaining ligament release in a deep-plane of dissection. Hamra[8] described deep-plane rhytidectomy, a ligamentous attachment release in the midface allowing for vertical suspension of the malar fat pad. Many facelift surgeons have adopted variations of this deep-plane technique and claim durable results, natural appearance, and decreased incidence of hematoma and flap compromise.

Although the evolution of facelift surgery generally involved more aggressive surgery involving deeper planes of dissection, there was a predictable counter-movement in the late 1980s towards less invasive techniques. Less invasive surgery offered less operative time, shorter convalescence, and reduced surgical risks as primary advantages. Less invasive procedures included short-scar facelifts, minilifts, the S-lift, the minimal access cranial suspension (MACS) lift, and minimally invasive threadlifting.

Facial volumization has recently become a popular adjunct to facelift surgery, particularly in the midface. Implants, alloplastic fillers, and autologous fat have evolved to address the facial deflation that occurs along with descent during aging. These techniques can have a profound impact on facial rejuvenation, especially when used in combination with rhyitidectomy.

Experts of facelift surgery have tended to be dogmatic in advocating their preferred technique. Much of the evidence supporting the available options has been anecdotal. This has led to significant controversy for decades. The interest in a best technique is substantial because aesthetic surgeons are always seeking better results by less invasive means. This would logically translate to improved patient satisfaction.

PATIENT CANDIDACY

Candidacy for facelift surgery is based on multiple factors. These factors include age, smoking status, history of inflammatory conditions, goals of surgery, and anatomic factors. Surgeon factors are also an important consideration. Skill with a given technique and prior experience should guide both patient and technique selection. Ideally, preoperative assessment of the face should include a statistically validated scale. This can allow for consistent comparisons and analysis of postoperative results. This has not been widely adopted although several tools exist.[9–11] Most surgeons rely on a nonstandardized general assessment of skin laxity, volume loss, and anatomic targets (midface, jowl, neck) during initial consultation.

There is no consensus regarding the optimal age for undergoing facelift and many patients tend to delay surgery until they display significant stigmata of aging. Contrary to common thought, a study by Friel and colleagues[12] found that patients younger than 50-years-old reported increased satisfaction with their procedure at both early and later times. Another study by Liu and Owsley[13] correlated increased self-reported patient satisfaction with improved objective results by photographic analysis in younger patient cohorts.

Patient smoking status is another important preoperative consideration. Active smoking is known to increase the risk of complications such as skin slough, tissue necrosis, and hematoma.[14,15] Most surgeons advocate smoking cessation before surgery, recommending a period of abstinence ranging from 2 weeks to 6 months.[16] A study by Parikh and Jacono[17] advocated use of the deep-plane technique in smokers. They demonstrated no increased risk of skin slough or healing complications in smokers compared with nonsmokers in their cohort. Other surgeons have supported this concept because the deep-plane flap is more robust and better vascularized.

INCISIONS

The facelift incision has multiple variations in both placement and length (**Fig. 1**). Opinions regarding optimal placement vary and consideration must be given to patient characteristics and surgical goals. Patients typically seek minimally invasive techniques with shorter and less visible scars. However, these do not always correspond with better outcomes.

The standard incision starts in the temporal region, extending preauricularly, beneath the lobule, onto the posterior concha, and postauricularly to the occipital region. Variations in placement of the temporal incision just below the temporal tuft hairline or within the hairline depend on patient factors. The amount of skin to be removed should be considered. Older patients or those with excessive skin laxity may require more excision. In this situation, incision placement below the temporal tuft prevents unnatural elevation of the temporal hairline. The potential disadvantage is more scar visibility, though meticulous tension free closure rarely leads to a suboptimal result.[18] If minimal skin excision is expected, placement within the temporal hairline with properly oriented beveling may be a better alternative.

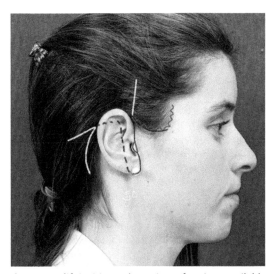

Fig. 1. Facelift incisions. The variety of options available for facelift incisions. The temporal incision can be placed below the temporal tuft (*red* and *blue lines*) or extend into the hairline (*yellow line*). The preauricular incision may be pretragal (*red line*) or retrotragal (*blue line*). The mastoid occipital component can follow the hairline or extend into it (*yellow lines*).

The preauricular incision can be pretragal or apical tragal. There is often a natural preauricular skin fold ideal for pretragal incision placement. This reduces scar visibility while preserving the pretragal notch and skin contour in this region. In men, a pretragal incision is often preferred given the adjacent hair-bearing skin that would look unnatural if extended into the external auditory canal. The apical tragal incision is advantageous because it is hidden on both frontal and lateral views. The pretragal dermis can be thinned and de-epilated to preserve natural skin contouring of the tragus and reduce unwanted hair growth. Some surgeons advocate placement of the incision on the tragal apex regardless of sex, citing scar concealment as a worthy tradeoff for the possibility of daily maintenance of displaced hair.

Usually the incision is continued around the lobule and postauricularly slightly onto the concha, allowing for scar relaxation into the natural postauricular sulcus. Extension onto the mastoid and occipital region is debated. Some surgeons extend the postauricular incision into the occipital hairline in a tricophytic fashion to allow hair growth through the scar to decrease visibility. Others make the incision just below the hairline or not following the hairline at all, with a 45° angle that veers off the overlying the mastoid to avoid an unnatural, notched appearance of the hairline.

Variations from the standard incision length described previously include the short-scar facelift described by Baker,[19] the S-shape incision advocated by Saylan,[20] and the incisions used in the MACS lift proposed by Tonnard and colleagues.[21] These incisions consist of a limited preauricular incision that extends to the lobule but is not continued postauricularly. They are shorter than standard incisions and associated with only a short segment of skin undermining.

FULL FACELIFT TECHNIQUES

Within the scope of a full facelift, techniques can be categorized by the plane of dissection, specifically in regards to management of the SMAS. The subcutaneous, supra-SMAS, and SMAS plication techniques do not involve incision or dissection of the SMAS, remaining superficial to this layer.

The subcutaneous technique, although a component of most facelifts, is seldom used alone in the modern era (**Fig. 2**). In thin, elderly patients in whom the problem is excessive skin laxity, or in revision situations in which the deep tissues remain adequately positioned, a subcutaneous-only dissection may accomplish the desired results. Most currently accepted techniques involve

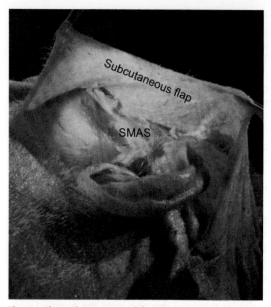

Fig. 2. The subcutaneous lift. The flap is raised in a subcutaneous plane leaving the SMAS unaddressed. The lift is in a vertical vector.

some manipulation of the SMAS because results with the subcutaneous technique have limited durability.

The supra-SMAS technique is an extension of the subcutaneous lift over the midface. The superficial fat and skin is raised as a flap, leaving the SMAS down. Dissection extends over the malar prominences, releasing all the dermal attachments of the SMAS to the nasolabial fold. The flap is suspended posterosuperiorly, often under tension. This allows correction of ptotic cheek fat and softens the melolabial fold, though there is a large potential dead space, increasing risk of hematoma. The undissected SMAS does not allow for improvement of the jowl.[22] There are also concerns regarding longevity because the SMAS is not manipulated.

Plication leaves the SMAS layer intact, using suture to fold the SMAS on itself. Typically, plication involves securing the mobile SMAS anterior to the parotid to the immobile preauricular SMAS, deep temporal fascia, and mastoid fascia.[23] The result is tightening of the SMAS layer with subsequent lifting. The vector of the SMAS lift should be vertical, whereas the overlying skin flap may be redraped in an aesthetically pleasing manner (typically superolateral). The principal author uses a variation of this technique, referred to as the buccal cerclage, which involves a series of 3 separate suspension sutures to lift the neck, lower face, and improve the jaw line (**Fig. 3**).[24–26] The main concern regarding plication is the ability

to maintain the lift long-term without the suture cheese wiring through the lifted tissue.

The remaining techniques all involve an incision through the SMAS. These include lateral SMAS-ectomy, sub-SMAS dissection, deep-plane dissection, and subperiosteal dissection. A lateral SMAS-ectomy[27] involves excision of a 1 to 2 cm strip of SMAS along the anterior border of the parotid, extending from the lower mandibular border obliquely toward the malar fat pad. No undermining is performed and the fascial layer is reapproximated. The vector of the lift depends on the design of the excision. Proponents of this technique argue the procedure is more rapid than a SMAS flap with less risk to the facial nerve. The main disadvantage is that this technique involves no ligamentous release, limiting mobilization of the malar fat pad.

Most SMAS techniques that do not include plication involve some degree of SMAS undermining and are referred to as imbrication techniques. The degree of undermining can be limited or extensive. Sub-SMAS dissection limited to the anterior border of the parotid is often generically termed SMAS rhytidectomy. This limited SMAS dissection theoretically poses less risk to the facial nerve. The SMAS rhytidectomy and its variations can rejuvenate the neck and jowl but usually provide minimal benefit to the midface and nasolabial fold.

To address the perceived shortcomings of limited SMAS dissection, more extensive techniques developed. The deep-plane rhytidectomy, introduced by Hamra[8] in 1990, aimed to achieve greater effacement of the nasolabial fold and elevation of the malar fat pad (**Fig. 4**). Another variation of the deep-plane rhytidectomy, termed the composite rhytidectomy, included elevation and suspension of the lower orbicularis oculi to better address the nasojugal and palpebromalar grooves. Disadvantages of the deep-plane facelift include the increased risk of facial nerve injury, long operative time, and prolonged recovery. With composite rhytidectomy, concerns for asymmetric palpebral fissures and weakening of the orbicularis oculi have made this technique less widely adopted.

Subperiosteal rhytidectomy is an even deeper plane of dissection, referring to elevation in a subperiosteal plane over the maxilla and zygoma. In 1979, Tessier[28] used his understanding of craniofacial principles, applying them to lifting of the facial tissues.[29,30] Later variations of the subperiosteal technique incorporated the endoscope and were often performed in conjunction with brow lifting. The approach for subperiosteal lifting can be transtemporal, transorbital via

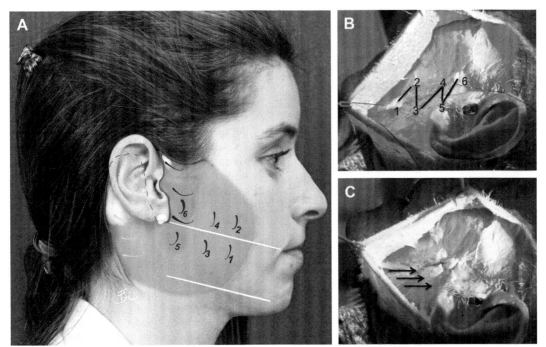

Fig. 3. Buccal cerclage technique. (*A*) A line is drawn from commissure to lobule and another along the inferior border of the mandible. Six bites of SMAS are taken using the lobular-commissure line as the central axis for each successive bite. The inferior bites remain above the inferior border of the mandible, avoiding marginal mandibular nerve injury. The final bite secures the plication to the immobile preauricular fascia. Two additional plication sutures are anchored to the deep temporal and mastoid fascia. (*B*) The stair step buccal cerclage plication in a cadaver. (*C*) Tightening of the buccal cerclage suture with the accompanying SMAS lift in the vertical vector (*arrows*).

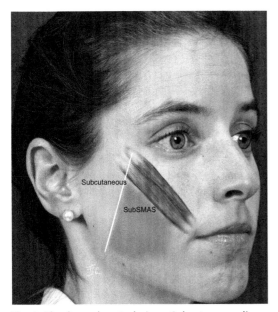

Fig. 4. The deep-plane technique. Subcutaneous dissection is performed to the point anterior to a line drawn from the lateral canthus to the mandibular angle. The dissection then proceeds sub-SMAS over the zygomaticus major and minor muscles with release of the malar fat pads and midface suspending ligaments to allow for midface lifting and nasolabial fold effacement.

blepharoplasty approaches, transoral through a gingivobuccal incision, or a combination. Subperiosteal techniques are helpful for midface rejuvenation but do not affect the jowl or upper neck. Often, standard rhytidectomy must be performed in conjunction.

LESS-INVASIVE TECHNIQUES

In contrast to the full facelift techniques previously described, several less-invasive techniques exist. Whereas full facelift techniques require more operative time, longer convalescence, general anesthesia, and increased surgical risk, the less invasive counterparts offer the opposite. The less invasive techniques were modifications of SMAS plication with a more limited dissection. In 1999, Saylan[20] described a short-scar technique termed the S-lift. The S-lift consisted of an S-shaped skin incision crossing the non–hair-bearing skin at the helical root, pre-excision of skin, and vertical purse-string sutures in the SMAS. The sutures were secured to the periosteum to achieve the lift. MACS was a modification of the S-lift first described by Tonnard and Verpaele[21] in 2002 (**Fig. 5**). The goal was a less invasive, long-lasting lift that could be performed with minimal

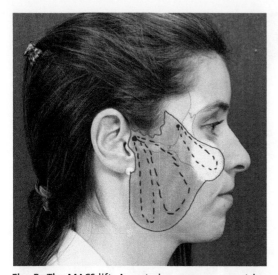

Fig. 5. The MACS lift. A posterior narrow purse-string suture is followed anteriorly by a wider purse-string suture placed at a 30° angle travelling obliquely through the SMAS. Both sutures are anchored to the deep temporal fascia. An additional anterior purse-string suture may be used to mobilize the malar fat pad. The suture for this loop is secured to the lateral orbital rim.

operative time under local anesthesia. The technique relied on SMAS plication with purse-string sutures lifting in a vertical vector.

IS THERE A GOLD-STANDARD TECHNIQUE?

With the numerous options available to the aesthetic surgeon, is there a single best technique? This is a source of significant controversy. No single technique completely fulfills the criteria for an ideal procedure. Such a procedure would be technically easy, require minimal operative and recovery time, have minimal risks and complications, provide a durable effect, and maximize patient satisfaction. Surgeon preference tends to guide practice because the available options fulfill some criteria and not others. Nonetheless, is there evidence in the literature that favors some procedures compared with others and that can guide surgical decision-making?

The deep-plane facelift has been widely touted to provide the most improvement and longest duration of results. Advocates specifically cite better improvement of the nasolabial fold and malar fat pad with lower complication rates compared with other techniques.[8] In an intraoperative analysis, Litner and Adamson[31] assessed the mean skin excess after SMAS plication, imbrication, and deep-plane lifting. Each procedure was performed in succession on the same side in 32 subjects. They found an increased amount of skin

excess with each subsequent technique, with the deep-plane having the most excess. They correlated this to a greater overall lift, although there was no further follow-up of patients to confirm improved results.

In 1996, Ivy and colleagues[32] performed a randomized controlled trial comparing lateral and standard SMAS lifting to composite and extended SMAS techniques. Procedures were performed on 21 subjects by 2 surgeons. On 1 side, subjects underwent conventional SMAS lifting. Composite or extended SMAS techniques performed on the other side. Three separate surgeons evaluated the results at 24 hours, 6 months, and 1 year, postoperatively. No discernable difference could be noted.

Kamer and Frankel[33] performed a retrospective review of SMAS versus deep-plane facelifting by a single surgeon using the rate of revision tuck-up procedures as a correlate of surgical efficacy. They found a significantly higher tuck-up rate in the SMAS facelift cohort (11.4%) compared with the deep-plane cohort (3.3%). They concluded that the deep-plane technique was more effective. Notably, the SMAS lifting technique was used earlier in the surgeon's operative career, whereas the deep-plane technique was performed after years of surgical experience. Logic would imply that tuck-up rates should improve with greater experience regardless of technique.

Becker and Bassichis[34] compared deep-plane techniques to SMAS plication in a retrospective review. Four blinded facial plastic surgeons rated the improvement in the nasolabial fold, jowl, and cheek areas, observing 6-month and 18-month postoperative photographs. They concluded that subjects undergoing SMAS plication had better overall scores, though subjects older than 70 years scored better with the deep-plane technique. This was 1 of the few studies that used statistical analysis in its methodology, although the study was limited by the lack of standardized objective measurements and subject input in regard to satisfaction.

Perhaps of most interest is the 2002, long-term, follow-up study by Hamra.[35] In his review, he noted that the deep-plane technique was not more effective in reducing the nasolabial fold. This is counter to one of the commonly perceived advantages of the deep-plane lift. The assertion that the deep-plane technique was the most efficacious with the most durable results was further challenged by a long-term prospective analysis of four different facelifting methods performed on two sets of twins.[36] A lateral SMAS-ectomy and composite lift was performed on one set of twins. An SMAS-platysma flap with bidirectional lift and endoscopic midface lift with open anterior platysmaplasty was performed on the other. Photographs of the subjects were taken at 1-, 6-, and 10-years postoperatively for evaluation and panel discussion at American Society of Aesthetic Plastic Surgery meetings in 1996, 2001, and 2005. There was consensus among the panel that even at 10 years after surgery, all subjects maintained good long-term results, looking better than they did preoperatively. One of the operating surgeons at the 10-year postoperative panel noted, "Finally deep plane and subperiosteal techniques have been demystified. All surgeons utilizing other techniques can feel relieved."

Other studies have also evaluated the less invasive techniques with interesting results. In 2006, Prado and colleagues[37] retrospectively analyzed subjects undergoing short-scar facelift either via MACS lift or lateral SMAS-ectomy technique. Two blinded facial plastic surgeons reviewed 24-month postoperative photographs and concluded there was no difference between the 2 groups, though 50% of subjects in both groups needed a revision tuck-up procedure. This suggested the short-scar facelifts may have less longevity.

None of the facelift techniques reviewed in the literature has proven to be superior in terms of efficacy or safety.[14,37–39] Regarding minimally invasive lifts, the evidence would suggest there is less durability. The lack of a proven gold-standard highlights the need for higher quality evidence. In a 2011 systematic review, it was noted that there were only 3 randomized controlled trials and 5 studies that attempted statistical analysis in the facelift literature. The studies also lacked standardized objective analysis measures.[40] In fact, the cited systematic review, to date, is the only of its kind. Higher quality research is needed that incorporates better methodologies with statistical analysis, incorporating standardized objective outcome measures. Subject satisfaction should also be considered using validated measures.

Management of the Midface and Volume Augmentation

Several changes to both the soft tissue and bony structures of the midface occur with aging. The orbital socket diameter increases, the maxilla resorbs, the overlying skin and SMAS develop elastosis, and the fat pads lipoatrophy. These changes manifest in the midface as tear trough deformities, malar hollowing, double convexity at the lip-cheek junction, and malar flattening and descent. Rohrich and Pessa[41] described the superficial and deep fat compartments in the midface, theorizing that volume loss and not descent was the primary contributor to the aging face. Creating a youthful appearance requires not only skin and soft tissue repositioning but also restoration of volume lost in the midface. Surgical approaches to midface volumization include malar implants or rhytidectomy techniques. Nonsurgical permanent techniques consist mainly of autologous fat transfer.

Rhytidectomy

The previously described deep-plane and subperiosteal techniques are the most common rhytidectomy approaches to the midface. As alluded to earlier, the long-term impact of the deep-plane technique on the midface is questionable.[35] However, using 3-dimensional imaging software, Jacono and colleagues[42] found that the deep-plane rhytidectomy added 3.2 mL of midface volume to each hemiface. They concluded that the deep-plane rhytidectomy may obviate adjunctive volumization techniques.

Implants

Alloplastic implants are a surgical alternative to rhytidectomy approaches for restoration of midface volume. Implants augment the midfacial skeleton, restoring volume and a youthful, heart-shaped appearance to the face.[43] Implant materials include silicone, expanded polytetrafluoroethylene (ePTFE), or high-density polyethylene. These allow for varying degrees of tissue ingrowth and implant stabilization. Implants are advantageous in that they are permanent, requiring a single operation. Disadvantages include implant displacement, deformation, extrusion, and infection.[44]

Autologous Fat Transfer

Autologous fat grafting is another alternative for volumization and many plastic surgeons are using this technique concurrently with rhytidectomy. A questionnaire by Sinno and colleagues[45] found that 85% of respondents have added autologous fat grafting as part of their surgical practice. The 2 most common regions augmented by survey respondents were the perioral and the deep malar compartments. Autologous fat grafting is advantageous in that it provides the large amount of volume needed for comprehensive midface rejuvenation (**Fig. 6**). This is something not possible with alloplastic fillers without considerable expense. Glasgold and colleagues[46] noted that only subjects receiving fat transfers to the cheek were satisfied with results, and recommended fillers only for isolated lip and nasolabial fold augmentation.

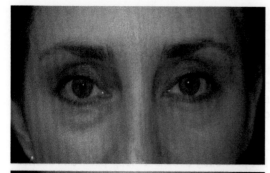

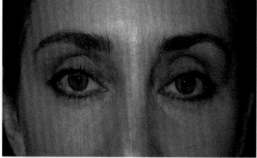

Fig. 6. (*Top*) Preoperative lower lid blepharoplasty and fat transfer to the cheek and tear-trough area. (*Bottom*) 3-year postoperatively.

Although autologous fat grafting has been found to be a useful technique, controversy exists regarding long-term viability and durability. Multiple studies evaluating the survivability of fat transfer differ in results, with reported volume retention ranging from 20% to 90%.

Meier and colleagues[47] evaluated the retention and longevity of autologous fat in the midface. They prospectively analyzed 33 subjects who underwent autologous fat transfer to the midface using 3-dimensional imaging software for quantitative volume measurements. They found that 32% of the injected volume remains at 16 months, and 25% of subjects required touch-up procedures.

Another question regarding autologous fat grafting is whether it is more effective than alloplastic fillers. A literature review by Winters and Moulthrop[48] suggested that poly L-lactic acid (PLLA) may be more advantageous due to the lack of need for overcorrection. However, this technique typically requires multiple treatments and with a potential complication of nodule or granuloma formation. Autologous fat avoids these complications and has potential for more durable benefits. However, because fat is subject to resorption, it often requires overcorrection. Occasionally, lumpiness and asymmetry may occur. Unfortunately, there is a lack of high-quality evidence to make any definitive conclusions or recommendations regarding the ideal injectable material.

Management of the Neck

A variety of techniques are available to address the neck, including liposuction, midline platysmaplasty, platysmal transection, direct excision of subplatysmal fat, and chin or prejowl augmentation. If submental skin laxity is the only problem, the skin removed during the rhytidectomy may be sufficient. Usually excessive submental fat or poor platysmal muscular tone is also found with excess laxity. Excess submental fat, whether subcutaneous or subplatysmal, should be removed. Suction-assisted lipectomy is commonly performed, with emphasis on medial excision in the central subplatysmal fat region. Lateral excision is limited because there is less fat in this region and aggressive lateral liposuction is associated with increased risk to the marginal mandibular nerve. Some surgeons advocate for subcutaneous and/or subplatysmal fat excision with scissors, under direct visualization, in the central region.

If the muscular sling of the platysma needs to be recreated or if platysmal banding must be addressed, midline sutures, platysmal excision, lateral suspension, transection, or a combination of these techniques are options. Some surgeons advocate for plication of the anterior edges of the platysma. Others excise a wedge of muscle, cut muscle in a transverse fashion at the level of the hyoid, or cut muscle in a vertical fashion. Proponents of imbrication suggest that excision of muscle helps break the continuity of the anterior platysmal bands, allowing for the more cephalad muscle to pull superiorly and contribute to a more defined cervicomental angle. Also, in elderly patients, a vertical excision may be required to allow a taut muscular sling. As evidenced by the variety of techniques available to address the neck, there is no consensus on which is optimal.

SUMMARY

Controversy exists regarding several aspects of facelift surgery. From patient selection to the varying methods of facial rejuvenation, there are differing opinions in regard to optimal management. The literature is unclear concerning the best practices. Much of the evidence supporting a particular technique is anecdotal. The limited studies directly comparing techniques have generally shown a lack of significant difference between compared procedures. What is clear is that further high-quality research is needed. The use of consistent methodologies, standardized preoperative assessments, and validated postoperative outcome measures can shed light on how best to manage the complex problem of facial aging.

REFERENCES

1. Hollander E. Die Kosmetische Chirurgie. In: Joseph M, editor. Handbuch der Kosmetik. Leipzig (Germany): Verlag von Veit; 1912. p. 688.
2. Lexer E. Die Gerante Wiederherstellungschirurgie, Vol 2. Leipzig: JA Barth; 1931. p. 548.
3. Bettman A. Plastic and cosmetic surgery of the face. Northwest Med 1920;29:205.
4. Adamson PA, Moran ML. Historical trends in surgery for the aging face. Facial Plast Surg 1993; 9(2):133–42.
5. Skoog T. Plastic surgery: new methods and refinements. Philadelphia: W.B. Saunders; 1974.
6. Mitz V, Peyronie M. The superficial musculoaponeurotic system (SMAS) in the parotid and cheek area. Plast Reconstr Surg 1976;58(1):80–8.
7. Furnas D. The retaining ligaments of the cheek. Plast Reconstr Surg 1989;83:11.
8. Hamra ST. The deep-plane rhytidectomy. Plast Reconstr Surg 1990;86(1):53–61 [discussion: 62–3].
9. Rzany B, Carruthers A, Carruthers J, et al. Validated composite assessment scales for the global face. Dermatol Surg 2012;38(2 Spec No.):294–308.
10. Carruthers J, Flynn TC, Geister TL, et al. Validated assessment scales for the mid face. Dermatol Surg 2012;38(2 Spec No.):320–32.
11. Narins RS, Carruthers J, Flynn TC, et al. Validated assessment scales for the lower face. Dermatol Surg 2012;38(2 Spec No.):333–42.
12. Friel MT, Shaw RE, Trovato MJ, et al. The measure of face-lift patient satisfaction: the owsley facelift satisfaction survey with a long-term follow-up study. Plast Reconstr Surg 2010;126(1):245–57.
13. Liu TS, Owsley JQ. Long-term results of face lift surgery: patient photographs compared with patient satisfaction ratings. Plast Reconstr Surg 2012; 129(1):253–62.
14. Grover R, Jones BM, Waterhouse N. The prevention of haematoma following rhytidectomy: a review of 1078 consecutive facelifts. Br J Plast Surg 2001;54(6):481–6.
15. Rees TD, Liverett DM, Guy CL. The effect of cigarette smoking on skin-flap survival in the face lift patient. Plast Reconstr Surg 1984;73(6):911–5.
16. McCollough EG, Perkins S, Thomas JR. Facelift: panel discussion, controversies, and techniques. Facial Plast Surg Clin North Am 2012;20(3):279–325.
17. Parikh SS, Jacono AA. Deep-plane face-lift as an alternative in the smoking patient. Arch Facial Plast Surg 2011;13(4):283–5.
18. Miller TR, Eisbach KJ. SMAS facelift techniques to minimize stigmata of surgery. Facial Plast Surg Clin North Am 2005;13(3):421–31.
19. Baker DC. Minimal incision rhytidectomy (short scar face lift) with lateral SMASectomy. Aesthet Surg J 2001;21(1):68–79.
20. Saylan Z. The S-lift: less is more. Aesthet Surg J 1999;19:406.
21. Tonnard P, Verpaele A, Monstrey S, et al. Minimal access cranial suspension lift: a modified S-lift. Plast Reconstr Surg 2002;109(6):2074–86.
22. Baker SR. Deep plane rhytidectomy and variations. Facial Plast Surg Clin North Am 2009; 17(4):557–73, vi.
23. Robbins LB, Brothers DB, Marshall DM. Anterior SMAS plication for the treatment of prominent nasomandibular folds and restoration of normal cheek contour. Plast Reconstr Surg 1995;96(6):1279–87 [discussion: 1288].
24. Wang TD. Rhytidectomy for treatment of the aging face. Mayo Clin Proc 1989;64(7):780–90.
25. Wang TD. Patient selection for aging face surgery. Facial Plast Surg Clin North Am 2005;13(3):381–2.
26. Wang T. Buccal cerclage. Presentation at AAFPRS winter meeting. October 1-3, 2015.
27. Baker DC. Lateral SMASectomy. Plast Reconstr Surg 1997;100(2):509–13.
28. Tessier P. Subperiosteal face-lift. Ann Chir Plast Esthet 1989;34(3):193–7.
29. Psillakis JM, Rumley TO, Camargos A. Subperiosteal approach as an improved concept for correction of the aging face. Plast Reconstr Surg 1988; 82(3):383–94.
30. De La Plaza R, Valiente E, Arroyo JM. Supraperiosteal lifting of the upper two-thirds of the face. Br J Plast Surg 1991;44(5):325–32.
31. Litner JA, Adamson PA. Limited vs extended face-lift techniques: objective analysis of intraoperative results. Arch Facial Plast Surg 2006; 8(3):186–90.
32. Ivy EJ, Lorenc ZP, Aston SJ. Is there a difference? A prospective study comparing lateral and standard SMAS face lifts with extended SMAS and composite rhytidectomies. Plast Reconstr Surg 1996;98(7): 1135–43 [discussion: 1144–7].
33. Kamer FM, Frankel AS. SMAS rhytidectomy versus deep plane rhytidectomy: an objective comparison. Plast Reconstr Surg 1998;102(3):878–81.
34. Becker FF, Bassichis BA. Deep-plane face-lift vs superficial musculoaponeurotic system plication face-lift: a comparative study. Arch Facial Plast Surg 2004;6(1):8–13.
35. Hamra ST. A study of the long-term effect of malar fat repositioning in face lift surgery: short-term success but long-term failure. Plast Reconstr Surg 2002;110(3):940–51 [discussion: 952–9].
36. Alpert BS, Baker DC, Hamra ST, et al. Identical twin face lifts with differing techniques: a 10-year follow-up. Plast Reconstr Surg 2009;123(3): 1025–33 [discussion: 1034–6].

37. Prado A, Andrades P, Danilla S, et al. A clinical retrospective study comparing two short-scar face lifts: minimal access cranial suspension versus lateral SMASectomy. Plast Reconstr Surg 2006;117(5): 1413–25 [discussion: 1426–7].

38. Rees TD, Barone CM, Valauri FA, et al. Hematomas requiring surgical evacuation following face lift surgery. Plast Reconstr Surg 1994;93(6): 1185–90.

39. Zager WH, Dyer WK. Minimal incision facelift. Facial Plast Surg 2005;21(1):21–7.

40. Chang S, Pusic A, Rohrich RJ. A systematic review of comparison of efficacy and complication rates among face-lift techniques. Plast Reconstr Surg 2011;127(1):423–33.

41. Rohrich RJ, Pessa JE. The retaining system of the face: histologic evaluation of the septal boundaries of the subcutaneous fat compartments. Plast Reconstr Surg 2008;121(5):1804–9.

42. Jacono AA, Malone MH, Talei B. Three-dimensional analysis of long-term midface volume change after vertical vector deep-plane rhytidectomy. Aesthet Surg J 2015;35(5):491–503.

43. Soares DJ, Silver WE. Midface skeletal enhancement. Facial Plast Surg Clin North Am 2015;23(2): 185–93.

44. Hopping SB, Joshi AS, Tanna N, et al. Volumetric facelift: evaluation of rhytidectomy with alloplastic augmentation. Ann Otol Rhinol Laryngol 2010; 119(3):174–80.

45. Sinno S, Mehta K, Reavey PL, et al. Current trends in facial rejuvenation: an assessment of ASPS members' use of fat grafting during face lifting. Plast Reconstr Surg 2015;136(1):20e–30e.

46. Glasgold M, Glasgold R, Lam S. Autologous fat grafting for midface rejuvenation. Clin Plast Surg 2015;42(1):115–21.

47. Meier JD, Glasgold RA, Glasgold MJ. Autologous fat grafting: long-term evidence of its efficacy in midfacial rejuvenation. Arch Facial Plast Surg 2009;11(1):24–8.

48. Winters R, Moulthrop T. Is autologous fat grafting superior to other fillers for facial rejuvenation? Laryngoscope 2013;123(5):1068–9.

Facial Transplantation

Jack E. Russo, MD, MS, Eric M. Genden, MD, MHCA*

KEYWORDS

- Facial transplantation • Composite tissue allotransplantation • Microvascular surgery
- Immunosuppression • Ethics

KEY POINTS

- Computed tomography angiography is helpful preoperatively for assessment of recipient vessel targets to plan for typically 2 arterial and 2 venous anastomoses to support the transplant.
- Skin is highly antigenic; acute rejection of facial transplants is common, if not universal, but chronic rejection is rare.
- Typical 3 drug immunosuppression exposes patients to risks of infection and development of malignancies, both of which can be deadly.
- Careful patient selection, thoughtful informed consent, and consideration of the psychosocial impact of facial transplant are necessary to keep the procedure ethically sound.

INTRODUCTION

Conventional approaches to facial reconstruction are largely dictated by the extent of the defect. Although smaller defects may be amenable to local flaps, more extensive defects often require free tissue transfer or large split-thickness skin grafts. These techniques may suffice to provide coverage and occasionally restore function. However, in terms of both cosmesis and functionality, traditional reconstruction options fall short for patients with the most severe whole face deformities, often resulting in a patchwork appearance that reflects the sometimes dozens of surgeries these patients endure in pursuit of the elusive goal of achieving an acceptable appearance and quality of life (**Fig. 1**).

Over the last 10 years, facial transplantation, a form of composite tissue allotransplantation (CTA), has emerged as a viable option for reconstruction of the most severe facial deformities in carefully selected patients. There have been 31 cases of facial transplantation reported in the world literature since the first case in 2005, with good results overall (**Table 1**). However, facial transplantation was controversial at its inception; despite growing experience with this procedure, significant controversies persist.

In this article, the authors focus on the current controversies, challenges, and questions that confront facial transplantation while highlighting the lessons learned and challenges overcome through experience thus far. The discussion focuses on 3 main topics: technical issues, issues of facial transplantation immunology, and ethical concerns.

TECHNICAL ISSUES

Facial transplantation is undoubtedly a highly technical and complex surgical undertaking that requires a cohesive team approach. Because of the complexity of the undertaking, only a handful of centers worldwide have the expertise and infrastructure necessary to perform facial transplantation. As the worldwide experience has grown over the last decade, technique has been refined, though some controversies and challenges remain.

Because facial CTA requires revascularization via microvascular anastomoses, a detailed understanding of the recipient vascular anatomy is

The authors have no financial disclosures.
Department of Otolaryngology – Head and Neck Surgery, Icahn School of Medicine at Mount Sinai, One Gustave L. Levy Place, New York, NY 10029, USA
* Corresponding author.
E-mail address: Eric.genden@mountsinai.org

Facial Plast Surg Clin N Am 24 (2016) 367–377
http://dx.doi.org/10.1016/j.fsc.2016.03.013

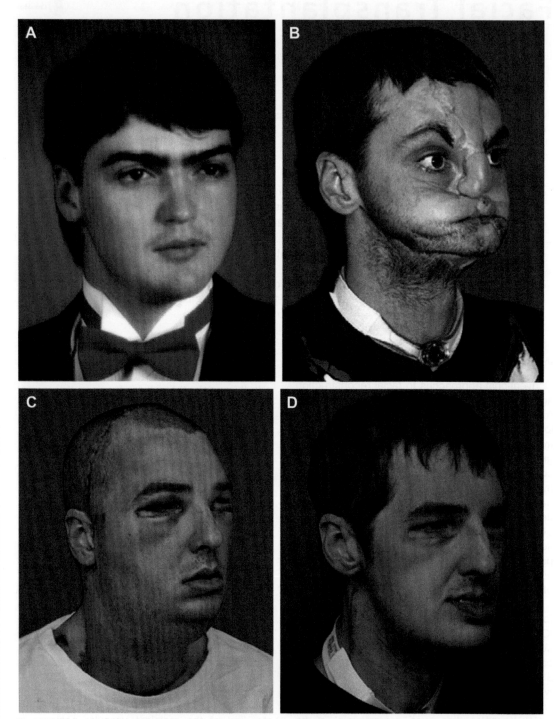

Fig. 1. A 37-year-old man before injury (*A*), before face vascularized composite allotransplantation (*B*), 6 days (*C*) and 7 months (*D*) following allotransplantation of the face. (*From* Murphy BD, Zuker RM, Borschel GH. Vascularized composite allotransplantation: an update on medical and surgical progress and remaining challenges. J Plast Reconstr Aesthet Surg 2013;66(11):1453; with permission.)

paramount to determine if a given individual is an acceptable facial transplantation candidate and, if so, to create a viable surgical plan. This understanding is especially important because most patients who are considered for facial transplantation have undergone numerous prior reconstructive surgeries, usually including prior free tissue transfer, which may limit the availability of viable recipient vessels and can make dissection of these vessels challenging and time consuming because of scarring and tissue fibrosis. Computed tomography (CT) angiography of recipients before facial transplantation is advocated to identify potential vascular targets and to better understand their relationship to other facial structures in the interest of shortening already long surgical times, minimizing intraoperative blood loss, and increasing the chances of having robust perfusion to the transplant.[1] CT angiography also helps to identify the specific branching patterns of the external carotid system and the caliber of these vessels for a given facial transplant candidate so that a specific surgical plan can be made preoperatively.

There has been controversy regarding the number of microvascular anastomoses necessary to support a face transplant. Each anastomosis increases surgical time and complexity, but loss of a CTA due to arterial insufficiency or venous congestion would be devastating; thus, redundancy in the feeding blood supply is typically sought. Studies have demonstrated that one vascular anastomosis is sufficient to perfuse a facial tranplant.[2] However, to minimize the risk of catastrophic graft lost, it is advisable to plan for at least 2 arterial and 2 venous anastomoses. Choosing recipient vessels with large caliber to ensure reliable flow is important. Caution must be exercised, however, when considering bilateral end-to-end anastomoses directly to the external carotid as ischemia of the hypopharynx and to the eyes (via loss of external carotid to ophthalmic collaterals) are potential complications.[1]

There are also questions on the donor side as to which vessels will adequately perfuse the transplanted tissue. The answer to this question undoubtedly depends on the specific tissues included in the transplant. There is evidence that the facial arteries alone can supply both the mandible through submental and periosteal perforators and the maxilla via perforators from the oral mucosa.[1,3] This allows for composite partial facial transplants of the midface and lower face, including bone, to be supplied by the facial arteries. The overarching principle is vascular supply via angiosomes in which particular territories of facial soft tissue are supplied predictably by certain vessels, with the understanding that there are often collaterals between angiosomes.[1] Although portions of the upper face and periorbital region are within angiosomes supplied by branches from the ophthalmic artery, itself a branch of the internal carotid system, full face transplants as well as partial face transplants of the upper face can be reliably supplied by

collaterals from the superficial temporal arterial system, which is fed by harvesting and anastomosing the external carotid.[1] It has also been advocated to leave the recipient's forehead skin intact until after the vascular anastomoses have been performed and the forehead portion of the CTA is observed to be well perfused (the most likely site of ischemia).[4] To standardize the transplant harvest and to maximize vessels available to robustly supply and drain a full face CTA, Lantieri[5] and his team routinely harvest 6 vessels (2 external carotids, 2 external jugular veins, and 2 thyrolingofacial trunks).

Most face transplants have been harvested from heart-beating, brain-dead donors, though harvest from non–heart-beating donors has also been performed. Coordination is required with other surgical teams who are harvesting solid organs from the same donor to determine the timing of facial harvest relative to harvest of organs, which will result in loss of perfusion to the remaining body tissues.[6]

Another potentially controversial aspect of harvesting of the face, as compared with other transplants, is the resultant external disfigurement to the donor. To lessen the impact that facial harvest will have on the families of donors, it is common to take a mold of the donor's face before harvest so that a painted resin mask can be fabricated during the harvest for placement on the donor before returning the body to the family[6] (**Fig. 2**).

One of the most important aspects of facial transplantation from a functional standpoint is restoration of facial movement. To achieve dynamic facial movement and static tone, anastomosis of the facial nerves must be performed. Some controversy exists as to the location of facial nerve anastomosis. Some advocate anastomosis of individual nerve branches as close to the target muscles as possible to prevent dyskinesis.[7] The counter opinion is that anastomosis should be made to the main trunk of the nerve on the donor tissue to prevent the need for an intraparotid dissection, which can compromise vascularity to the transplanted tissue.[5] Regardless, reported facial motor outcomes have been generally favorable, with most patients achieving improvement in facial expressivity and often a symmetric smile.[7,8] It is also known that nerve regeneration is enhanced by tacrolimus, which is a beneficial side effect of immunosuppression in these patients.[4,7]

FACIAL TRANSPLANTATION IMMUNOLOGY

As with any allotransplant, a central tenant of facial transplantation is the need for immunosuppression

Table 1
Facial transplants performed worldwide to date

Number	Month/Year	City & Team Leader	R Sex, Age (y)	D Age (y)	Indication	Type	SD (h)
1	11/2005	Devauchelle, Amiens, France	F, 38	46	Animal attack	Partial myocutaneous	15
2	04/2006	Guo, Xian, China	M, 30[a]	25	Animal attack	Partial osteomyocutaneous	13
3	01/2007	Lantieri, Paris, France	M, 29	65	NF 1	Partial myocutaneous	11
4	12/2008	Siemionow, Cleveland, United States	F, 45	44	Gunshot injury	Partial osteomyocutaneous	22
5	03/2009	Lantieri, Paris, France	M, 27	43	Gunshot injury	Partial osteomyocutaneous	19
6	04/2009	Lantieri, Paris, France	M, 37[a]	59	Burns	Partial myocutaneous	13
7	04/2009	Pomahac, Boston, United States	M, 59	60	Burns	Partial osteomyocutaneous	17
8	08/2009	Lantieri, Paris, France	M, 33	55	Gunshot injury	Partial osteomyocutaneous	16
9	08/2009	Cavadas, Valencia, Spain	M, 42[a]	35	Radiotherapy	Partial osteomyocutaneous	15
10	11/2009	Devauchelle, Amiens, France	M, 27	—	Burns	Partial osteomyocutaneous	19
11	01/2010	Gomez-Cia, Seville, Spain	M, 35	30	NF 1	Partial myocutaneous	22
12	04/2010	Barret, Barcelona, Spain	M, 31	41	Gunshot injury	Full osteomyocutaneous	—
13	07/2010	Lantieri, Paris, France	M, 37	—	NF 1	Full myocutaneous	14
14	03/2011	Pomahac, Boston, United States	M, 25	48	Burns	Full myocutaneous	17
15	04/2011	Lantieri, Paris, France	M, 45	—	Gunshot injury	Partial osteomyocutaneous	—
16	04/2011	Lantieri, Paris, France	M, 41	—	Gunshot injury	Partial osteomyocutaneous	—
17	04/2011	Pomahac Boston, United States	M, 30	31	Burns	Full myocutaneous	14

#	Date	Surgeon, Location	R (sex, age)	D (age)	Cause	Transplant type	SD
18	05/2011	Pomahac, Boston, United States	F, 57	42	Animal attack	Full osteomyocutaneous	19
19	01/2012	Özkan, Antalya, Turkey	M, 19	39	Burns	Full osteomyocutaneous	9
20	01/2012	Blondeel, Gent, Belgium	N/A	N/A	N/A	Partial osteomyocutaneous	20
21	02/2012	Nazir, Ankara, Turkey	M, 25	40	Burns	Full face transplant	—
22	03/2012	Özmen, Ankara, Turkey	F, 20	28	Burns	Partial face transplant	—
23	03/2012	Rodriguez, Baltimore, United States	M, 37	21	Gunshot injury	Full osteomyocutaneous	36
24	05/2012	Özkan, Antalya, Turkey	M, 27	19	Burns	Full face transplant	—
25	01/2013	Pomahac, Boston, United States	F, 44	—	Burns	Full myocutaneous	15
26	05/2013	Özkan, Antalya, Turkey	M 27	19	Gunshot injury	Partial osteomyocutaneous	27
27	07/2013	Maciejewski, Warsaw, Poland	M, 33	42	Crush trauma	Partial osteomyocutaneous	—
28	07/2013	Özkan, Antalya, Turkey	M, 27	—	Ballistic trauma	Full osteomyocutaneous	—
29	08/2013	Özkan, Antalya, Turkey	M, 54[a]	—	Ballistic trauma	Partial osteomyocutaneous	—
30	12/2013	Özkan, Antalya, Turkey	M, 22	—	Ballistic trauma	Partial osteomyocutaneous	—
31	12/2013	Maciejewski, Warsaw, Poland	F, 26	—	Neurofibromatosis	Full myocutaneous	—

Abbreviations: D, donor; F, female; M, male; N/A, not applicable; NF 1, neurofibromatosis type I; R, recipient; SD, surgery duration.

[a] Patient died.

Data from Smeets R, Rendenbach R, Birkelbach M, et al. Face transplantation: on the verge of becoming clinical routine? Biomed Res Int 2014;2014:1–9; and Roche NA, Blondeel PN, Van Lierde KM, et al. Facial transplantation: history and update. Acta Chir Belg 2015;115(2):99–103.

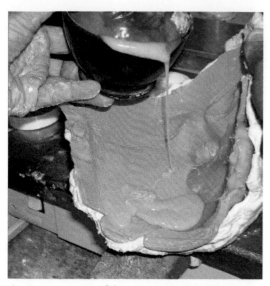

Fig. 2. Preparation of the resin mask after obtaining an alginate donor mold. (*From* Infante-Cossio P, Barrera-Pulido F, Gomez-Cia T, et al. Facial transplantation: a concise update. Med Oral Patol Oral Cir Bucal 2013;18(2):e267.)

to avoid rejection of the transplanted tissue. Achieving a safe and effective regimen of immunosuppression remains one of the biggest challenges in facial transplantation. Unlike other common solid tissue transplants, such as kidney and liver, facial transplants are histologically heterogeneous and contain tissue components that express different antigenic forms. Therefore, allotransplantation mandates substantial lifelong immunosuppression to prevent rejection. Failure of or noncompliance with the regimen could lead to devastating results, including the loss of the transplanted face.[9,10]

Facial transplants typically contain a large component of skin, which is known to be one of the most antigenically reactive tissues.[11] Episodes of acute rejection are common and considered almost inevitable in facial tranplantation.[5] Review of the first 28 cases of facial transplant showed that all patients had experienced episodes of acute rejection within the first year.[7] Because the transplanted skin is external and, thus, highly visible, episodes of acute rejection can be picked up quickly and treated. This ability may partly explain why chronic rejection has only been reported in one facial transplantation despite the high incidence of acute rejection, though this could also be due to the relatively short follow-up time for most cases so far.[7,9] Acute rejection can typically be managed with adjustment to immunosuppression medications (**Fig. 3**).

A typical immunosuppression regimen for facial transplantation includes antilymphocyte induction in the operating room followed by standard triple therapy that includes a calcineurin inhibitor (tacrolimus), antiproliferative agent (mycophenolate mofetil), and corticosteroids.[5,7,11] This regimen has proven effective but requires close monitoring and patient compliance. This type of multidrug immunosuppression also puts patients at significant risk for infections, development of malignancies, and even death. Among the first 28 face transplant patients, at least 11 experienced infectious complications.[7] Two patients have received simultaneous face and bilateral upper extremity transplants; both developed sepsis postoperatively and one died of this complication, whereas the other lost the extremity grafts. Additional complications have included development of B-cell lymphoma, chronic renal insufficiency, new-onset diabetes, tumor recurrence in a patient with head and neck cancer, and death from presumed grade 4 rejection (**Table 2**).[7] In total there have been 5 deaths reported in face transplant patients thus far, caused by noncompliance with immunosuppression, recurrent malignancy, sepsis, suicide, and multiorgan failure.[10]

Because of these serious risks of immunosuppression and the risks of transplant rejection without immunosuppression, current efforts are focused on achieving lasting tolerance in patients toward the transplanted tissue, though it is debated whether this is realistically achievable.[12] Efforts have involved using bone marrow transplants from the facial transplant donor to induce stable chimerism.[5,13] Vascularized transfer of bone marrow with the CTA may have a similar effect when portions of the mandible and less likely the maxilla (with its smaller marrow space) are transferred to the recipient.[5] Research has also been directed toward nonhematopoietic efforts to induce tolerance, such as using UV radiation or chemotherapy to push T cells to a tolerogenic phenotype.[5]

Whether to use a sentinel flap, that is, a second free flap transferred from the same donor and inset elsewhere on the body, to monitor and test for episodes of rejection is debated. Although the facial transplant remains highly visible, making monitoring for rejection straightforward, biopsies are often needed to confirm episodes of rejection and grade their severity. Repeated biopsies on the transplanted facial skin can lead to scarring and compromise the aesthetic outcome as well as be a nidus for infection. Thus, a sentinel flap, such as a radial forearm free flap transferred to an extremity that is antigenically similar to the facial transplant, can serve this purpose. A side benefit is that the sentinel flap can be used to reconstruct defects elsewhere on the body, as

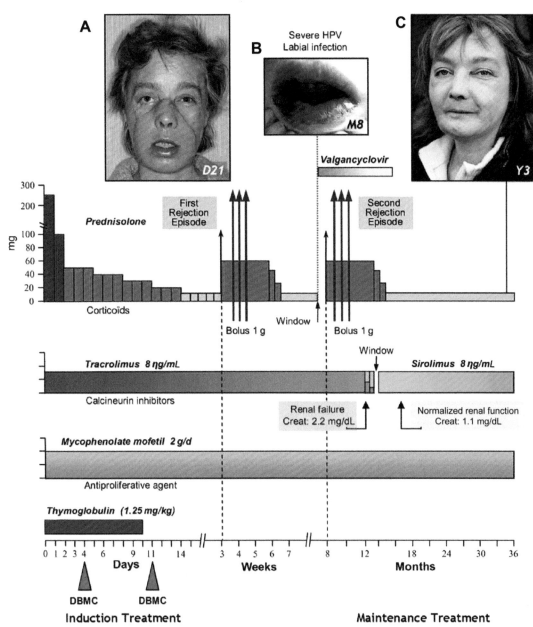

Fig. 3. Immunologic outcomes of the first partial face transplant. Color rectangles indicate the relative doses of immunosuppressants used to prevent graft rejection and arrowheads show the 2 infusions of donor bone marrow cells (DBMC) given during induction treatment. Vertical dotted lines show the 2 rejection episodes. (*A*) Erythematous aspect of the graft during first rejection. (*B*) Severe human papillomavirus (HPV) labial infection, just before the second rejection episode. Arrows indicate steroid boluses given to control both episodes. At month 12, a transient renal failure complicated the immunosuppressive treatment but disappeared when tacrolimus was stopped and replaced by sirolimus. Maintenance treatment is characterized by low doses of immunosuppressant drugs. (*C*) Appearance at 3 years. (*From* Lengelé BG. Current concepts and future challenges in facial transplantation. Clin Plast Surg 2009;36(3):513, with permission.)

these patients often have injuries in addition to their facial deformity.

Another significant benefit of sentinel flap use is the ability to distinguish between rejection and local facial skin-specific processes, such as

dermatitis. A notable example of this came from the Boston series in which a patient developed an erythematous appearance to the face transplant skin in the early posttransplant period, which did not respond to pulsed steroids. There was a

Table 2
Complications of immunotherapy in first 27 face transplant cases

Immunotherapy Complications	n
Infections	
Viral (CMV, HSV, EBV, and poxvirus)	8
Bacterial (*Pseudomonas*, staphylococcal, and others)[a]	7
Fungal (*Candida*)	3
Rosacea	1
Metabolic	
Acute rejections	14
Renal failure	2
Glucose intolerance/diabetes mellitus	2
Transient leukopenia	1
Severe rhabdomyolysis	1
Neoplasia	
Cervical dysplasia	1
Monoclonal B-cell lymphoma	1
Secondary squamous cell carcinoma[a]	1

Abbreviations: CMV, cytomegalovirus; EBV, Epstein-Barr virus; HSV, herpes simplex virus; n, number.
[a] Complication leading to death.
Adapted from Smeets R, Rendenbach C, Birkelbach M, et al. Face transplantation: on the verge of becoming clinical routine? Biomed Res Int 2014;2014:6; with permission.

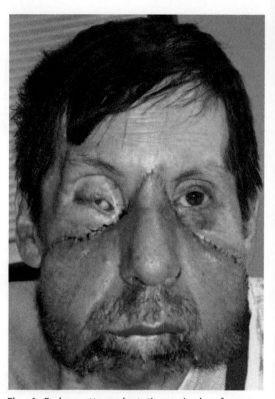

Fig. 4. Early posttransplantation episode of rosacea with diffuse erythema in the facial allograft. (*From* Kueckelhaus M, Fischer S, Lian CG, et al. Utility of sentinel flaps in assessing facial allograft rejection. Plast Reconstr Surg 2015;135(1):252; with permission.)

discordance between the facial skin and the sentinel flap, with the sentinel flap not showing signs of rejection. Dermatologic evaluation of the facial skin revealed findings consistent with rosacea, and the erythema resolved with topical metronidazole therapy[14] (**Figs. 4** and **5**).

One potential concern with the use of sentinel flaps is the possibility that the transfer of additional tissue would require higher dosages of immunosuppression, though this has not been found to be the case.[14] Opponents have also postulated that the different tissue composition of the sentinel flap may make it more or less susceptible to rejection than the facial transplant, but Kueckelhaus and colleagues[14] found a high correlation in degree of rejection between the sentinel flap and CTA based on repeated biopsies.

ETHICAL ISSUES

Much has been written about the ethics of facial transplantation and ethical issues remain arguably the most controversial aspect of the procedure. Using the standard framework of ethical discussion, ethical issues in facial transplantation can be broken down into issues of autonomy, beneficence, dignity, justice, and nonmaleficence.

Autonomy refers to the patient's right as an individual to make independent decisions for him or herself. With regards to facial transplantation, preserving autonomy involves adequate informed consent and central to the issue of informed consent is an understanding of the potential risks. Facial transplantation should be considered an experimental procedure and patients should be informed that there are likely risks which are yet

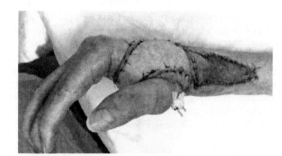

Fig. 5. Early posttransplantation episode of rosacea with no erythema in the sentinel flap. (*From* Kueckelhaus M, Fischer S, Lian CG, et al. Utility of sentinel flaps in assessing facial allograft rejection. Plast Reconstr Surg 2015;135(1):253; with permission.)

unknown. However, 10 years after the first facial transplant, outcomes data are now starting to emerge. Known risks of surgery include long surgical and anesthesia times with potentially large blood loss. These risks should be familiar to the head and neck reconstructive surgeon, if somewhat more significant in the case of facial transplantation.

Most of the nonsurgical risks, however, stem from the need for high-dose, long-term immunosuppression, which can lead to serious complications anytime from the immediate postoperative period to years after the surgery. The need for immunosuppression has been a central topic in the ethical debate surrounding facial transplantation. Available outcomes data from the first decade of facial transplantation have shown that most facial transplant patients have developed opportunistic infections, including cytomegalovirus activation, herpes simplex, herpes zoster, Epstein-Barr virus, candidal, staphylococcal, enterobacter, and pseudomonas infections.[11] Metabolic derangements are also possible; new-onset diabetes, acute renal failure, rhabdomyolysis, transient leukopenia, transient thrombocytopenia, and transient steroid-induced confusion have also been reported[11,15] (see **Table 2**). Even more concerning are the reported cases of posttransplantation cancers, including one case of cervical dysplasia requiring hysterectomy and 2 cases of lymphoma.[11] The most troubling fact, however, is that 5 deaths have been reported following facial transplantation after review of the first 31 cases.[10] This finding puts the mortality rate on par with solid organ transplantation but raises the ethical question of whether this is an acceptable risk to assume to fix a problem that is not life threatening.

The next ethical issue to consider is the principle of beneficence, which refers to the responsibility of the facial transplantation team to act in the best interests of the recipient and the donor's family, with honesty and disclosure of conflicts of interest. The transplant team needs to ensure that the necessary expertise and infrastructure are in place to safely perform facial transplantation and to support the recipient medically as well as provide social and psychological support, security to protect privacy and safety, and legal advice as necessary in the postoperative period.

Dignity refers to the idea of preservation of honor, value, and self-esteem. In many ways, preservation of dignity is a central goal of facial transplantation, that is, to provide patients with an appearance that allows them to assimilate into society and feel less self-conscious. The psychological impact of facial transplant has

been an area of concern. Systematic psychosocial evaluation of the first 3 face transplant patients performed in Boston showed decline in their physical quality of life in the 3 months immediately after surgery but significant improvement by 6 months.[16] There was also significant improvement in patients' mental health 6 months after surgery as compared with preoperatively. Interestingly, self-esteem remained normal to high throughout the evaluation period, and there was no change in the quality-of-life measures. The psychosocial outcomes were also studied over the first 3 years for the first US face transplant patient.[17] This patient was found to have improvements in self-rating of appearance and quality-of-life measures and decreases in anxiety regarding body image, the facial anxiety score, depression, and chronic daily pain. These results suggest facial transplantation has an overall positive psychosocial impact, though data are still lacking.

Nonmaleficence should be familiar to all physicians as it is embodied by the dictum, *first do no harm*. However, it is also one of the most controversial aspects of the ethical debate surrounding facial transplantation. Potential harm can come in the form of psychological or emotional risks. Not all patients with severe facial disfigurement are good candidates for facial transplantation; thus, it is important to be honest and direct with patients, many of whom have already experienced significant psychological stress from their injury, so as not to engender false hope. Potential facial transplantation patients have often had previous blood transfusions and potentially cadaveric skin grafts, which can cause presensitization, making it difficult or even unrealistic to find an HLA-matched donor.[5] In these instances is it important to set realistic expectations for patients.

For patients who are deemed acceptable candidates for facial transplantation, the principle of nonmaleficence would dictate that one should plan for a viable salvage or backup plan if the transplant were to fail. This plan may include skin grafting, free tissue transfer, local flaps, or most likely a combination. Determining a specific salvage plan preoperatively and leaving sufficient tissues and recipient vessels intact at the time of surgery helps ensure that patients can be kept safe even in the case of transplant loss.

Significant harm can also result as a consequence of immunosuppression, and this issue alone has led some to suggest that facial transplantation is not ethically sound enough to pursue.[18] At a minimum, patient selection is important to maximize benefits and minimize risks. Patients should be chosen who stand to have a functional gain as well as a cosmetic improvement from the transplant. Patients with medical conditions, such as history of malignancy, human immunodeficiency virus, severe cardiac disease or diabetes, traumatic brain injury, or psychiatric illness, may be poor candidates for facial transplantation as these factors can increase the risk of perioperative complications, immunosuppression-related malignancies and infections, and/or noncompliance with immunosuppressive regimens.[15]

The final ethical principle is that of justice, which refers to the equitable distribution of resources and dictates that scarce donor tissue should be given to patients who have the potential for the most gain with a low risk of transplant failure or death. This issue brings the discussion back to careful patient selection.

The ethics surrounding distribution of resources among potential facial transplant candidates can be extended to the health care system as a whole when studying the cost-effectiveness of the procedure. The cost of the first US facial transplant performed in Cleveland was found to be $349,959, which was very similar to the $353,480 the patient's prior 23 reconstructive surgeries were estimated to have cost.[19] Billing data from the first 4 facial transplant cases in Boston were used to estimate a 1-year cost of facial transplant of $337,360. Data from patients who had undergone conventional reconstruction was used to calculate a 1-year cost of $70,230. However, when adjustments were made to account for the severity of injury, those costs increased to $184,061.[20] The authors also point out that face transplants so far in the United States have been experimental; funding has, therefore, either come from institutional support or grants. It is unclear whether institutions will maintain this support after initial excitement and publicity wane and whether insurance companies will deem the procedure worthy of coverage. There are also ongoing costs of immunosuppressive medications, which have been estimated at around $14,000 per year depending on the regimen.[21] It is vital to ensure immunosuppression will be covered for the life of patients with facial transplants before undergoing surgery.

SUMMARY

Facial transplantation has graduated from theory and proof of concept to an evolving, yet still new endeavor. Although the procedure must still be considered experimental and true long-term follow does not yet exist, there are now several centers throughout the world that have demonstrated the ability to safely and reliably perform the procedure. Many technical issues have been refined, and facial transplant centers have developed and shared effective protocols. Controversies remain, however, particularly in the areas of immunology and ethics. The ethical question of whether we should try this has been answered; but a procedure as complex, risky, and expensive, and involving anatomy as important as the face, will continue to incite ethical debate. Advances in transplant immunology may lead to safer immunosuppression regimens or potentially obviate their need, thus eliminating one of the main technical challenges, medical risks, and ethical concerns, allowing facial transplantation to flourish.

REFERENCES

1. Soga S, Pomahac B, Wake N, et al. CT angiography for surgical planning in face transplantation candidates. AJNR Am J Neuroradiol 2013;34(10): 1873–81.
2. Nguyen JT, Ashitate Y, Venugopal V, et al. Near-infrared imaging of face transplants: are both pedicles necessary? J Surg Res 2013;184(1):714–21.
3. Alam DS, Chi JJ. Facial transplantation for massive traumatic injuries. Otolaryngol Clin North Am 2013; 46:883–907.
4. Pomahac B, Bueno EM, Sisk GC, et al. Current principles of facial allotransplantation: the Brigham and Women's Hospital experience. Plast Reconstr Surg 2013;131(5):1069–76.
5. Lantieri L. Face transplant: a paradigm change in facial reconstruction. J Craniofac Surg 2012;23(1): 250–3.
6. Infante-Cossio P, Barrera-Pulido F, Gomez-Cia T, et al. Facial transplantation: a concise update. Med Oral Patol Oral Cir Bucal 2013;18(2):e263–71.
7. Khalifian S, Brazio PS, Mohan R, et al. Facial transplantation: the first 9 years. Lancet 2014; 384(9960):2153–63.
8. Fischer S, Kueckelhaus M, Pauzenberger R, et al. Functional outcomes of face transplantation. Am J Transplant 2015;15(1):220–33.
9. Petruzzo P, Kanitakis J, Testelin S, et al. Clinicopathological findings of chronic rejection in a face grafted patient. Transplantation 2015; 00(00):1–7.
10. Wo L, Bueno E, Pomahac B. Facial transplantation: worth the risks? A look at evolution of indications over the last decade. Curr Opin Organ Transplant 2015;20(6):615–20.
11. Siemionow M, Ozturk C. Face transplantation: outcomes, concerns, controversies, and future directions. J Craniofac Surg 2012;23(1):254–9.
12. Leonard DA, Kurtz JM, Cetrulo CL. Achieving immune tolerance in hand and face transplantation: a realistic prospect? Immunotherapy 2014;6(5): 499–502.

13. Leonard DA, Gordon CR, Sachs DH, et al. Immunobiology of face transplantation. J Craniofac Surg 2012;23(1):268–71.

14. Kueckelhaus M, Fischer S, Lian CG, et al. Utility of sentinel flaps in assessing facial allograft rejection. Plast Reconstr Surg 2015;135(1):250–8.

15. Coffman KL, Siemionow MZ. Ethics of facial transplantation revisited. Curr Opin Organ Transplant 2014;19:181–7.

16. Chang G, Pomahac B. Psychosocial changes 6 months after face transplantation. Psychosomatics 2013;54(4):367–71.

17. Coffman KL, Siemionow MZ. Face transplantation: psychological outcomes at three-year follow-up. Psychosomatics 2013;54(4):372–8.

18. Kiwanuka H, Bueno EM, Diaz-Siso JR, et al. Evolution of ethical debate on face transplantation. Plast Reconstr Surg 2013;132(6):1558–68.

19. Siemionow M, Gatherwright J, Djohan R, et al. Cost analysis of conventional facial reconstruction procedures followed by face transplantation. Am J Transplant 2011;11:379–85.

20. Nguyen LL, Naunheim MR, Hevelone ND, et al. Cost analysis of conventional face reconstruction versus face transplantation for large tissue defects. Plast Reconstr Surg 2015;135(1):260–7.

21. Westvik TS, Dermietzel A, Pomahac B. Facial restoration by transplantation: the Brigham and Women's face transplant experience. Ann Plast Surg 2015; 74(Suppl 1):S2–8.

Injectables in the Nose
Facts and Controversies

William Walsh Thomas, MD[a], Lou Bucky, MD[b], Oren Friedman, MD[a],*

KEYWORDS

- Injectable • Filler • Nasal reconstruction • Hyaluronic acid • Triamcinolone • Rhinoplasty

KEY POINTS

- All injectable types have been reported to cause rare but serious ocular and cerebral complications; exercise even greater caution following nasal surgery because the altered blood supply may increase risk.
- Hyaluronic acid is commonly used to smooth out minor irregularities following nasal surgery; hyaluronidase may be used to minimize the severity of complications. Hyaluronic acid lasts longer in the nose compared with other areas of the face.
- Autologous fat is commonly injected into the post-rhinoplasty nasal deformity, particularly when significant volumes are needed.
- Steroid injections may be used to reduce edema and scarring following nasal surgery and nasal reconstruction.
- Skin resurfacing can improve scars, and is especially useful for full-thickness skin grafts and paramedian forehead flaps.

INTRODUCTION

The use of injectable fillers has soared over the past 10 years. The American Society of Plastic Surgeons reports an increase from 650,000 filler procedures in 2000 to 2.3 million procedures in 2014.[1] As with many new technologies and medications, increased experience by physicians has led to "pushing the envelope" and using the materials for ever-increasing indications.[2–5] Before the current era, medical-grade silicone injections had been used for many years to correct thousands of postrhinoplasty deformities with good success; however, the use of this product was not specifically US Food and Drug Administration (FDA) approved for the nose, was associated with several complications, and its use was therefore controversial.[6] Safe new injectable biomaterials

have fueled the current surge in use, but none of them are FDA approved for the nose. Despite this fact, nonsurgical primary, revision, and reconstructive injectable rhinoplasty has gained popularity. This article discusses the use of injectable fillers in the nose. In addition, it examines the use of autologous fat injections as well as the use of dermabrasion in nasal reconstruction.

THE NEW RECONSTRUCTIVE LADDER

The goal of facial and nasal reconstruction is to allow patients to return to their premorbid condition with as little stigma from the deficit as possible. As with every reconstructive situation, strong consideration should be given to the least invasive but appropriate method first, and then clinicians may consider other options from

Disclosure: The authors have no financial interest to declare in relation to the content of this article.

[a] Department of Otorhinolaryngology-Head and Neck Surgery, University of Pennsylvania, 3400 Spruce Street, Philadelphia, PA 19104, USA; [b] Division of Plastic Surgery, Hospital of the University of Pennsylvania, 3400 Spruce Street, Philadelphia, PA 19104, USA
* Corresponding author. 3400 Spruce Street, Attn: Otorhinolaryngology, Philadelphia, PA 19104.
E-mail address: orenfriedman@hotmail.com

elsewhere on the reconstructive ladder (**Fig. 1**). Surgery remains the gold standard for safe, long-term correction of nasal abnormalities, both functional and aesthetic. The role of fillers in the nose continues to be explored, and is not considered standard of care for the long-term management of nasal defects. This article presents controversies associated with the use of different types of injectables in the nose, different injection techniques, side effects, complications, and histologic findings.

OVERVIEW OF NASAL INJECTABLES

The term nasal injectable in this article is used to mean any substance injected into the nose to physically alter the appearance of the nose. This use differs from medications injected into the nose, such as corticosteroids or botulinum toxin, that alter the healing or functional properties. **Table 1** represents a background classification of the basic characteristics and functional properties of injectables, which is essential to understanding the ideal uses of the different injectables.

INJECTABLE FILLERS
Hyaluronic Acids: Restylane, Juvaderm, Belotero

Hyaluronic acid (HA) products (Restylane, Juvaderm, Belotero, and others) have been used

as adjuncts following rhinoplasty or nasal reconstruction to adjust minor deformities. In addition, they have been used as stand-alone tools for primary injectable rhinoplasty and nasal reconstruction. The most commonly reported applications of HA fillers include the correction of tip ptosis, dorsal irregularities, dorsal hump camouflage, and saddle deformity. These irregularities may occur as a result of prior trauma or genetic predisposition, or may be iatrogenic following nasal surgery.

To address a drooping, ptotic nasal tip, which is commonly seen in Asian women, Han and colleagues[3] described multiple injections at the supraperiosteal, supraperichondrial, intramuscular, and subcutaneous layers. Layering the HA in multiple planes was thought to prevent the dorsal widening that can be seen with supraperiosteal injections alone. In addition, the investigators speculated that the use of both sharp needles and blunt cannulas may help minimize the risk of intravascular injection in higher-risk vascular regions. Han and colleagues[3] used EME (Love II), a different HA than is used in the United States and that requires the use of larger gauge needles and cannulas as it is more viscous, has a higher N', and contains more HA per milliliter relative to Restylane and Juvaderm. In their series of 280 patients, there are no reports of skin necrosis or ocular complications.[3]

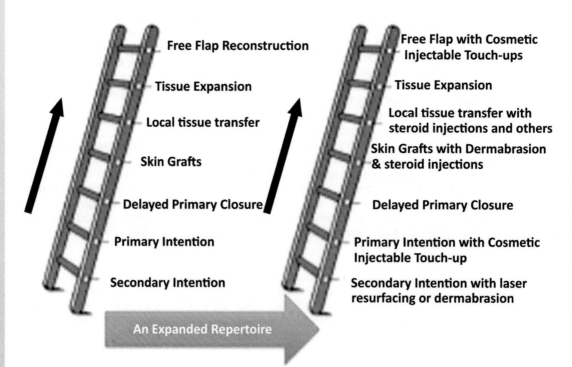

Free Flap Reconstruction

Tissue Expansion

Local tissue transfer

Skin Grafts

Delayed Primary Closure

Primary Intention

Secondary Intention

Free Flap with Cosmetic Injectable Touch-ups

Tissue Expansion

Local tissue transfer with steroid injections and others

Skin Grafts with Dermabrasion & steroid injections

Delayed Primary Closure

Primary Intention with Cosmetic Injectable Touch-up

Secondary Intention with laser resurfacing or dermabrasion

An Expanded Repertoire

Fig. 1. The new reconstructive ladder.

Table 1
Paradigm of injectables and their physical attributes G′ and N′

G′: elasticity coefficient. Ability to resist deformation from pressure; higher indicates more lift with less volume	—	N′: viscosity coefficient. Ability to resist sheering forces; less diffusion into tissue
High G′ and high N′	Medium G′ and N′	Low G′ and N′
CaHA: Radiesse	CaHA with lidocaine and HA: Restylane, Perlane, Restylane SubQ, Restylane Lyft	HA: Juvederm Ultra, Juvederm Ultra Plus, Juvederm Voluma, Belotero Balance
Less diffusion; precise sculpting	—	More diffusion; improved blending
Less volume needed for lift	—	More volume needed for lift

Data from Sundaram H, Voigts B, Beer K, et al. Comparison of the rheological properties of viscosity and elasticity in 2 categories of soft tissue fillers: calcium hydroxylapatite and hyaluronic acid. Dermatol Surg 2010;36 Suppl 3:1859–65; and Sundaram H, Cassuto D. Biophysical characteristics of hyaluronic acid soft-tissue fillers and their relevance to aesthetic applications. Plast Reconstr Surg 2013;132(4 Suppl 2):5S–21S.

Redaelli[7] addresses the drooping tip with a combination of HA and botulinum toxin injections (**Fig. 2**). Botulinum toxin type A (1.5 units of Vistabex) was injected into each depressor septi nasalis muscle in 45% of the reported patients. Preventing motion of the depressor septi muscle limits the nose's tendency to droop with smiling and perioral animation, and provides a stable platform for HA

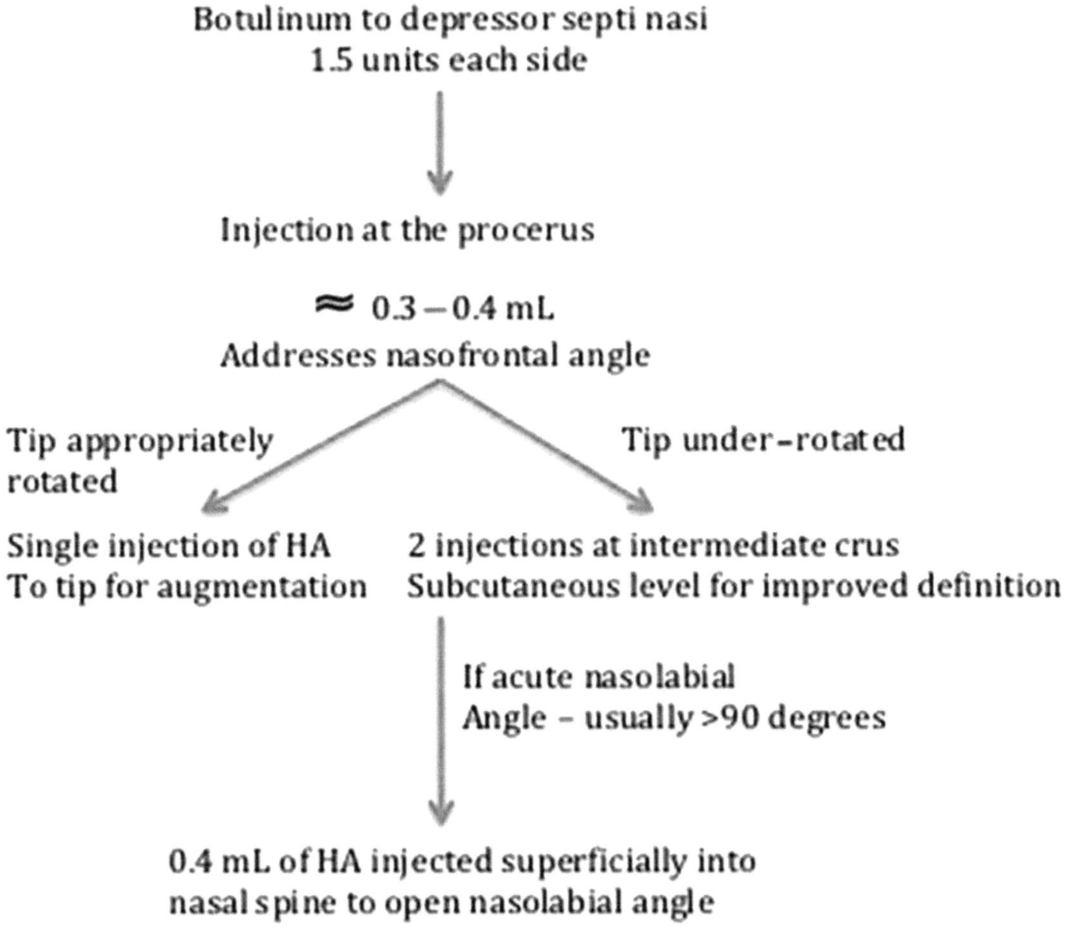

Botulinum to depressor septi nasi
1.5 units each side

↓

Injection at the procerus

≈ 0.3 – 0.4 mL
Addresses nasofrontal angle

Tip appropriately rotated   **Tip under-rotated**

Single injection of HA   **2 injections at intermediate crus**
To tip for augmentation   **Subcutaneous level for improved definition**

↓

If acute nasolabial
Angle – usually >90 degrees

↓

0.4 mL of HA injected superficially into
nasal spine to open nasolabial angle

Fig. 2. Redaelli's[7] algorithm for drooping nasal tip. (*Data from* Redaelli A. Medical rhinoplasty with hyaluronic acid and botulinum toxin A: a very simple and quite effective technique. J Cosmet Dermatol 2008;7(3):210–20.)

layering. Depending on the extent to which the nose drooped, injections were performed in a stepwise sequence. Ninety-five patients are presented in the series and no significant complications were encountered. These principals of injection rhinoplasty can also be applied to the reconstructed nose; however, care must be taken to avoid intravascular or pressure ischemia–induced necrosis caused by the altered and less predictable blood supply patterns.[7]

The literature contains many reports of injectables used in the nose, but not every article should be accepted as evidence for safe or appropriate clinical practice. Liapakis and colleagues[8] report that HA can provide aesthetic improvements in postrhinoplasty patients for the temporary postrhinoplasty defects caused by asymmetrical soft tissue edema. Eleven patients were seen 1 month following standard surgical rhinoplasty for asymmetry that was presumed to be associated with asymmetrical postoperative soft tissue edema. A variety of injectable techniques were used to insert Juvederm into the nose to correct the asymmetrical edema. No complications were reported, but 7 of the 11 patients required secondary HA injections within 2 weeks to correct residual deformities. Despite the reported success of this publication, the idea of injecting the nose at such an early postoperative period must be seriously questioned. Clearly, following rhinoplasty, edema may persist for a year or more. Variations in the amount and location of edema in the early and even later postoperative periods may be caused by something as simple as the patient's sleeping position, and is not likely to alter a well-constructed nose's long-term symmetry. At the same time, the long-term effects of healing and persistent edema that may be induced by filler injection at 1 month following surgery are unknown and may themselves cause long-term asymmetries and complications. The suggestion of filling the nose with an HA product to create postoperative symmetry at 1 month after surgery should be seriously doubted as a reasonable approach, and the authors warn against incorporating this as a standard practice.

The use of HA in the treatment of saddle nose deformity is a useful technique that can provide patients with improved cosmetic appearance in place of, or preceding, definitive surgical nasal reconstruction. Bennett and Reilly[9] present a case of Restylane injection to correct a significant saddle nose deformity in a 22-year old woman with antineutrophil cytoplasmic autoantibodies (ANCA)-associated vasculitis, who was shown to have continued improvement in appearance at 6 months postoperatively. They point out that this patient will also have an improved appreciation of what to expect following definitive surgical reconstruction.[9] Vogt and colleagues[10] report 4 cases of successful 42-month mean follow-up after definitive surgical nasal reconstruction of saddle nose deformity with an L-shaped cartilage rib graft. These patients were in remission from granulomatosis with polyangiitis (ANCA-associated vasculitis) at the time of surgical rhinoplasty, but they were continuing to receive immunosuppressive medication. Although the data are limited, it is suggested that patients with granulomatosis with polyangiitis with saddle nose deformity can undergo cosmetic nasal filler during active disease states with temporizing injectable fillers, and once in remission they may safely undergo definitive surgical repair.

Calcium Hydroxyapatite: Radiesse

Significant controversy exists regarding calcium hydroxyapatite (CaHA) in nasal reconstruction and to a lesser degree as a form of injection rhinoplasty. Postrhinoplasty, CaHA offers a longer duration; its effects can be expected to last 12 to 18 months compared with 6 to 12 months with HA products. Stupak and colleagues[11] reported their experience with 13 patients. At least 3 months following rhinoplasty or trauma, Radiesse was injected to treat sidewall depressions, overly deep supratip breaks, alar asymmetries, and dorsal irregularities. Injections were performed with 27-gauge and 30-gauge needles and patients were evaluated for appearance, complications, and pain. Fifteen of 17 injection sites were graded as improved; 8 of 13 patients considered their outcome excellent, with 2 patients considering their outcome good. There was 1 minor complication of self-limiting dorsal erythema. Pain was tolerable for all patients. This series suggests that the feasibility and outcomes of CaHA nasal augmentation are similar to what has been presented with fat and HA.

In contrast, Kurkjian and colleagues[12] discourage CaHA use for primary injection rhinoplasty and for secondary nasal reconstruction. The arguments against CaHA are 3-fold: clinicians cannot correct injection imperfections because of a lack of an equivalent hyaluronidase analog, HA products can last up to 2 to 3 years in the nose (not inferior to CaHA), and thin nasal skin can lead to palpable nodularity. These same principles are magnified in postrhinoplasty patients with the added caveat that the blood supply to the skin is fundamentally compromised and so the risk of irreparable complication is increased. There is limited clinical evidence to suggest that CaHA presents a higher risk of complication with injectable rhinoplasty. Bernd Schuster[13] reports on 46 patients (26 undergoing CaHA injections and 20 undergoing HA injections) with 88 treated areas, with 6 patients experiencing complications, all of whom were treated with CaHA. Mild complications included 2 visible hematomas and palpable subcutaneous nodules. Moderate complications included an erythematous nasal tip, treated effectively with topical steroids and cefuroxime. Serious complications included extensive facial cellulitis, and, in a postrhinoplasty patient, a displaced Medpor implant, nasal tip abscess, and skin necrosis. The abscess was drained and the implant repositioned. Given these complications, Dr. Schuster no longer performs CaHA injection rhinoplasty.[13] CaHA is a controversial injectable material to use following nasal reconstruction. Surgeons should be aware of the risks, and exercise their best judgment to ensure optimal results.

AUTOLOGOUS FAT

Autologous fat transfer can be used as a stand-alone nasal augmentation procedure or as a touch-up following nasal reconstruction or rhinoplasty. The donor site should be easily camouflaged and highly lipogenic, with common sites including the abdomen or outer thighs in women and the flanks in men.[14] Fat harvest is achieved through a small incision with a 3-mm suction cannula and 10-mL syringe for suction. The aspirated fat is centrifuged and prepared for injection. Some practitioners freeze the remaining fat, store it in personal freezers, and then thaw it for subsequent injections. This practice is not standard and should cease, because the storage of any part of a human body in a non–tissue bank setting should be avoided because of disease transmission, other health-related factors, and legal implications. Various injection techniques are listed in **Table 2**.

Following rhinoplasty, the skin–soft tissue envelope may be highly distorted by scar, thereby impeding fat placement and often requiring greater force for injection. Clinicians should avoid higher-risk areas for intravascular injection, such as the glabella.[15] As the authors have observed in other body areas, there is variability to the amount of fat that survives transplant. A recent study showed a good to high rate of satisfaction in 80% of fat-injection rhinoplasty patients.[15] This same report commented that fat grafts are useful in conditions of nasal scarring and tight thin skin. Autologous fat grafts seem to create space between densely adherent skin and the underlying nasal skeleton, helping to camouflage deformities and making secondary procedures and subsequent dissection significantly easier.[15]

Indications for fat injection following rhinoplasty or nasal reconstruction include correction of dorsal irregularities, inverted V deformities, stairstep deformities, and saddle nose deformities. In Baptista and colleagues'[16] series, lipofilling was performed at least 1 year after each patient's most recent rhinoplasty. Only a small volume of fat reabsorption was noted so only 2 patients required secondary injections. Two patients also required subsequent surgical procedures to ultimately correct their saddle nose deformity and asymmetric osteotomies respectively. From a technical standpoint, this series showed improved postoperative edema and greater surgical precision in fat graft placement when using the smaller 0.8-mm microinjection cannula.

Autologous fat can also be used for subtler dorsal irregularities that may accompany even the most elegant rhinoplasty. In a series by Cardenas and Carvajal,[17] autologous fat was prophylactically injected to cover and soften the various cartilage grafts placed on the bony structure. Of the 78

Table 2
Reported techniques for fat injection with or without rhinoplasty

	Injection Equipment	Injection Plane	Injection Technique
Baptista et al,[16] 2013: 20 postrhinoplasty	21-gauge needle then 21-gauge cannula	At the periosteum and in the SMAS	Cross-hatched layers
Cardenas & Carvajal,[17] 2007: 78 at rhinoplasty	Via 5-mm incisions as closing rhinoplasty	Subcutaneous, onto bone and cartilage grafts	Directly onto structures of nose
Monreal,[15] 2011: 15 at rhinoplasty, 18 postrhinoplasty	1.2–1.4-mm blunt-tip cannulas; 18-gauge needles for adherent or fibrous tissues	In the SMAS and subcutaneous planes	Direct injection without cross-hatching
Erol, 2014[33]: 313 no rhinoplasty	22–24-gauge cannula	Intradermal or subcutaneous	Directly on to deformities

Abbreviation: SMAS, superficial muscular aponeurotic system.

rhinoplasty procedures performed, 61 were primary and 17 were revisions; the investigators noted no differences between the two procedures. Their results showed a 99% satisfactory rate and an 88% excellent rate. Weaknesses of the study were that there were no independent or blinded observers and their cohort had no control group.[17] Autologous fat injections can also be used in larger nasal reconstructions involving microvascular free tissue transfer. In the series presented by Haddock and colleagues,[18] more than 200 cosmetic autologous fat injections were performed. Most of these procedures, involving nasal reconstruction, were small-volume injections to augment the nasal ala as late refinements to more subtle defects.[18]

Other Injectables Used in Nasal Reconstruction

There are multiple other injectable fillers that can be used in nasal reconstruction. Examples include silicone, both liquid and solid/sheet form; Artecoll, which is bovine collagen; and polymethyl methacrylate (PMMA). Liquid silicone has a long history and numerous applications in cosmetic facial injections; one of the largest and earliest case series documenting outcomes of postrhinoplasty augmentation injections was performed by Webster and colleagues[6] and published in 1986. This series reported on 347 patients who received 1937 liquid silicone touch-up treatments following rhinoplasty. Most patients underwent multiple injections with small volumes of 0.03 to 0.08 mL of silicone injected to improve postrhinoplasty nasal asymmetries and depressions (**Table 3**). Silicone causes an inflammatory response of varying severity, so the technique to correct nasal asymmetry involved the following: first undercorrect the defect and then reassess every 6 to 12 weeks with subsequent injections as needed until the defect was satisfactorily corrected.[6]

The histology of the inflammation induced by liquid silicone injections has been shown to be no different in in-vivo animal models compared with implantation of autologous cartilage or silicone sheets. The durability of the inflammatory response is associated with durability of correction of the nasal defect. The resulting inflammation from liquid silicone is a low-grade and long-term response caused by the highly inert nature of liquid silicone.[19] In a comparison of the silicone implants Artecoll and Restylane, nasal height was found to regress back to baseline significantly after 6 months following injection rhinoplasty using Restylane only. This study also showed that at 12 months the Artecoll injection patients had resorption and

replacement of the bovine collagen component with autologous collagen but the PMMA component of the injectable persisted. This study additionally showed that silicone implants are susceptible to complications such as infection, hematoma, extrusion, displacement, and telangiectasia, which are not seen commonly with injectable fillers.[20] Solomon and colleagues[21] reported on Artecoll injections in 26 individuals who had undergone rhinoplasty at least 12 months earlier; only asymmetries of the upper one-third of the dorsum were treated and injections were subperiosteal. A standard 0.2 mL of product was injected in each patient and there was 100% patient satisfaction with 2-year follow-up. Artecoll is a more permanent injectable filler than can be used to treat nasal deformities following nasal reconstruction.

Complications of Nasal Injections

All injections to the face carry the risk of intravascular injection; the nose is particularly sensitive, because its vascular supply has anastomoses with vessels from the branches of the internal carotid, such as the ophthalmic artery. In 80% of participants, Saban and colleagues[22] showed that the ipsilateral ophthalmic artery supplies the nose with blood if the ipsilateral facial artery is occluded. In addition, given the rich supply of nasal vascular anastomoses, the patient is unlikely to have cutaneous necrosis even if there is an ophthalmic or cerebral complication. Blindness and cerebral ischemia are the most serious complications of injectable filler use, and have been reviewed in the literature extensively.[23,24]

Box 1 highlights the findings of a literature review by Lazzerie and colleagues[23] and **Box 2** highlights their tips for avoiding intravascular complications. In a national survey of retinal specialists in South Korea, between December 2013 and May 2013, 44 cases of ophthalmic artery occlusion associated with filler injection were presented. **Table 4** presents the data from that survey, comparing autologous fat–related and HA-related complications. Both fat and HA injections ophthalmic and cerebral complications are very unlikely but, when they occur, fat complications tend to be more serious. This phenomenon is likely related to the larger volumes and higher pressures associated with fat injections.[24]

STEROID INJECTIONS

Unlike the aforementioned injectables, with which direct contour manipulation is the goal, the injection of corticosteroids into the nose following nasal surgery is to control edema and the healing process in order to optimize the final cosmetic

Table 3
Case series injectable frequency and revision

Series	Primary Injection or Reconstruction	Secondary Injection or Injection Postreconstruction	% Touch-up or % Requiring Injection	Note
Lipakis 2013	11	7	64	Postrhinoplasty - HA
Han et al,[3] 2015	280	9	3	Asian primary injection rhinoplasty; HA
Redaelli,[7] 2008	95	21	22	HA and Botox; all drooping nose deformity primary
Baptista et al,[16] 2013	20	2	10	Postrhinoplasty; fat
Cardenas & Carvajal,[17] 2007	61: primary open rhinoplasty	17 revision rhinoplasty	NA	Fat injected at time of 1 or revision rhinoplasty; no touch-ups reported
Hanasono et al,[26] 2002	127	92	72	Postrhinoplasty: triamcinolone, specifically for pollybeak
Stupak et al,[11] 2007	13	5	38	Postrhinoplasty: CaHA
Quatela et al,[28] 1995	32 PMFF	5 requiring injection	16	Post-PMFF: triamcinolone for edema
Tan et al,[29] 2014	186 FTSG	14 requiring injection	8	Post-FTSG: triamcinolone for edema and thickness
Collar et al,[30] 2011	72 nasal reconstructions	16 requiring injection	22 overall 50 of bilobe reconstruction 71 of PMFF reconstruction	Post–nasal reconstruction; various methods, corticosteroid for pin-cushioning

Touch-up injections are not a complication or unexpected. Surgeons attempt to treat as conservatively as possible and multiple injections can be assumed to be part of a comprehensive treatment regimen.

Abbreviations: FTSG, full-thickness skin graft; NA, not applicable; PMFF, paramedian forehead flap.

outcome. One well-known example is the use of triamcinolone to correct a relative convexity of the supratip following rhinoplasty. Hanasono and colleagues[26] reported their experience with supratip triamcinolone injections following rhinoplasty; in the immediate 1-week to 2-week postoperative period, 0.1 to 0.2 mL of 10 mg/mL triamcinolone was injected. Subsequent injections were performed as indicated every 4 weeks. For cases of established supratip scar in the late postoperative period, higher doses of 4 to 8 mg of triamcinolone were used every 4 weeks, as needed. In their series of 173 patients who underwent rhinoplasty, 127 received a triamcinolone injection at 1 week postoperatively and 92 patients received a second injection. No complications were encountered. The pollybeak deformity may represent a temporary postrhinoplasty edema in the supratip region,

which can be optimally controlled with taping or postoperative triamcinolone. Over time, the edema may turn into permanent irreversible scar tissue. By administering the triamcinolone early in the postoperative period, inflammation and fibroblast stimulation and migration are reduced, thereby minimizing the risk of a permanent soft tissue pollybeak. Injection of corticosteroids into the supratip has risks; too high or too frequent a dosing may result in dermal atrophy, depigmentation, and rarely necrosis, ulceration, or blindness.[26,27]

Corticosteroids can also be used following nasal reconstruction. Quatela and colleagues[28] presented a case series of 32 paramedian forehead flaps (PMFF) for the reconstruction of Mohs defects. Five of these patients required triamcinolone injections for prolonged edema and tissue thinning and no complications of injection were reported. Injections were performed following separation of the pedicle and final thinning of the flap as needed. Similarly, full-thickness skin grafts (FTSGs) used in nasal reconstruction may also benefit from corticosteroid injection. Tan and colleagues[29] reported the use of triamcinolone injections in 26 of 186 FTSGs applied to Mohs defects in order to reduce persistent graft swelling at 6 weeks postoperatively. Injections were performed in the center of the graft with subsequent direct pressure and massage and no complications were reported. In a retrospective review and comparison of FTSG, PMFF, bilobed flap, and adjacent tissue transfer, Collar and colleagues[30] used corticosteroid injections in 16 of 72 patients requiring Mohs nasal defect reconstruction. Of the 16 patients receiving corticosteroid injection, 6 had undergone bilobe reconstruction and 10 had undergone PMFF reconstruction. The 6 bilobe patients requiring corticosteroid injection represented 50% of all bilobe reconstructions[9] and likewise the 10 PMFF reconstruction patients represented 71% of the forehead flaps[11] in the series. The average time to corticosteroid injection was 2.4 months. The investigators cite aggressive use of corticosteroid injection to prevent flap pin-cushioning, also known as the trapdoor deformity. In this series, 1 PMFF patient had to undergo a corrective Z-plasty for persistent trapdoor deformity.[30] There is little controversy that corticosteroid injections can be useful in managing postoperative swelling and fibrosis following nasal reconstruction. Surgeon preference dictates the frequency with which patients are offered the injections, but largely the indications for injection are uniform among surgeons.

Table 4
Fat compared with HA injectable complications

	Fat	HA	P-value
Extent of occlusion: diffuse	86%, 19 of 22	39%, 5 of 13	.007
Best correct visual acuity (log conversion of Snellen chart) (SD)	2.6 (0.8) Higher is worse	1.4 (1.4)	.01
Long-term vision loss	100%, 9 of 9	43%, 3 of 7	.02
Cerebral lesions	46%, 10 of 22	8%, 1 of 13	.03
Site of injection	Glabella: 13 Nasolabial fold: 7 Dorsum: 2	Glabella: 9 Nasolabial fold: 2 Dorsum: 5	Not significant
Number of injections in study	22	13	Not significant
Annual incidence of cosmetic injections	20,000	90,000	Not tested; ISAPS survey on aesthetic procedures[25]

Abbreviations: ISAPS, International Society of Aesthetic Plastic Surgery; SD, standard deviation.
Data from Park KH, Kim YK, Woo SJ, et al. Iatrogenic occlusion of the ophthalmic artery after cosmetic facial filler injections: a national survey by the Korean Retina Society. JAMA Ophthalmol 2014;132(6):714–23.

DERMABRASION AND OTHER RESURFACING TECHNIQUES

All surgical interventions for nasal reconstruction leave a visible external scar. Even when adhering to the principal of aligning scars within nasal subunits or along the subunit borders, scars can be disfiguring and unsightly. Dermabrasion is frequently used as an adjunct to nasal reconstruction to improve skin contours, color match, and to decrease scar visibility. One of the classic reviews

Table 5
Dermabrasion (Dab) usage and recommendations

Author	Type of Reconstruction	% With Dermabrasion	Notes
Tan et al,[29] 2014	FTSG to Ala	36%, 67 of 186	Dab: not related to patient age, sex, tumor type or size
Quatela et al,[28] 1995	PMFF to various subunits	47%, 15 of 32	Dab- to forehead and entire nasal unit 4–6 wk post inset
Fader,[34] 2000	Muscle hinge flap and FTSG	42%, 5 of 12	Spot Dab done 4–8 wk postop
McCluskey,[35] 2009	FTSG to lower one-third nasal reconstruction	34 of 55, 62%, 1 tx; 14 of 55, >2 tx	Dab done rotary diamond at 6 wk only graft and scar
Collar et al,[30] 2011	72 patients: 41 FTSG, 14 PMFF, 12 bilobe, 5 local flap	18 of 72	No significant difference in Dab per type of repair; mean 20 wk postreconstruction
Zimbler,[36] 2000	Dorsal nasal flap review	Offered to all patients	6 wk at incisional interface only
Rohrick,[37] 2004	1334 patients: 532 PMFF, 369 nasolabial flap, 213 dorsal nasal flap	Nearly all patients	DAB or CO_2 laser at initial surgery or division and inset of PMFF
Ammirati et al,[32] 2001	74: FTSG or secondary intention	100% laser resurfacing: 3 CO_2 lasers or 1 Er:Yag laser	Improved wound contour and healing for convex subunits: tip and alar with secondary intention healing, hypopigmentation more with older CO_2 laser

Abbreviations: Er:Yag, erbium: yttrium aluminum garnet; tx, treatment(s).

of dermabrasion, by Richard Farrior,[31] advocates its use particularly in the lower third of the nose during primary laceration repair before placement of the most superficial sutures. In addition, dermabrasion can be used to improve supratip swelling following rhinoplasty. However, there should be at least a 6-month delay between the primary procedure and dermabrasion.

FTSGs and PMFFs benefit greatly from dermabrasion because the grafted skin is not as closely matched with native nasal skin as a local skin flap and dermabrasion helps to blur the lines of demarcation. There is considerable variability concerning the timing and extent of dermabrasion (**Table 5**). In addition, laser resurfacing can be used as a replacement or complementary procedure. Laser resurfacing at the time of reconstruction after Mohs resection improved wound contour and scar appearance, even for those wounds left to heal by secondary intention. The benefit was most apparent on convex surfaces, which typically granulate poorly.[32]

SUMMARY

There are a variety of novel tools that may improve nasal appearance following nasal surgery, including injectable fillers, fat, HA, and silicone. There are also several outstanding, tried and true, adjuvant procedures such as dermabrasion and laser skin resurfacing that are essential for long-term scar optimization. There is no definitive evidence to discount any one injectable or procedure as inappropriate for use in the nose. However, injectable fillers have also not become an indispensable part of the repertoire for nasal reconstruction or rhinoplasty, and should continue to be studied for their safety and efficacy. The appropriate enthusiasm for bioengineered materials and new technological advances must be tempered by the reality of what is known to work, and what is in the patient's best long-term interest. Interventions should always place the needs of the patient first, and should always aim to minimize complications and maximize outcomes. Although there is clearly an important emerging role for injectables in rhinoplasty and nasal reconstruction, they are not a replacement for nasal surgery. By continuing to improve surgical skill and maximize surgical outcomes, it may be possible to reduce the need for potentially harmful adjunctive camouflaging tools such as fillers. There is no substitute for a well-thought-out and executed rhinoplasty or nasal reconstruction. The more established and safe adjunctive procedures, such as dermabrasion and steroid injection, are essential tools for scar management. Nasal injectable filler seems to represent a fairly safe tool that is continuing to be explored as a temporary means to alter the nasal shape.

REFERENCES

1. American Society of Plastic Surgeons. Plastic surgery statistics report. Arlington Heights (IL): American Society of Plastic Surgeons; 2014.http://www.plasticsurgery.org/Documents/news-resources/statistics/2014-statistics/plastic-surgery-statsitics-full-report.pdf.
2. Jasin ME. Nonsurgical rhinoplasty using dermal fillers. Facial Plast Surg Clin North Am 2013;21(2): 241–52.
3. Han X, Hu J, Cheng L, et al. Multiplane hyaluronic acid (EME) in female Chinese rhinoplasty using blunt and sharp needle technique. J Plast Reconstr Aesthet Surg 2015;68(11):1504–9.
4. Tanaka Y. Oriental nose occidentalization and perinasal shaping by augmentation of the underdeveloped anterior nasal spine. Plast Reconstr Surg Glob Open 2014;2(8):e197.
5. Moradi A, Watson J. Current concepts in filler injection. Facial Plast Surg Clin North Am 2015;23(4): 489–94.
6. Webster RC, Hamdan US, Gaunt JM, et al. Rhinoplastic revisions with injectable silicone. Arch Otolaryngol Head Neck Surg 1986;112(3):269–76.
7. Redaelli A. Medical rhinoplasty with hyaluronic acid and botulinum toxin A: a very simple and quite effective technique. J Cosmet Dermatol 2008;7(3): 210–20.
8. Liapakis IE, Englander M, Vrentzos NP, et al. Secondary rhinoplasty fixations with hyaluronic acid. J Cosmet Dermatol 2013;12(3):235–9.
9. Bennett HS, Reilly PG. Restylane–a temporary alternative for saddle nose deformity in nasal Wegener's granulomatosis–how we do it. Br J Oral Maxillofac Surg 2011;49(4):e3–5.
10. Vogt PM, Gohritz A, Haubitz M, et al. Reconstruction of nasal deformity in Wegener's granulomatosis: contraindication or benefit? Aesthetic Plast Surg 2011;35(2):156–61.
11. Stupak HD, Moulthrop TH, Wheatley P, et al. Calcium hydroxylapatite gel (Radiesse) injection for the correction of postrhinoplasty contour deficiencies and asymmetries. Arch Facial Plast Surg 2007;9(2):130–6.
12. Kurkjian TJ, Ahmad J, Rohrich RJ. Soft-tissue fillers in rhinoplasty. Plast Reconstr Surg 2014;133(2): 121e–6e.
13. Schuster B. Injection rhinoplasty with hyaluronic acid and calcium hydroxyapatite: a retrospective survey investigating outcome and complication rates. Facial Plast Surg 2015;31(3): 301–7.

14. Donofrio L. Autologous fat transplantation. In: Kaminer MS, editor. Atlas of cosmetic surgery. Philadelphia: Saunders; 2009. p. 309–21.

15. Monreal J. Fat grafting to the nose: personal experience with 36 patients. Aesthetic Plast Surg 2011; 35(5):916–22.

16. Baptista C, Nguyen PS, Desouches C, et al. Correction of sequelae of rhinoplasty by lipofilling. J Plast Reconstr Aesthet Surg 2013;66(6): 805–11.

17. Cardenas JC, Carvajal J. Refinement of rhinoplasty with lipoinjection. Aesthetic Plast Surg 2007;31(5): 501–5.

18. Haddock NT, Saadeh PB, Siebert JW. Achieving aesthetic results in facial reconstructive microsurgery: planning and executing secondary refinements. Plast Reconstr Surg 2012;130(6): 1236–45.

19. Hizal E, Buyuklu F, Ozdemir BH, et al. Long-term inflammatory response to liquid injectable silicone, cartilage, and silicone sheet. Laryngoscope 2014; 124(11):E425–30.

20. Chen L, Li SR, Yu P, et al. Comparison of Artecoll, Restylane and silicone for augmentation rhinoplasty in 378 Chinese patients. Clin Invest Med 2014;37(4): E203–10.

21. Solomon P, Sklar M, Zener R. Facial soft tissue augmentation with Artecoll(®): a review of eight years of clinical experience in 153 patients. Can J Plast Surg 2012;20(1):28–32.

22. Saban Y, Andretto Amodeo C, Bouaziz D, et al. Nasal arterial vasculature: medical and surgical applications. Arch Facial Plast Surg 2012;14(6):429–36.

23. Lazzeri D, Agostini T, Figus M, et al. Blindness following cosmetic injections of the face. Plast Reconstr Surg 2012;129(4):995–1012.

24. Park KH, Kim YK, Woo SJ, et al. Iatrogenic occlusion of the ophthalmic artery after cosmetic facial filler injections: a national survey by the Korean Retina Society. JAMA Ophthalmol 2014;132(6): 714–23.

25. International Society of Aesthetic Plastic Surgery. ISAPS international survey on aesthetic/cosmetic procedures performed in 2011. Columbus (OH): Industry Insights; 2011.

26. Hanasono MM, Kridel RW, Pastorek NJ, et al. Correction of the soft tissue pollybeak using triamcinolone injection. Arch Facial Plast Surg 2002; 4(1):26–30 [discussion: 31].

27. Shafir R, Cohen M, Gur E. Blindness as a complication of subcutaneous nasal steroid injection. Plast Reconstr Surg 1999;104(4):1180–2 [discussion: 1183–4].

28. Quatela VC, Sherris DA, Rounds MF. Esthetic refinements in forehead flap nasal reconstruction. Arch Otolaryngol Head Neck Surg 1995;121(10): 1106–13.

29. Tan E, Mortimer N, Salmon P. Full-thickness skin grafts for surgical defects of the nasal ala - a comprehensive review, approach and outcomes of 186 cases over 9 years. Br J Dermatol 2014; 170(5):1106–13.

30. Collar RM, Ward PD, Baker SR. Reconstructive perspectives of cutaneous defects involving the nasal tip: a retrospective review. Arch Facial Plast Surg 2011;13(2):91–6.

31. Farrior RT. Dermabrasion in facial surgery. Laryngoscope 1985;95(5):534–45.

32. Ammirati CT, Cottingham TJ, Hruza GJ. Immediate postoperative laser resurfacing improves second intention healing on the nose: 5-year experience. Dermatol Surg 2001;27(2): 147–52.

33. Erol OO. Microfat Grafting in Nasal Surgery. Aesthet Surg J 2014;34(5):671–86.

34. Fader DJ, Wang TS, Johnson TM. Nasal reconstruction utilizing a muscle hinge flap with overlying full-thickness skin graft. J Am Acad Dermatol 2000; 43(5 Pt 1):837–40.

35. McCluskey PD, Constantine FC, Thornton JF. Lower third nasal reconstruction: when is skin grafting an appropriate option? Plast Reconstr Surg 2009; 124(3):826–35.

36. Zimbler MS, Thomas JR. The dorsal nasal flap revisited: aesthetic refinements in nasal reconstruction. Arch Facial Plast Surg 2000;2(4):285–6.

37. Rohrich RJ, Griffin JR, Ansari M, et al. Nasal reconstruction–beyond aesthetic subunits: a 15-year review of 1334 cases. Plast Reconstr Surg 2004;114(6):1405–16; discussion 1417-9.

Index

Note: Page numbers of article titles are in **boldface** type.

A

Facial Plast Surg Clin N Am 24 (2016) 391–404
http://dx.doi.org/10.1016/S1064-7406(16)30052-9
1064-7406/16/$ – see front matter

Printed and bound by CPI Group (UK) Ltd, Croydon, CR0 4YY

08/05/2025

01864686-0017